INTO THE BREACH

INTO THE BREACH

A YEAR OF LIFE
AND DEATH WITH EMS

J. A. KARAM

ST. MARTIN'S PRESS   NEW YORK

Design by Phil Mazzone

ISBN 0-312-30617-2

Printed In The U.S.A.

For Walter, Danny, and Gerald

CONTENTS

FOREWORD

Not everything that can be counted counts,
and not everything that counts can be
counted.

—ALBERT EINSTEIN

*T*wenty-five years ago I made a discovery that would alter my life's direction. Early in my formative years I had the normal fascination with emergency services and vehicles. Family members do not hesitate to reminisce (and bust my chops) about my frantic dash to the apartment windows as a toddler to watch the passing parade of vehicles and personnel en route to an emergency.

As I grew older, my interest in emergency response and management intensified. In the early 1970s, while in grade school, I discovered the emerging world of Emergency Medical Services and paramedics only to have my appetite for helping people and the excitement of "the job" increase. By thirteen, I was certified in CPR and advanced first aid. My parents supported the youthful exuberance, but I think they also believed that this would pass like many childhood interests.

Alas, as a seventeen-year-old high school senior I would burden them again with being driven twice weekly for six months to the College of Medicine and Dentistry of New Jersey in Newark to attend emergency medical technician training. What a great experience! The people I met have influenced my personal and professional life for decades. Individuals like Judd Fuller, UMDNJ

EMS director and course coordinator, who took a chance on a kid by allowing me to attend the program; Battalion Chief Al Freda, of the Newark Fire Department, who no matter how tough the call would always remind you that "compassion is as important as proficiency of skills"; and Keith Holtermann, M.B.A., M.P.H., Dr. P.H., who would continue to push each student to achieve excellence both in and out of the classroom—they have all become lifelong friends and encouraged me to continue to progress in this exciting and demanding profession.

At eighteen, I found myself successfully completing the entry requirements to become a member of New York City Emergency Medical Service, the oldest, finest, and busiest EMS organization in the nation. I also became a paramedic, the coveted training I sought through NYC★EMS. As the years progressed, I rose through the ranks to the position of deputy chief. My professional experiences in New York have been the most exciting and rewarding, and I cherish each minute and the people I have met over the years.

But this book is not about me; it is about the trials and tribulations of EMS and my colleagues across the river in Newark, New Jersey, where my EMS aspirations started many years ago.

EMS is the toughest job you'll ever love. It requires the strong back of a construction worker, the compassion of a clergyman, the guts of a soldier, the patience of a parent, a cast-iron stomach, and supportive family and friends if you are going to succeed.

Many times EMS takes more than it gives. Family and social functions are often interrupted by the call of duty. Holidays and special celebrations are frequently rescheduled owing to rotating work schedules. The effects of cumulative stress from the numerous horrific emergency scenes all detract from the glamour portrayed on TV and enhance the recruitment and retention problems we in EMS continue to experience today.

EMS is a family. We fight with each other, we laugh with each other, and we cry with each other. All differences aside, when an EMT or paramedic is in trouble and calls for help, all members of the team drop everything and run to assist their brother or sister in danger. A good day is going home . . . a great day is going home in one piece.

But there is a public dimension to all of this. Without question, when the public needs emergency medical help they call 911, and 911 calls EMS to remedy the problem. In many instances this means the difference between life and death.

Members of the EMS community place their lives on the line daily, responding to thousands of emergencies and disasters throughout the United States. In high-volume urban systems such as Newark, New Jersey, the crews often have little time to use the rest-room facilities, not to mention thinking about sitting down on a tour of duty to eat a meal like a human being. These brave men and women are often confronted with responding to violent emergencies such as shootings, arriving on the scene before the police and while the shots are still flying.

EMS members have frequently been assaulted and subjected to harassment, verbal abuse, infectious diseases, and constant thoughts of their peers who have been killed in the line of duty throughout the nation. In most cases, these dedicated members of society take on EMS employment fully knowing that the wages they will earn are just above that of a fast-food or retail worker, but they do so to help people. So the next time you think about those "brave men and women," also think about the fact that they rarely receive recognition or remuneration for the responsibilities that they have or the risks the public expects them to take on their behalf. Perhaps this book will allow you to develop a better understanding and respect for what my "brothers and sisters" across the nation stand ready to do for you twenty-four hours a day.

Nevertheless, the book and my preface are not supposed to be a sounding board for the myriad of issues we continue to work through as a profession. Remember that Emergency Medical Services, as a contemporary profession, is only thirty-five years young (a mere infant by most professional and historical standards).

After many rigorous educational programs and clinical internships, you are allowed to "hit the streets" with your newly acquired knowledge so you can start to learn how to apply these skills in the austere and often complex environment of prehospital medicine and rescue. But the learning does not stop there. You learn every day. Every shift the "job" changes, and there is no time to become sloppy or stale. In this business, if you misplace a decimal point you can kill someone.

We are required to "sing for our supper," as we call it. Every two to three years, depending on certification and licensing bodies, we must recertify or relicense. Failure to successfully complete this process can result in our termination. How many professions can you think of that have to worry about continued employment based upon these stringent requirements?

The stress can be overwhelming at times. For instance, if you execute a rescue incorrectly you can kill your patient, your partner, or yourself. Clearly, this job is not for the fainthearted or the meek. Knowing yourself, knowing your partner, and being confident in your knowledge under fire are essential. Without those the results can be catastrophic.

At times I sit and think about what my peers and I are called upon to do and the obstacles we must overcome daily. With great respect I ponder the talents required to be successful, the sacrifices made to be dedicated, and the commitment needed to stay optimistic. But then I reflect not on the hardships of the job but on the great experiences that many will never know. Being the first person to hold a newborn infant you have just helped into the world (I have had this privilege more then twenty times in my career), for instance. Or the gratification you have when you have successfully resuscitated a patient, and the relief you see on the family's faces. Even in the worst of times—such as the last decade, where we have been called to the scenes of disasters and terrorist attacks—I am inspired by the professionalism, bravery, dedication, and humanity exhibited by my fellow EMS members across the country. Clearly, it is EMTs and paramedics who are on the front lines of defense for America.

In closing: J. A. Karam's attempt at providing the world an inside glimpse of EMS is to be commended. This area is often overlooked by the mainstream media and misrepresented by the entertainment industry via TV shows and movies.

She presents the real and gritty world of being an EMT and paramedic in modern society. While her travels chronicle a large urban EMS system, the stories and lessons she illustrates could easily be from a manicured suburb or a bucolic rural setting. Emergencies remain essentially the same: people get sick and they need help; accidents happen and people need help; disasters occur and communities need help. It is EMS that supplies a major component of that help every time. By choosing to utilize UMDNJ EMS, she selected one of the finest EMS organizations in the nation. The people who work there are some of the best our business has to offer. Keep an open mind and heart, and when you have concluded reading this book, I am sure, you will have developed a newfound respect for the profession, the trials and tribulations, and the people of EMS.

I wish you and my entire EMS family many days of coming home in one piece.

Paul M. Maniscalco, M.P.A., Ph.D.(c), EMT/P
Past President—National Association of Emergency Medical Technicians
Deputy Chief—Paramedic New York City

INTRODUCTION

EMS aficionados trace the profession's roots back to the biblical Good Samaritans,[1] but modern Emergency Medical Services (EMS) has evolved over the past thirty-five years as high-speed highways began crisscrossing the continent and high-impact car accidents began shattering lives on a daily basis. At the time, volunteer rescue squads covered a few parts of the country in their low-slung Cadillac ambulances or Chevy Suburban high-tops, but funeral homes provided almost half of the nation's emergency transports.[2]

In the late 1960s, young Dave Garmon, now an EMS educator at the University of South Alabama, dreamed of becoming a doctor. When Garmon was a teen, his dad sent him to work for the Perry Funeral Home in Centre, Alabama, to see if he could handle the sick and the dead. "Everybody listened to scanners," Garmon remembers. "If you heard of an accident, you'd take off and whoever got there first would take over the scene." Untrained mortuary attendants rushed to calamities, parting traffic with detachable bubble lights that flashed brightly atop their somber black hearses and earsplitting sirens mounted under the hoods. Depending on victims' conditions, Garmon and hundreds like him would shuttle their charges to the hospital or the morgue. Highway casualties in the U.S. were more likely to die of injury than soldiers hurt on Vietnamese battlefields halfway across the globe.[3]

In the mid-1960s, President Lyndon Johnson asked the National Academy of Sciences to study why tens of thousands of people were dying on the nation's roads each year. Its 1966 report, *Accidental Death and Disability: The Neglected Disease of Modern Society*, identified trauma as a scourge responsible for more deaths among people of ages one to thirty-seven than any other factor. It also made several proposals to address the epidemic and is credited as the catalyst for contemporary EMS. For example, to help correct widespread deficiencies in emergency medical care it suggested standardized training and equipment for ambulance attendants. At the time, there was no emergency-medicine specialty for physicians, much less a national curriculum for field responders.

Also in 1966, the Highway Safety Act directed the Department of Transportation to create an EMS program. Three years later, the first EMT curriculum was published, although training and certification procedures were inconsistent from one place to another. Over the next several years, government and foundations made millions of dollars available for EMS demonstration projects in several states.

By the early 1970s the City of Newark had experimented with ambulance services run by its fire department and its hospital. Each of the city's five wards staffed volunteer ambulances to supplement municipal service, too. University Hospital EMS Chief Mario Piumelli, then a prematurely tall and husky teen, remembers being pressed into the service by a citizens' committee. "You'd be good on the ambulance squad," one of the committee members told him. Piumelli, who wanted to be a fireman, had no such inclination and said so. When the committee member suggested he join or get his legs broken, Piumelli says, he was persuaded. "*No one* said no to the committee."

"Back then, *no one* took blood pressures," Piumelli recalls. " 'Look, kid,' they'd say, 'don't try none of that doctor shit!' Or, 'Put that thing (stethoscope or blood-pressure cuff) away, you're no doctor!'

"Old-timers found it hard to accept change. Here I was, a fifteen- or sixteen-year-old kid whose training was based on the Boy Scouts' first aid, a defensive-driving course, and CPR. Liter flow (on the oxygen tank) was like— you listened." Back then, just hearing the oxygen hiss was good enough. Now crews set flow meters to a specific number of liters per minute depending on the patient's condition and the type of oxygen-delivery system used. "Stretchers were 'sticks.' " The primary patient-carrying device was a battlefield holdover made from a swath of canvas slung between two sticks. EMS has always borrowed ideas from the military—from Native Americans to Napoleon to Roman campaigns. "We had no KEDs or short boards"—devices that help stabilize and protect noncritical trauma patients from additional injury during extrication and transport—"no Reeves, no backboards, no hare traction"—a special splint for thigh fractures. "Everything was dispatched by the police. They'd just give a call, and we'd pick the patient up and take them to the hospital. There were no communications with the hospital. There was no early warning. And there were no run sheets, no charts—just verbal reports."

With the EMS Systems Act, in 1973, came $300 million and federal guidelines for EMS research and development. The National Highway Transportation and Safety Administration (NHTSA), a Department of Transportation division, developed first-aid curriculum guidelines. Soon hearse drivers, firefighters, and enthusiastic volunteers transformed themselves into the first generation of emergency medical technicians (EMTs).[4]

About the same time, cardiologists were experimenting with defibrillation and cardiac pulmonary resuscitation (CPR) to reverse sudden death in the field. Both trauma surgeons and cardiologists found they had something in common. *Bringing* skilled care *to* the critically ill and wounded could save lives. Previously, the concept was limited mostly to the battlefield.

Since the mid-1970s, government agencies, health-care providers, and private enterprise have been enriching EMS training and scope of practice. Now NHTSA estimates that between one and two million EMS workers do everything from rescue breathing to treating the consequences of terrorism on American soil. The quality and quantity of EMS varies from state to state, however, in part because the Omnibus Budget Reconciliation Act of 1981, which provided some of the last substantive, federal financial support, channeled monies for EMS through state block grants.

Six years ago, a coworker and I walked from a downtown Manhattan meeting to our offices, where we worked on children's television programming and products. New York was still digging out from back-to-back blizzards, its curbs buried beneath four-foot piles of snow. From the corner of my eye, I saw a car hit a bicyclist. I watched as he soared through the air and smacked headfirst into the car snowed in beside me. The dull thud was sickening. I scrambled over the snowbank to spy a crumpled heap lying in a bed of cold slush. "Call 911!" I shouted to my colleague, and crouched beside the man to help. Then it dawned on me: I had no idea what to do.

I searched my memory for anything helpful that I might have seen on television. Nothing came to mind. All I could think to do was to keep the man still and warm. I draped my coat over him, knelt beside him, and, although he seemed to be in shock, talked in what I hoped was a soothing voice. All the while, blood poured from his ears and his skull; it steamed in the frigid air. I held him steady and prayed for an ambulance.

I don't know how much time passed before I realized I was eye-level with several pairs of black boots. Looking up, I saw police controlling a growing crowd. "Where's the ambulance?" I asked anxiously.

"It's coming," an officer replied, arms crossed in front of his chest.

Some forty minutes later, the ambulance arrived. EMS workers loaded the man on their stretcher. Before driving off to a trauma center, one suggested I get an AIDS test. That surprised me until I noticed that my hands were bloodied, as were my clothes.

When I returned to the office, my boss gave me the rest of the day off, but I was too shaken to be alone. I cleaned up, phoned the hospital, and befriended one of its public-relations officers. I persuaded her to keep me informed of the man's condition. She called me every hour for twelve hours, while neurosurgeons operated. When it was clear that he would survive and his condition was stable, she arranged a visit.

A Middle Eastern civil servant with a family to support overseas, the man had come to America to find his fortune. He worked as a delivery man for a New York restaurant while studying English and hoping to become an accountant.

The injuries caused permanent neurological damage. I might have kept in touch with him, but his lawyer began phoning and trying to persuade me that a city bus had caused the accident. As far as the vehicle that struck him—I did not get much in the way of a description. But it was no bus. The man was in dire financial straits and I was sympathetic. Nevertheless, I resented his apparent intent to sue the city to better his situation.

The bloody episode changed my life. I enrolled in a community first-aid class near my home in New Jersey. EMTs taught the class. One of the instructors, a retired engineer who had been volunteering on the town's emergency squad for thirty years, tried recruiting me. *I am* not *ready for that!* I thought. The collision disturbed me, but, having taken the short course, I felt somewhat better prepared.

As I went about errands in town, however, I spotted recruitment posters pleading the need for members. I saw placards at the bank, supermarket, and train station. I had never before considered the people who staff ambulances. Now I wondered, *How well trained are they? And why does it take so long?* When I discovered that our town of seventeen thousand residents delegated its emergency care to volunteers, I wanted to know more.

I phoned the number on the poster and learned that the squad was a nonprofit organization whose crews were professionally trained and state-certified.

The next thing I knew I was one of those volunteers, taking the 120-hour basic EMT course at an area hospital. I learned how to evaluate patients, treat shock, stop bleeding, splint broken body parts, and deliver babies as well as how to document crises on charts, package patients for transport, even how to protect and care for people trapped in car wreckage or those contaminated by hazardous materials.

The course also required a ten-hour ER internship. Watching ER technicians wheel in trauma victims with their raw and meaty wounds, hearing the shrill screams of terrified children, restrained so plastic surgeons could neatly stitch their soft skin back together, I sometimes found it hard to stay cool. Literally. When the sights and sounds became too much, I overheated and became dizzy. Our instructor warned us against fainting and creating extra effort for an already overworked ER staff. It was not uncommon for classmates to collapse and become patients themselves! So I headed for fresh air and orange juice when I felt lightheaded.

At first, the EMT course and its unfamiliar material intimidated me. I had a lifelong aversion to all things bloody and had long since dismissed any notions of becoming a doctor or veterinarian—besides, high-school algebra left me dazed and confused and I could never manage to balance equations. Several squad members had Ph.D.s. *How would I ever get through it?*

Again, I lucked out. My new friends on the crew encouraged and coached me. My EMS classroom instructors were patient, thorough, and not at all hesitant to shove me out of my comfort zone. In the end, I was pleased to graduate. Best of all, I discovered that my loathing of blood had evaporated—as long as I was dealing with someone else's blood. It was simply a matter of realizing that people needed my help more than I needed to be frightened. Now when I encounter people who say, "I could never do that," I assure them that it's possible. Opportunity usually knocks on the right door.

The chance to help people in real time, as opposed to slogging away for stockholders, was refreshing. I discovered colleagues whose priorities I admired—even if it meant being startled awake by the pager's sharp tones and racing through the town's dark streets at 0400 hours. (In keeping with EMS practice, this book generally reflects time on the twenty-four-hour military clock.)

Our squad had a captain, lieutenants, and line officers as well as an administrative board and about thirty members. To meet the town's needs, we divided into teams (two, three, or four EMTs), each of which worked one twelve-hour shift per week plus one weekend shift per month. To help the duty crew, which sometimes was expected to be in two places at once, we kept our pagers on and responded to as many other calls as possible.

My first crew chief came from Romania by way of Israel. A retired mathematician with a Ph.D. from Berkeley, he was an impressive athlete with a wicked sense of humor. My two other crewmates had advanced degrees in nursing. One hailed from Scotland and the other from Hong Kong. Under their tutelage, I learned a lot. On Tuesday nights at 1845 hours we would gather at headquarters, inspect our trucks, have coffee, practice some of our skills, and visit. In so doing, we became good friends. Others on the squad, ages twenty to eighty, included a retired Fortune 500 vice-president, a mail carrier, travel and real-estate agents, a youthfully retired investment banker and a liquor distributor, a church secretary, housewives, and myriad others.

As I developed a taste for EMS, the bicyclist's catastrophe continued to motivate me to reconsider what I was doing with my life. I left the corporate world in favor of consulting projects that interested me and made time to explore EMS. The more I learned, the more I wanted to know.

On the squad, I began noticing that our performance was sometimes less than it should have been. However well intentioned, crews were sometimes too rusty or too tempted to use their discretion instead of following protocol. Such shortcomings did not reflect on our squad members' intelligence or innate capabilities, but they did point to a lack of expertise. Smaller towns in many places suffer similarly. Comparatively few calls result in limited experience. Complacency, a reluctance to invest time in drills, and fear of failure and criticism only make things worse.

New Jersey's Department of Health and Senior Services does not regulate volunteer ambulance services, which experts say provide more than eighty-five percent of New Jersey's basic life support (BLS) services. At their option, squads can belong to the nonprofit, self-regulating First Aid Council, whose members police themselves. The FAC publishes equipment guidelines and conducts inspections, and each district publishes an annual report. But, apart from steadily raising the bar for members and notifying municipalities when members fail to meet standards, it has no enforcement authority. No independent experts audit volunteer performance, credentials, or equipment suitability.

Although our squad was devoted, I thought more hands-on training could improve our execution and volunteered to be training officer. (In our town, the training-officer position *did not* mean I trained everyone. I lacked the experience to do that.) We were fortunate to live and volunteer in an affluent and generous area. Our coffers were full and we could afford to reach out and hire experts to teach us about various subjects, from Do Not Resuscitate orders to caring for near-drowning victims. (We held that class in the township pool, where one of our students accidentally cracked the instructor on the head with a body splint. As his blood stained the water, twenty EMTs hell-bent on rescuing him practically sank him instead.)

I hoped that we would also drill for the bus accident, the train derailment, the bridge collapse, the school shooting, or one of the other calamities that seem to occur wherever there is ubiquitous denial and the fervent belief that it can't happen "here." Several years previously the squad had hosted a drill that did not go as well as members would have liked. They were hesitant to try again. In time, though, they agreed and sent me to EMS Today, an annual conference sponsored by the *Journal of Emergency Medical Services* (*JEMS*), where I spent long, information-packed days learning about mass casualty incidents and how to organize drills. As a marketer, I had produced complex celebrity-studded special events and international product launches. Yet I never imagined what would be necessary to competently manage even a small-scale disaster.

The seminars covered everything from tabletop exercises to preplanned escalation tables that showed how to draw EMS resources from surrounding areas without stripping the region bare. The instructors raised one taxing logistical question after another. How would we organize triage teams and treatment areas? How many patients could we assess and treat before becoming overwhelmed? How effective were our plans and systems for summoning aid from neighboring communities, the state, and the federal government? Would our tools and equipment be compatible? (Surprisingly often, they are not.) How would we distribute patients among area hospitals without besieging their ERs? What were our plans for giving rescue workers the rest and refreshment they would need to serve throughout physically and emotionally trying events?

Battle-tested instructors demonstrated how to keep track of which patients went to which hospitals. They shared strategies for coordinating drills with police, firefighters, and area hospitals, as well as media, local politicians, government officials, and their resources, too. They pointed out possible complications arising from interrupted power supplies and inadequate radio and cell-phone frequencies. Would our assumptions stand up to all kinds of weather and regional disasters that might decimate our neighboring communities, too? They suggested setting up letters of credit with local vendors, utilities, and telecommunications companies so supplies and materials could be readily acquired if needed. *Who knew?*

Years earlier, I had earned a master's degree in International Affairs with a concentration in international security from Columbia University, and so I could not resist Paul Maniscalco's lecture on EMS and terrorism. I sat next to Matthew Streger, who turned out to be a bright and amiable young paramedic who had once worked at University Hospital, was a fellow New Jerseyan, and was a former intern of Maniscalco's.

Maniscalco's presentation was riveting, illuminating, and motivating. I clearly grasped how superior community-EMS is the foundation for the responsiveness our nation needs in the event of terrorist attacks and other large-scale calamities.

Having seen our squad's sometimes less-than-efficient response to multi-car collisions, I doubted whether we had the skill and experience to be truly useful at any mass casualty. Although some of my volunteer colleagues consistently outperformed some paid EMS workers whom I eventually came to know, I could not help but compare my fellow volunteers to the gung-ho pros I met at EMS Today. Although I did not know it at the time, I had stepped into a muddy area of EMS, where paid professionals and volunteers debate their relative merits and weaknesses, each group thinking the other leaves much to be desired.

Volunteers tend to assert that their passion for EMS, their concern for community, and their gift of time are hallmarks of sincerity and devotion. They sometimes view paid EMS workers as mercenaries. Paid EMS caregivers, almost all of whom began their EMS careers as volunteers (at least in New Jersey), often dismiss their volunteer counterparts as "siren-heads," people who use EMS to feel important; bored retirees and clueless housewives; wannabe firefighters and police officers; and adrenaline junkies. Both volunteers and paid professionals have their pros and cons, but the public is often too ill informed to evaluate its local resources, much less influence performance.

For all its flaws, I saw, and still see, EMS as an invaluable gem—precious and sufficiently strong to withstand scrutiny. I wanted to study it and raise its profile. As long as I was setting goals, I decided to change my profession. What I liked most about marketing was my exposure to idea people—writers, artists, scientists, etc. So I stopped consulting, returned to Columbia University, and earned a second master's degree, this time in journalism. At Columbia, I first began writing about EMS. Through Matt Streger I had met Paul Maniscalco. In turn, through Paul, and later Daniel Gerard, I met dozens of distinguished and dedicated EMS workers who also inspired me to undertake this book.

This book's goal is to show how members of one team in a busy, urban system allocate emergency resources; where EMS workers tread; the demands of the job; and what type of people are drawn to the profession and are able to perform. Although EMS is a young profession, still in its earliest stages of development, it is far too complex for this book to cover in its entirety. I chose an agile, well-reputed service as a lens. Approximately 273,500 people live in Newark, America's third-oldest city. Many thousands more work here. Each year, tens of millions use Newark International Airport, the world's eighteenth busiest; its Pennsylvania Station, with 450 trains, forty-five bus lines, and subway; the New Jersey Marine Terminals, the largest mechanized container port in the U.S.; and the city's multiple highways. What plagues the people of Newark plagues people everywhere, and that means everything from the cockroaches lodged in the ear and diabetic comas to severe lacerations and family violence.

As part of my research, I attended professional conferences, which gave me the chance to meet EMS workers who toil in vastly different territories, from the Grand Canyon and New Orleans to Vermont, which has less than one hundred medics, and Australia. I learned that the travails suffered by people in Newark are suffered by others. "Birmingham has drug abuse and crime, too," Alabaman Dave Garmon admits, stressing that today's problems are omnipresent. "The big cities sometimes get a bad rap. People are people wherever they live." Tennessean John Fitzsimmons, an EMS veteran from the earliest days who sits on the board of the National Association of Emergency Medical Technicians (NAEMT), concurs. The major difference between large cities and suburban and rural areas is volume, Fitzsimmons says, not the type of call.

Where I live, in white-picket-fence territory, young adults die from heroin overdoses, too. Occasionally, someone will slaughter his or her family or commit suicide or fall in a shower and be scalded to death. One emotionally disturbed resident dropped his drawers in public, regularly. Alcoholics waste away in large, fancy homes. EMS, wherever it is practiced, can feel like a horror peepshow that runs 24/7.

University Hospital in Newark, New Jersey, is a 466-bed teaching hospital affiliated with the University of Medicine and Dentistry of New Jersey, the largest health-science university in the U.S. It is also the primary trauma center for the two million people who live in Newark's immediate metropolitan area.

In August 2001, Communications Coordinator Robert Resetar reported that the E-911 medical dispatch center was handling roughly 300,000 incoming calls; and this was prior to September 11, when volume soared owing to the EMS Department's efforts to aid victims and coordinate emergency responders throughout New Jersey.

Newark's EMS workers are among the country's most productive. On average, dispatchers handle hundreds of calls per shift. Each two-person EMS crew responds to between twelve and twenty-five emergencies *each* twelve-hour shift.[5] In 1999, basic life support (BLS) crews transported 42,743 patients, advance life support (ALS) transported 10,158 patients, and the air medical division transported 558 patients, for a total of 53,459. The total *does not* include visits to people who ultimately refuse medical aid, deceased patients, or those who have disappeared when EMS arrives (or never existed).

The department runs four EMS teams in Newark. The day teams are busier, and their challenges are more visual. For example, one day I accompanied a crew to a job nearby quarters. Medics opened a squeaky, rust-coated gate to climb the front steps of a sagging row house. Weather-beaten and misshapen by age and neglect, the decrepit old building itself looked to be in pain. Someone had taken the trouble, though, to paint the front steps with high-gloss, bloodred paint, which screamed in the sunlight. The porch was festooned with red velour tulips and fluorescent silk plants stuffed into cracked plastic pots. A Caribbean-accented, turbaned woman answered the door whispering and rolling her eyes: "The whole house is filled with crazy."

Backing into her kitchen, she pointed toward a dark, narrow staircase. "Get him out. I can't stand it no more." Cautiously, the EMS workers coaxed a famil-iar mental patient, who wore rose-colored glasses, into their truck. At night, the same house blends innocuously into the backdrop, one of several such houses that have huddled together for generations.

Ultimately, I chose to ride with the B team, which works overnight. It is known for fierce camaraderie, irreverence, and immense skill. And its members prefer working with less direct supervision from management, which stays on call, but from the comfort of home. During my year at University, I rode with BLS EMTs, ALS paramedics, rescue specialists, and supervisors. I also inter-viewed air medical crews and spoke with physicians, psychiatrists, social work-ers, and EMS managers.

At shift change, about 1845 hours, I showed up at headquarters, where the crews swiped in, signed for their duty radios, and climbed on their designated buses. (EMS pros say "bus" or "truck" instead of "ambulance." They *do not* call the ambulances "rigs," a dead giveaway to one's volunteer status.)

Often I stashed an overturned milk crate on the floor between the driver's and copilot's seats so that I could ride up there with them. (In retrospect, although this afforded tremendous access to the EMS workers, I was lucky to emerge from my year unharmed, and it was not very bright. The high rate of ambulance accidents, an industry-wide phenomenon, is a life threat itself.) When patients were in the bus, the cramped box in back was center stage, and I sat, stood, kneeled, and crouched there. Otherwise, I wanted to ride shotgun.

University EMS-worker uniforms are shades of blue: navy, slate, and sky, enlivened by silver shields, black trim, and the occasional gold accent. To blend in, I wore blue, too. I carried no hospital identification or any of my own EMS credentials, because I was not permitted to treat patients. I held a reporter's notebook and took notes. No one, except the occasional detective and one patient's daughter, asked who I was. When I explained that I was writing a book about EMS workers, no one complained or showed any interest. Aqeed Al-Atiyat, Iyad Al-Atiyat, and police officer Debra Conte are patients who wanted to share their stories and help people understand the vital nature of EMS. They permitted me to use their names. Similarly, the EMTs and paramedics whose names I feature all gave their consent. Although the events and people I have written about are real, I have changed all other patient names and some minor identifying details.

I stayed on the buses and followed the EMS workers on call after call, many nights for the entire twelve hours. If I was deeply exhausted, I could get off and go home. They could not.

The fatigue and constant exposure to sick people wore me down. "You'll either get used to this or you'll have a psychotic break," my EMS sherpas predicted. In fact, I never got fully accustomed to the arduous hours. I felt so weary after the marathon shifts that I had to roll down my car window, crank up the radio, and slap my face, unpleasantly often, to stay awake on my thirty-mile ride home. Tangerine-and-raspberry sunrises, although spectacular, were not sufficiently stimulating. I suffered more colds and viruses in one year than I could count, including a rare one that took months to resolve and forced me to consult a specialist.

Like many of the overnight EMS workers, I developed a profound sleep disorder, still troublesome months after I stopped reporting. The over-the-top weariness made me marvel at their stamina and wonder: *How do they do it?* I have never seen people will themselves beyond the limits of human exhaustion night after night, year after year, decade after decade.

The B team teased me without mercy, although it could have been *much* worse. My attire screamed hospital employee, not EMS. I was too slow, too clumsy, too emotional, too sympathetic. Worse, if I visited the bathroom *twice* during a busy shift, they would invoke the nickname they assigned to my bladder: "Peanut." That changed when I got an infection on my arm. Then I became "Ebola Girl."

I interviewed anyone and everyone, sometimes oblivious of danger. The crew's hard-won street smarts allowed me to feel at home (sort of). And they protected me. One night at a motorcycle club's rally, a man fractured his leg so badly the bones protruded through his skin. EMT and rescue specialist Eugene "Geno" O'Neil had to yank me from conversation with the group's sergeant-at-arms. "That's the job they give to the toughest guy with the most weapons," he growled under his breath.

The classic EMS response has an anatomy that helps impose order on turmoil. The components are often executed simultaneously; the order can change. EMS is dynamic and flexible, but the best practitioners don't overlook these basics. This book harnesses this archetypal structure to show readers the ins and outs of day-to-day EMS. Chapter 1 throws readers into the action, showcasing a typical crisis. Successive chapters break the continuum into sections: dispatch, scene safety, rescue, assessment, treatment, transport, documentation, and some of the side effects of a career in EMS.

Although the book was complete when terrorists turned September 11, 2001, into a day Americans will never forget, I added a section to illustrate aspects of the department's initial response. Sad, devastating, life-altering, it was still just a day on the job—one of the most dangerous, challenging, and little-known jobs one can have. Alleviating others' pain and distress, often under grueling conditions, and sometimes at the cost of one's life, is the EMS worker's daily bread.

Once more unto the breach, dear friends, once more;
Or close the wall up with our English dead!
In peace there's nothing so becomes a man
As modest stillness and humility;
But when the blast of war blows in our ears,
Then imitate the action of the tiger:
Stiffen the sinews, summon up the blood,
Disguise fair nature with hard-favoured rage;
Then lend the eye a terrible aspect.

—WILLIAM SHAKESPEARE, *HENRY V*, III.i.

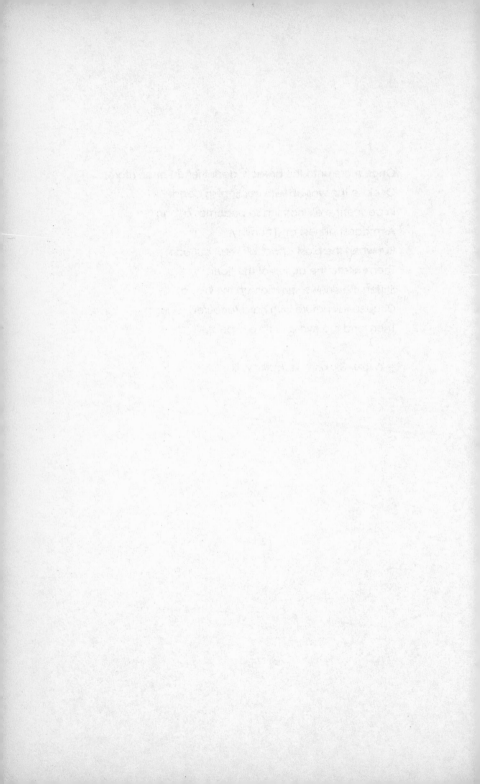

INTO THE BREACH

1   *DUSK*

Spring showers have rained down on Brick City and soaked its streets for seven days straight. The sun is setting and the deluge has abated, leaving steam rising from the many brick buildings that crowd Newark, New Jersey's Central Ward. Tonight, members of University Hospital's EMS B team will fight to control urban trauma and medical emergencies under a severe thunderstorm watch. Eugene "Geno" O'Neill has come to work early, as usual. Crews who ride the Rescue truck do. The reciprocal courtesy means that when 6:45 rolls around, whether A.M. or P.M., relief is on campus, and the duty shift can walk away without another thought.

Between ominous clouds, streaks of apricot sunlight wash over O'Neill's oblong face, squared off at the top with a tight buzz cut and at the bottom by a strong chin. He sports a soldier's trim build with skin as weathered as an ace bombardier's flying jacket. Because he works at night, however, his face is an incongruous shade of cotton-candy pink. O'Neill flips open his box of Marlboro Lights, and taps it hard against his fist until a butt slides out. He has rolled up his uniform sleeves and cuffed them below his elbows. The muscular cords of forearms flex with even the simplest movement. After lighting up, he stuffs the pack in his pocket and squares his stance on the tarmac outside EMS headquarters.

Against the backdrop of a squat, one-story building with flaking blue paint and a corrugated tin roof the EMT and rescue specialist straightens his spine, rests a wrist on the small of his back, and pinches the cigarette between his thumb and forefinger before taking a long, deep drag. He sucks in the tar and nicotine, and his clear blue eyes close to slits. An agile and tightly wound man, at thirty-four O'Neill has been involved in emergency health-care more than half his life. A severe Catholic-school education took the edge off his propensity for defiance, but O'Neill's parents made additional efforts to keep him out of trouble. When he turned fourteen, they had him volunteering at a local hospital.

Between drags, he pensively rolls the cigarette between his thumb and index finger. He smokes, and admires the sunset through the compound's chain-link fence, which separates quarters from the Georgia King Village garden apartments and other area residences. The soft hues of dusk do little to diminish the staccato sounds, screaming sirens, and troubling sights around him. There is no sign that the city is bedding down for the night.

A paramedic, passing O'Neill on her way to swipe in for duty, remarks casually, "This city never sleeps; all it does is get dark out. It's like an eclipse or something. It just keeps going."

EMS administrators have been angling for a structure better suited to house its crews, fleet of vehicles, dispatchers, instructors, and paper-pushers for more than ten years; they predict five more years will pass before that vision is realized. For now, their roost is a secondhand "temporary" building, erected in the 1960s with concrete blocks and a prefabricated metal shell. Prior to EMS's occupancy, the medical examiner conducted business here; the floors inside slope slightly toward drains designed to draw excess blood and fluids.

O'Neill has already clocked in, signed for his radio, and taken a quick tour through quarters. Inside, the top portion of the concrete-block walls is painted vanilla. The bottom third is raspberry-colored. But the building is anything but appetizing. Glass-shielded bulletin boards line the halls. Floors are scuffed. The day's detritus spills off crowded counters and overflows from garbage pails onto the kitchen floor. O'Neill stashed a snack in the refrigerator, hung an extra uniform in his locker (it pays to be prepared), hit the head, and checked his mail in the perpetually darkened TV room. A few day-teamers, aka day-pukes, lounge there, lumps on coffee-colored couches, their feet propped on a square brown table along with remnants of lunch. A sheet lies crumpled in a corner of a couch, defying a recent management decree that EMS workers shall not use linen for personal comfort.

A computer junkie, O'Neill has stowed his personal digital assistant and laptop in the Rescue office, a cramped Pepto Bismol–pink space stuffed with desks, awkwardly juxtaposed cabinets, and a gallery of children's artwork.

More day-pukes camp around a rickety picnic table outside HQ, slugging soda and finalizing last-minute paperwork. Billy "the Squirrel" Heber, O'Neill's partner, is already putting the 38,000-pound Rescue truck, aka "the Beast," through his nightly meticulous inspection. He examines tool after tool, more than 375 of them. A burly German-American with wavy chestnut hair and a dusting of freckles, Heber drove trucks before joining the service nineteen years ago.

Back then, EMS here was still in its infancy. Paramedics were still new to New Jersey and few in number. Heber and a partner worked the ambulance and routinely handled twenty-five to thirty jobs during their eight-hour shifts. Budgets were tight, and sometimes supplies ran short. A colleague remembers. "We'd find ourselves asking, 'Is this patient sick enough for me to use one of my four-by-fours [bandages]?' Whereas with Heber, it was never a problem 'cause he always had plenty of everything squirreled away in little hiding places." Dashing between hectic ERs, Heber might borrow a spare box of bandages here, a few surplus cravats there. He'd be quick to claim equipment abandoned at accident scenes. He'd stuff every nook and cranny on his bus with every conceivable supply and tool. In a pinch, colleagues soon realized, Heber was the best and fastest source for whatever they needed. They dubbed him "the Squirrel," and his resourcefulness became legendary.

Paramedic Vincent Francis "Fester" Cisternino, a twenty-nine-year-old colossus of German-Italian descent, swipes in and tromps outside to the picnic bench, where he greets O'Neill, "Hey, meat." At six feet, one inch and 270 pounds, Cisternino dwarfs the wiry O'Neill. He's not kindly disposed to the day-scum either; he finds them careless with the equipment—prone to overstuffing his bus's med bag with catheters and sticking trauma dressings inside the airway kit.

Each spring, as a sign of spiritual renewal, Cisternino shears his thick, curly brown locks to reveal a blue-white scalp. Six years ago, he converted from Catholicism to Buddhism. He carries a crimson strand of hand-carved rosewood prayer beads that a Buddhist monk gave him. He secretes a miniature Tibetan flag in his pocket and a miniature Cartman, the roly-poly, cheeky character from TV's *South Park*. He's had an elaborately detailed and colored dragon of his own design tattooed on his body. It bursts through a violent sea on his shoulder, rides his right chest, soars over his scapula, and wraps its tail around an ornate cherry tree on his biceps. Cisternino says it reflects his dual nature: fierce and gentle.

East Asian studies is one of two majors Cisternino doggedly pursues in his decade-long quest to complete his college degree. He would have finished it years ago but for the fact that he didn't know much about budgeting, and, at eighteen, tried to finance tuition, books, and living expenses on his first credit card. It took him years to pay off the debt, which he has done while attending school and juggling three or more jobs on the same 168-hour week as the rest of the world. It has been a tough haul, even for the colossus Cisternino, who has since perfected the art of piling each minute high with activity. He first cultivated this ability in high school. In addition to classes and a full-time job as an office/shipping clerk, the teenager worked as a bouncer and a lifeguard. He also lifted weights two hours a day to sculpt a fifty-four-inch chest and thirty-eight-inch waist and biceps that bulged like bowling balls. In his spare time, he volunteered as an EMT for a Pallisades Park emergency squad.

From behind his Oakley polarized Straight Jackets, Cisternino grins at O'Neill, who holds court at the picnic table with others who have begun to assemble. Cisternino wears his University baseball cap backward; it displays his nickname, "Fester," in neat embroidery. When he smiles, the impish six-year-old he must have been once is briefly visible. One hardly notices his tongue bar. He lights a cigarette and takes a seat.

Those who dare greet the ascetic O'Neill with a dulled "Good morning." Although it is twilight, their day is just beginning. Others, eyes downcast or straight ahead, squeak by hoping not to draw attention. If O'Neill and his buddies are not otherwise engaged, they might focus on a passerby. It's part instinct, one medic explains. Whenever they shake hands with someone, they subtly check out the veins and assess how easily they could slide a catheter in. A fat person walks by; they're a potential case of congestive heart failure. A *really* fat person waddles across the road, another quips, "Basically, he died three years ago. He just hasn't lied down yet." And work-related romances or "knocking boots," no matter how secret the parties imagine them to be, are fair game for ridicule, too. Nothing is sacred.

Cisternino, O'Neill, and a few others compose the Council of Elders, which they characterize as "a nondescript government agency loosely affiliated with the Foundation for Urban Combat Survival Systems," a fantastical entity they have nicknamed FUCSS University or FUCS U. Why waste the effort they placed into Y2K preparations? they joke—explaining FUCS U as an alternative to wilderness survival programs. It's harder to endure the hostile and austere conditions of a large urban center than to crash-land in the Peruvian jungle, O'Neill says. "For a thousand bucks, we train Americans and select foreign nationals in the nuances of not only surviving, but flourishing, unarmed, in an environment that most people won't admit exists."

O'Neill discusses an upcoming camping trip. Cisternino checks out a camouflage-colored water-storage device that one of the other medics received as a birthday gift. The two, and a few other blue-shirts, have taken several FNGs (fucking new guys) under their wing. Through ambitious outdoor excursions, hazing, and errands only eager-to-please pledges could endure, the veterans hope to toughen their charges, improve their street smarts, and shape their perspective to the team's benefit. The B team considers itself a fraternity; most members have at least ten years' experience, and they are close on and off the job. They try attracting EMS workers with a similar mind-set, but they don't control assignments. They do have some say, however unofficial, as to who makes the cut. The waiting list is reputedly long. And openings, which are infrequent, are no guarantee that newcomers will find a home.

Smart neophytes used to keep their mouths shut, work, and speak when spoken to. Eventually, those who hung on the longest would improve enough to be folded into the pecking order. Cisternino and his partner, Tracey Ann Fazio, say more than a year passed before anyone spoke to them conversationally. But something in the culture has changed of late. The FNGs are still too timid to sit at the table when veterans are present, but now they talk too much.

For example, one of the new hires yaps about a job he went to earlier. He found a quadriplegic locked inside a room. Caretakers had left the man flat on his back on top of a bare and filthy mattress. They had torn a hole in the bedding beneath his buttocks. When the man defecated, his waste splashed into a bucket below. Maggots infested his flesh. The medic was appalled, but no B-teamer within listening range broke a sweat. War stories do not impress them; they say they see more in two months than most EMS workers see in a lifetime. O'Neill, for instance, has seen patients whose bodies burst apart from contact with downed electric wires. He has witnessed child abuse, hostage takings, disembowelments, dismemberments, and other grotesque atrocities. He has watched fire-eaten roofs buckle under coworkers minutes after he descended. In his twelve years on the job, O'Neill says he has buried four team members. Talk *is* cheap. B-teamers think of themselves as "hard-core, bad-to-the-bone rescuers." They pride themselves on eating their young.

The Council of Elders has tasked the FNGs with a precamping exercise to shut them up and engage them in proving their worthiness. O'Neill orders them to construct a twenty-item survival kit inside an Altoids' tin. At minimum, he barks, they should have twenty feet of parachute cord, a biohazard bag, six feet of electrical tape, thirty feet of waxed dental floss, twenty feet of snare wire, a wire saw, safety pins, a button compass, a razor, cotton, sewing needles, four windproof candles, four waterproof matches, fishing weights, finger cots, cotton balls, anti-inflammatory pills, and a whistle.

"On a kit like this, my dad survived two weeks in the jungle," a seasoned EMS worker says about his mud marine father. O'Neill nods knowingly. As a five-year-old, he watched with awe the first time he saw his dad rifle through the first-aid kit he used as an army medic in Korea's demilitarized zone and parts of Indochina.

As the FNGs scramble to comply, Patricia Vogt rests a foot on the rescue truck's bumper and lights a cigarette. The only B-teamer who is also a grand-mother, Vogt once managed an auto body shop. Her boyfriend became an EMT first, and she joined him. Surprised to find EMS a relief from stress at the shop, she changed careers.

"Last night it was chicken noodle," Chief Paulie Visoskas mutters to himself in a veteran smoker's gravelly voice. He strolls toward the group and lights up. "Tonight, it's probably cream of chicken." He knows a popular nearby diner's menu by heart, and recites it aloud as he considers what to eat for breakfast. "It's pea soup on Thursday, and Sunday is chicken corn chowder. Or is that Friday?" No one answers.

While O'Neill lectures, one of the Elders approaches an escaped stretcher, twists a lever, and converts it into a chair. Next, he whips out his set of hair clippers and slaps the back of the chair, which causes O'Neill to pause his lesson and take a seat. O'Neill wraps a sheet around himself with a flourish and submits to the clippers.

"After the fall of society, we're going into the barber business," O'Neill declares, rising from the chair totally bald but for a faint velvet brush on the top of his head. "Jesus Christ, I love being a man among men. This is fucking fab-ulous." He polishes his newly shorn skull. "You can't get this in the corporate world!"

"Yeah, they're not giving high-and-tights in the Prudential building," someone chimes in.

Then Cisternino gets up from the table and steps into the chair with a wicked smirk.

"But he's bald already!" someone shouts.

"Let me do your eyebrows," the amateur barber begs. "And then I'll file your teeth into points!"

Enjoying the moment, Cisternino nods a greeting to his partner and friend of many years, paramedic Tracey Ann Fazio. A curvaceous five feet, eleven inches, with cascading hair the color of raging flame, Fazio parks herself at the table, opens her cosmetics case, and inserts her contact lenses. Next, she applies mink dark mascara, and glosses her lips with raspberry tint. Her lips, sometimes rose-petal pink, tomato, or berry, are often the only bright spot on the neutral canvas that is Newark at night—a dim palette of cream, shades of gray, dusky blues, and muted greens enlivened by scattered, twinkling lights. It's doubtful that any other female on the team could get away with such fastidious attention to appearance, but the twenty-nine-year-old Fazio has proven her mettle during her eleven-year tenure, and no one messes with her. "I'm like Ma Barker and these are my boys," she says with a wry smile and a faint lisp.

Ignoring the high jinks around her, she leafs through *Bride* magazine; her wedding to a fellow paramedic is just a few months away. The magazine rests on a pile of patient-care reports (charts), which an administrator has evaluated and stuffed in her mailbox to review.

Fazio also fell into EMS while in high school, after accepting a dare from EMT classmates she had teased because they wore uniform jackets, with patches and pagers, to school. "You couldn't do it," they challenged her. Fazio had been around "old-time ambulance folks forever," because her mother worked as an ER nurse and Fazio sometimes accompanied her. She decided to prove her classmates wrong. She volunteered for her municipal squad and worked for an ambulance transport company in college. That's where she met the air medical paramedic who persuaded her to work at University.

For years Fazio held a second job at another area hospital, where she sometimes worked with Cisternino. She convinced him to come to "the dark side," one of their nicknames for University. During their time together, she says, she has seen him transition through several phases, from a "dapper, Mr. L. L. Bean, GQ type" to the cowboy-hat-and-boots look to his current incarnation: bald head, surgical-steel body jewelry, and penchant for tattoos.

Although her coworkers are colorful, working the graveyard shift can be grim. Still, Fazio wouldn't trade it. *We definitely have the better part of the night,* she thinks, watching day-team stragglers head out to their cars. *I like it when the sky is half indigo and full of stars, and the other half is lit by the sun, and the two compete with each other.*

Then the city wakes up and it all turns to shit again.

She has a talent for finding the silver lining in any situation, even if she has to force it. *The nice thing about pollution is that it makes the colors go in really nice layers,* she muses as garish streaks of lemon and lavender striate the evening sky. Fazio is observant that way. As a second job, she designs online environments for fantastical computer worlds. She is a natural storyteller, attentive to the big picture and to the details, too. She can synthesize and structure large chunks of complex information in her mind and then deliver a rapid-fire analysis with gravitas and stunning precision. Her handwriting is exquisite. Administrators at other institutions have written EMS managers to compliment Fazio's reports. But she senses that the charts stacked beneath her bridal magazine are riddled with criticism.

Fazio has always been proud of her chart-writing skills, but there is new quality-assurance system in place, which has been tripping her up, nipping at her heels. She's supposed to review the charts, sign them to acknowledge that she understands the administrator's comments, and return them promptly. With a sigh and a drag on her cigarette, she sets the magazine aside and stares at one chart until she remembers the job all too well.

She had arrived at an apartment to find her patient deceased, absolutely unsalvageable. With a doctor's permission, which she obtained by radio, she pronounced the man dead, and checked off the "Dead at Scene" box on the chart. She filled in the hundreds of other tiny boxes, wrote a clear, succinct narrative, and attached the patient's flatline ECG (electrocardiogram). The manager declared the chart unacceptable, because Fazio didn't also mark the boxes labeled "unconscious," and "respiratory arrest," and "cardiac arrest." *"Dead at Scene" should be sufficient*, she thinks as her brows knit with exasperation. *If the patient is dead, he is neither conscious nor unconscious.* And what is dead if not a persistent lack of heartbeat and breath?

Fazio copes with her disappointment and wounded pride by lashing out with blazing indignation. Many of her charts go unscathed, but because she treats a lot of sick people and uses aggressive procedures,[1] her charts come up for inspection more often. "The QA process here has no human element," she complains as others around the table nod in agreement. Spirited invective concerning the administrator they've dubbed "the Chart Nazi" follows.

Discouraged and frustrated, she stays on the job nevertheless. The pull of the pension is part of the reason. And, like several of her comrades, she's enmeshed in a powerful love-hate relationship with EMS. The job's autonomy, the inherent responsibility, and the B team's brand of camaraderie are magnetic in their appeal even though her patients' lives can be profoundly depressing and the blue-shirts are constantly engaged in a no-win battle with bureaucracy. "We have a bit of combat mentality," Fazio explains. "We despise our surroundings and circumstances, but we muddle through and try to have a good time doing it."

Paramedic Tommy Opperman is especially grateful to Fazio. Recently, his mother died at home after carotid-artery surgery. He found her in the bathroom, and admits the grief he felt as a mourning son overpowered all his instincts as a medic. He struggled through the funeral and returned to work. At the time he was partnered with Fazio. Coincidentally, Dispatch sent them to a female patient who had died in her bathroom. When they arrived, Fazio told him, "I'll get this." Opperman figured, *She's a good medic. She can do the pronouncement. I don't have to double-check her.* A week later, he says, it dawned on him that she deliberately spared him a flashback.

One of several siblings in his large half-Irish, half-Hungarian family, Opperman also became an EMT as a teen. He despised the Catholic school he attended, where nuns cracked rulers over his knuckles. He felt much more at home with friends on the local emergency squad. A thirty-eight-year-old, Opperman has worked the B team for nearly twenty years. Not long ago, he switched from the overnight shift to the noon-through-midnight tour in order to have more time with his wife and daughter.

He has discovered that Newark has a different face at night. For the most part, the ubiquitous graffiti disappear. Caved-in fences melt into the background. Dark shapes glide along dark sidewalks. Toddlers and parents roaming the streets in the wee hours seem grossly out of context; parading whores are obscenely cliché. The bleak despair that cries out from worn, sunlit buildings is muffled by shadow except for chunks of neglect spotlighted by the occasional harsh peach-and-silver glare of security lights. "At night you kind of blindly drive by it all," Opperman says. "During the day, you can see it. It's a pretty depressing town."

At the edge of the tarmac near Littleton Avenue, EMT Benny Cardona uses an arm-length scrub brush and a barrel of suds to scrub down Bus No. 103. His usual vehicle, Bus No. 108, is under repair. The brakes failed while the bus was sailing through a thunderstorm the other night. But it is always out of service, it seems. The other day, he and a team of corrections officers helping to transport an inmate found roaches scurrying about. He's not sure whether they came aboard with the ninety-nine-year-old patient who spent the drive to the hospital crying that the insect in her ear was eating her brain. Cardona hates roaches. He sent the bus, which his partner, Vince Callahan, dubbed "a straight-up ghetto truck," to be fumigated.

Cardona keeps his bus spit-shine clean. He puts his muscular shoulders to the task. Black sunglasses shield his eyes from the setting fireball. Toasty breezes blow. Spraying off the residual foam with a hose, he makes the white truck gleam. Its distinctive orange and yellow stripes encircle the vehicle, interrupted by hot yellow blazes streaking down the sides.

Meanwhile, Callahan stocks it with gauze, tape, cravats, linen, sterile water, saline, dressings, and other supplies. A B-team veteran of eighteen years, like "the Squirrel," Callahan remembers the early days, too. He *never* takes a full supply cabinet for granted.

Tonight, the two almost rush through their ritual, eager to get on the road.

They towel off the truck, and Cardona wipes himself down, too. At 1850 hours it is ninety degrees in Brick City.

Prior to his foray into EMS, Cardona worked armed security. By arguing that the guards would be better assets if they could defibrillate cardiac-arrest victims, he persuaded his employer to train the force in first aid. To his surprise, he found he had a knack for it. When layoffs ensued, he became an EMT. That's how the partners met. Callahan's mother suffered an allergic reaction to shrimp and EMTs rushed her, in anaphylactic shock, to the closest hospital. Cardona was working there as an ER technician. He helped stick a tube down her throat to prevent it from constricting, arranged an oxygen-pumping machine to assist her breathing, and hooked up a nitroglycerin drip to reduce her skyrocketing pressure. A year later, Cardona went to work for University and, to their mutual surprise, the two became partners.

Callahan, age forty-one, protects the twenty-nine-year-old Cardona as a big brother would. "They all pick on him because he wants to be a cop," Callahan says. "But he's the best partner I ever saw." And he's seen his share of EMS workers. Callahan was eighteen when a friend invited him to come along as he explored options at an Army recruiting station. The recruiter tested Callahan, too, and offered him a surprising variety of choices. The next thing he knew, Callahan was an Army medic.

At 1855 hours, Walter Joseph "the Commander" Drivet, a bald and bespectacled thirty-nine-old, walks briskly across the compound, determined to clock in before the shift officially begins at 1900 hours. The picnic-table crowd and others on the tarmac crisply salute the team's de facto leader. Most everyone looks up to Drivet, because of his knowledge, stability, and professional demeanor.

A sought-after lecturer, Drivet also teaches extensively at home and abroad. He works a second medic job, too, in Elizabeth, New Jersey, another busy urban center. And he commands a team of tactical medics who back up law-enforcement officers on SWAT missions. In fact, he just returned from leading a cadre through recertification at an elite SWAT school. There, he trained with an arsenal of weapons, from submachine guns to sniper weapons systems, and allowed police to assault him and spray him with Mace while he defended his weapon.[2] "I'm like a white Anglo-Saxon Protestant who can't even take spicy food!" Drivet cracks. "This was like having Tabasco sauce thrown in my eyes."

An avid and expert skier, Drivet discovered that he could get more time on the slopes and free lift tickets by getting his first-aid credentials and joining the ski patrol, which is how he came to join his local volunteer rescue corps at age sixteen. Now he helps oversee ski-patrol operations at a posh resort. This, his nth job, doesn't pay much, but it still affords him the chance to ski a few days each week throughout the winter.

Drivet became a paramedic while in college. No longer willing to live at home, he opted for self-sufficiency and fell headlong in love with EMS. His campus studies paled by comparison, and he drifted away. But Drivet's family wanted more for him. (People often think of EMS as a way station on the road to police work, firefighting, traditional medicine, or other opportunities.) For years, they pushed and pleaded with him to finish his degree and give the family business, a school lunch program, a chance. Drivet complied. He earned better money, but after a decade as an urban medic he found the challenge of getting children their Friday-afternoon pizza anticlimatic and returned to the streets.

In his heart, he has always wanted to be a Navy SEAL. At the Defense Department, where he has trained to fight the effects of terrorism, Drivet met and befriended a bunch of SEALs and made them laugh with characteristic self-deprecation. Over a few beers, the portly would-be military man called himself the Navy's *real* secret weapon: a Navy walrus.

Despite his rotund physique, Drivet has ramrod-straight posture. He spends far more than the department's $250-a-year wardrobe allowance keeping his uniform sharply pressed, his black patent-leather shoes shined, and his silver name tag and shield polished. With a black stethoscope draped over his shoulders and his blue canvas briefcase tucked under his arm, Drivet resembles the Navy man he always wanted to be.

Cisternino says Drivet approaches his job "like a child headed for recess." When Drivet walks into any one of Newark's hospitals, nurses will stop what they are doing to hug and kiss the chubby charmer. Doctors discuss unusual cases with him. Drivet is a diplomat, too. He remembers the hospital staff's birthdays. He buys the card, obtains team-member signatures, and makes his partners look good by suggesting they present it. His savior faire is palpable. Patients—from gangbangers to psychotics—relax and let him take charge.

When the Commander exits the building after swiping in, everyone at the picnic table quickly shuffles to make room. Drivet sits and switches his stylish Oakley Frogskins to a pair of bifocals so he can review the marked-up charts he, too, found stuffed into his mailbox. Ironically, he held the administrator's job for two years but, admittedly, did not fit into the "corporate culture." Despite the advantages the white-collar slot offered, Drivet did not enjoy being a "carpet-dweller," his term for the administrators whose offices have the luxury of industrial carpet. He found he was spending more time than he wanted to on budgets, disciplinary actions, investigations, and operations. He accomplished a number of goals, such as helping to launch Newark's tactical medic support team and drafting a memorandum of understanding between New York and New Jersey in the aftermath of the 1993 World Trade Center bombing. But he missed the challenge of patient care under pressure and returned to the line.

Ensconced among his teammates, Drivet buries himself in a medical textbook. Soon enough, Dispatch will call or his partner will want to get breakfast. He doesn't go out of his way to acknowledge any of the FNGs or outcasts, but he doesn't snub them either. Colleagues have confided in him that walking the gauntlet, past the packed picnic table and its irreverent blue-shirts, is the hardest part of the job. That says a lot, considering that they also have to spend twelve grueling hours a night working in a city their *Policies and Procedures Manual* describes as "one of the most violent in the United States."

Founded in 1666, Newark has a distinguished pedigree. The crews take pride in knowing the city's rich history and which fascinating stories took place from one corner of Newark to another. For example, they know where Thomas Edison labored, where Abraham Lincoln spoke, where Civil War–era jails housed Confederate prisoners, where celluloid film was discovered, where beer magnate Peter Ballantine lived.

But Newark has also struggled with socioeconomic problems for decades. After World War II, city planners discovered that Newark had been declining for years. The city had hemorrhaged jobs and industry. Property values had been eroding. The tax rate had increased but revenues had fallen more than twenty percent. The hospital was overcrowded. Streets had deteriorated. Schools were dilapidated. A third of its housing was characterized as below "the generally accepted minimum standards of health and decency."[3] Thousands lived without private toilets, baths, or central heating. Hundreds lived without electricity and running water. Half of the city's blacks, who had come to Newark to work in the war-related manufacturing plants, lived in "unhealthful and unwholesome quarters" and paid slumlords handsomely for the privilege.[4]

Although periods of prosperity and revitalization followed, Newark never satisfactorily addressed its problems, particularly housing. By 1967, a brew of despair, racial divisiveness, and political corruption poisoned the climate. People were displaced in the name of urban development. With whole neighborhoods already on edge, an incident between police, a taxi driver, and a crowd ignited race riots. Angry residents smashed windows with bottles and bricks, looted storefronts, and set the city ablaze.[5,6]

The 1967 uprising was not the first the illustrious city sustained, but it may have been the most damaging. For decades since, Newark has struggled to heal itself. Much of its business district is well scrubbed and thriving. The Newark Bears' shiny new minor-league stadium is colorful, well lit, and drawing crowds.

Its New Jersey Performing Arts Center attracts top acts and packed houses. Restaurants entice patrons from outlying areas. A $355 million YankeeNets stadium is the talk of the town. And, the potential to turn the sagging, toxic riverfront into a development property similar to Baltimore's Inner Harbor is a hot topic, too.

Chocolate-box town houses have replaced high-rise public housing projects turned towering slums. Although some of the picturesque new buildings are lovingly maintained, EMS workers see evidence that they may ultimately fail, too. Inside some, the walls and floors are so smeared with filth, one has to wonder what goes on behind the tidy white fences, miniature lawns, and closed doors. Studies say residents from the poorest neighborhoods feel excluded from the most recent urban-renewal thrust. Much infrastructure remains in grave disrepair even as infusions of cash flow in. Cisternino follows Newark real-estate transactions, politics, economics, and scandals. He points out when local politicians do the Jersey version of "the Potomac two-step" and goads his colleagues into discussing the meaning of persistent urban decay. Many wonder whether the much-ballyhooed renaissance will ever trickle down to the back of the ambulances where patients still wrestle with mundane, but deadly, problems such as malnutrition.

The mayor's administration has adopted laws to reduce pollution and protect the environment but has not compelled the citizenry to pick up after themselves. Garbage plasters pockets as far as the eye can see. Newark's Central Ward, where University Hospital sits, remains visibly depressed, although a $200 million neighborhood project is under way just blocks from the campus. Charred and boarded-up buildings, crumbling sidewalks, and abandoned storefront churches surround the medical complex, a forty-six-acre sprawl of putty-colored concrete buildings and prefabricated shelters that vary in height and breadth. With shifts lasting twelve arduous hours, and overtime to boot, this is the B team's home away from home.

An urban-policy expert once described parts of Newark, walking distance from "glittering new office buildings," as having "some of the worst conditions in America, like Dresden (Germany) after World War II."[7] Barbed wire, floodlights, aggressive dogs, and prolific violence are just some of the reasons EMS workers here compare Newark to Saigon.

2 TAG, YOU'RE IT!

*N*obody wants pizza on the Fourth of July, Iyad Al-Atiyat thinks, after eight boring hours in his Newark, New Jersey, pizzeria. It's the year 2000. He has owned the pizzeria and the grocery, a small store next door, for the past five years. Neither is as lucrative as he had hoped, even with him toiling sixteen hours a day, up to seven days a week. Robbers have hit the stores several times, once as recently as last week.

No deliveries today, just pickup. So the strapping twenty-four-year-old with soft brown eyes opens the restaurant later than usual. And he gives his brother Aqeed, a lanky twenty-two-year-old with a Clark Gable smile, the day off. Still, there isn't enough to keep Iyad busy. He might as well close early. Sometime after 6:00 P.M., Iyad phones Aqeed and asks for a ride to a cousin's party.

Aqeed's wife wants to come along. But the eighteen-year-old just gave birth to their first child. "Stay home," Aqeed instructs. "I'll be right back and we'll all go together." For the Al-Atiyats, family is everything. Iyad and Aqeed are two of ten brothers and eight sisters.

When Aqeed arrives at the Broadway storefront, the brothers share orange

15

juice, Pepsi, and cigarettes. They talk business, or the lack thereof, and they talk security. Weapons are too dangerous to have on hand. But they can't fight guns with their fists. *Maybe we should get out of this business altogether?* Iyad muses. They might try importing clothes or joining another brother in his fledgling electronics store. As they debate their options, the phone starts ringing. Now everyone in Newark is hungry for crispy, hot tomato pies. Order after order floods the small pizzeria. Suddenly, the brothers find themselves hustling to meet the demand.

Finally, the crush of orders slows and stops just after 11:15 P.M. Fifteen minutes later they're cleaning up. Iyad pulls the metal security gate down over the plate-glass window and locks the door. Aqeed goes into the kitchen to clean the deep fryer. If they hurry, they'll still have time to join their wives and relax at the party.

When Iyad hears a knock on the door, he looks up from the cash register. A bony black woman in her mid-twenties stands outside, barely visible through the protective metal honeycomb. Holding curled fingers to her mouth, she gestures that she wants something to drink. Iyad shakes his head no and mouths, "We're closed." Shrugging her shoulders helplessly, she mouths the word "Please?" Then she cradles her arms, rocks them side to side, and shouts: "It's for my baby!"

Iyad relents. *It's almost midnight in Newark, on a holiday, and the woman has a baby. Where is she to go?* The tough neighborhood in the city's North Ward has an abundance of drug dealers, but Iyad knows all the characters and consciously treats everyone kindly. Prayers that honor Allah, in graceful Arabic script, hang on the pizzeria's stucco walls beside oversized, airbrushed graphics of pizza, hot dogs, and a New York City skyline. Iyad spends most of his waking hours here; the prayers are a comforting reflection of his faith as well as a visible reminder to show respect to everyone.

Stepping from behind the waist-high white tile counter, he crosses the front portion of the restaurant, between two booths. He opens the glass door and pulls the gate up a few feet so the woman can duck inside. Before he gets anywhere near the soda case, however, three black men materialize and scramble inside, too. Stockings pulled over their heads mash and distort their features. Iyad is six feet tall and 230 pounds, yet he thinks the thugs, who tower over him, huge.

"What you want, guys?" he asks nervously.

"We want money!" one barks.

"OK, OK," Iyad agrees, "Take it easy." He pulls a wad from his pocket— three thousand dollars in cash. Handing it over, he hopes it will placate them. Normally he wouldn't be so flush, but he had intended to meet his accountant the next day to pay his rent and taxes.

"Open the register!" one thug commands.

Iyad walks back to the register, opens the drawer, and extracts the four hundred dollars inside. "OK, OK," he gushes as he hands it over. "Here's the money."

Meanwhile, Aqeed hears voices in the front. *Iyad must have opened for one of his friends*, he thinks. He pays no mind and goes about cleaning the machinery. The robbers hear him puttering around in the kitchen, but do not know what to make of the sound. Seeing confusion grip them, Iyad yells to Aqeed, "*Kahlehk wara! Kahlehk wara!*" In Arabic, this means: "Stay back! Stay back!"

But that only panics the crooks. One of the muscle-bound men pulls a .22-caliber out of his pocket and stalks towards the kitchen. Iyad can't stand the thought of his youngest brother in danger. Lunging at the man, he struggles for the weapon. But before Iyad can reach him, two of the gunman's accomplices clobber him. Suddenly, he is in the fight of his life, unable to help his brother, much less himself.

The armed man barrels into the kitchen, confronts Aqeed, and attacks him. Between the pizza ovens, the refrigerators, the deep fryer, the counter, and the sinks, there is little room to brawl. Aqeed, half the size of his assailant, can't toss him. Instead, the scrappy young man tries desperately to stand and gain control of the robber's gun-holding hand. *I have to go see my brother*, he thinks as he shoves the robber with all of his strength and rams him into a sharp table corner.

Scraped, the thug curses and squeezes off a shot. It bounces off a steel counter and pings off the pizza oven. Aqeed is still wrestling for control of the weapon when the gunman shoots again. Bullets fly. Two pierce the refrigerators' metal doors. A fourth smacks into the still-steaming grill. And two more rip through Aqeed's left lower leg. So tense is the scene that he doesn't even feel it. The robber is still coming at him, so Aqeed staggers to the back door connecting the pizzeria and the grocery, hoping to get to a phone and summon help.

Iyad hears the shots and his temper explodes, but he can't overpower the two toughs who are beating and tossing him about the store, smashing the soda cases, crushing the phone, and fracturing the lights. He's still struggling when he takes a blunt and heavy chop on the back of his head. Stumbling into the wall, Iyad hears his brother scream as he slumps heavily to the floor.

With blood spurting from his leg, Aqeed throws his shoulder against the back door. It won't budge. If he stays here, he'll be cornered. Weaving his way through the back of the kitchen, he leaves a slick of blood in his wake. Aqeed sees Iyad's feet sticking stiffly out from behind the counter. *My brother is shot*, he thinks numbly. *My brother is dead.* He could drop and die of grief right there, but for the image of his month-old son, which pops into his mind and urges him on. *I can't leave him fatherless*, Aqeed thinks, as his blood leaks onto the floor.

He spies one of the hoods ducking out the door. Another jostles Aqeed and squeaks out through the opening. By now Aqeed is crawling. He pushes himself out of the restaurant and drags himself toward the pay phone just a few feet away. Automatically, he dials his eldest brother. But no one answers. Next, he calls 911. A female operator picks up.

"I got shot! I got robbed," he gasps into the receiver. Having come to the U.S. from Jordan only two years ago, he still has an Arabic accent as thick as Turkish coffee. "My brother, I think, died inside."

She asks him where he is and promises to send police right away. Jamaican neighbors who live in a pale gray clapboard house next door peek out the window in response to the commotion. Seeing Aqeed on the ground bleeding and calling for help, they rush downstairs. The woman tells him to elevate his leg as the blood pools around him on the sidewalk and he sinks into shock. Her husband calls the police. It seems to Aqeed that the couple calls and calls. As he lies on the sidewalk, his blood pumps onto the street and he begins to shiver.

Jimmy Smith, a loading-dock worker turned EMT turned dispatcher, is on duty tonight at University Hospital's E-911 Dispatch Center. (E stands for *enhanced*; E-911 technology captures information about callers and their locations.) The Dispatch Center occupies almost half of the fourth floor of the old Martland Hospital, which University absorbed and now uses for administration. The tall, blond brick building sits on Bergen Street, a main drag that crisscrosses the 334-year-old city. From its perch, the Dispatch Center overlooks dark city streets snaking out over twenty-four square miles. Inside, air-conditioning keeps the staff and roughly $1 million of telecommunications equipment comfortably cool and dry. Outside, however, people swelter in the summer night's heat. Just after midnight, the city is still celebrating the Fourth of July, and the calls for help flood the center nonstop.

The pace doesn't faze Smith, though. A self-professed "pure Newark thoroughbred," Smith has been a dispatcher since the service began, in 1974. Prior to that, he rode the streets for nearly five years providing first aid. When the phone rings again at 0016 hours, the fifty-eight-year-old father of two glances at his computer screen and sees that the call originates from a Newark police precinct. He presses a flashing button, one of hundreds on the console before him, and speaks hoarsely into his headset: "Emergency medical?"

"Yes. Hi. This is Communications Division at the police department calling," a woman says before giving her badge number. "Someone has just been shot at 119 Broadway."

EMS prefers that police transfer 911 medical emergencies directly to them so the call takers can get a better idea of what resources to send. But that doesn't happen as frequently as it should. Smith confirms the data, and types the shooting and address into his computer. Automatically, the software categorizes the event as an immediate life threat. It accesses a global positioning satellite—GPS—which identifies the nearest available, appropriate ambulance and recommends the assignment. "D" or Delta priority, pops up in white type against a bloodred background, at the top of the emergency queue signaling a life threat. It makes an eye-catching statement against the monitor's black screen, where active jobs stack up.

Seated a few consoles away, his stiff silver hair flying out behind him like Superman's cape, dispatcher William "Buzz" Busby spots the new crisis as it materializes on one of the many displays he monitors. The entire dispatch team can see every call in the system simultaneously. And, because they are cross-trained, they can take calls, assign missions, patch through radio communications, coordinate air medical flights, and wear any number of other hats. Still square and stocky from his days as a high-school football hero, Buzz checks unit availability. Delta priority merits instant, advanced-level attention, but all the advanced life support (ALS) units are busy. The busy urban system is overstretched, a problem that plagues suburban and rural areas, too.

Paramedic Walter Drivet is dropping off a patient at Beth Israel, a hospital near the southern tip of the city, miles from the shooting. *Still, he's the patient's best bet,* Buzz thinks. He awards the job to Drivet, Unit 2202, and then pages a field supervisor, Unit 401, which is standard operating procedure for violent incidents.

"401, 2202," Buzz broadcasts in the mellow, matter-of-fact tones that have made him a favorite among the EMS workers on the street.

Two supervisor units and nine University ambulances patrolling the streets of Newark and neighboring Orange and East Orange hear the call. But after a few years, most of the EMS veterans have learned to listen selectively to radio chatter—tuning in to unit numbers and code words that mean chaos is afoot. It takes a whopper to make these busy professionals, who handle more than 130,000 missions each year, to sit up and take notice.

Buzz relates the facts in smooth, resonant tones: "119 Broadway. On the outside. Possible shooting."

"119 Broadway. Roger," Paulie Visoskas, field supervisor, Unit 401, replies. He crushes a cigarette onto the asphalt carpet outside EMS headquarters and climbs into one of the big, white Ford Expeditions that supervisors drive. Heading straight to the pizzeria, he tunes in to the police frequencies to see what he can learn en route.

* * *

Meanwhile, emergency medical technicians (EMTs) Vince Callahan and Benny Cardona are driving their ambulance back to headquarters. Their last patient refused medical assistance. Riding through Brick City, so named for its myriad brick housing projects and tenements, they spot clusters of people on tenement stoops, sitting with wet towels draped on their heads. Others spread through the stifling streets in search of a breeze or other distraction. The dearth of air-conditioning turns the brick buildings into ovens, with withering room temperatures exceeding 120 degrees. Callahan and Cardona grew up in two such housing projects. They know just how cooked the people feel and thank God that their bus's air-conditioning is working tonight. (The air-conditioning at quarters "rocks," too, the B-teamers say, because the medical examiner had installed powerful refrigeration to keep its corpses chilled.)

It's just after midnight when Cardona overhears Buzz assign the shooting. It's right down the street. *I'd rather have four to five good traumas and decent saves than nineteen bullshit jobs,* the trauma junkie thinks. Cardona, who is halfway to his degree in criminal justice and once worked armed security, wants to be a Newark cop. Eager to jump the job, he turns to Callahan and says, "Let's take that!"

Callahan nods.

Snatching the radio microphone from its cradle, Cardona radios Buzz. "1202," he reports, identifying his unit number. All radio communications employ unit numbers. First names are usually saved for special occasions, such as subtle ways to alert the team to hostage situations.

"1202," Buzz acknowledges.

"We're a straight shot up Broadway from that shooting and can take it if you like," Cardona offers hopefully.

"All right, 1202," Buzz replies, updating the computer. As EMTs, Cardona and Callahan are no substitute for paramedics, which is why the computer didn't assign them the job. However, when Cardona takes the initiative, with the medics still busy and relatively far away, it strikes Buzz as a sensible stopgap. Although Cardona and Callahan are lesser-trained, they are close by. They can patch wounds and take other preliminary steps to stabilize the patient before the medics arrive. Moreover, they can make the decision to transport immediately and let the medics catch them en route.

A Pepsodent smile breaks through Cardona's meticulously trimmed black Vandyke beard, and his dark eyes sparkle. Leaning into the dashboard, he flips on the light bar and twists the siren knob. The bus showers the streets with amber, red, and electrifying white strobes. Warning wails shriek through the loudspeaker. Callahan accelerates and they speed south.

Cardona knows firsthand what it feels like to be shot. One summer afternoon, five years ago, he stood in front of his Newark home with a young cousin. Cardona had his bicycle out; his cousin was lacing up in-line skates. The two planned to go for some exercise. Cardona's intuition sparked as a wiry, bare-chested man sauntered by with a T-shirt wrapped around his head. The man slowed, spun around, pulled a handgun, and demanded Cardona's thick gold necklace. A firearm connoisseur, Cardona first thought, *That little silver automatic is a poor excuse for a gun.* When he worked armed security, he owned a GP100 Ruger .357 Magnum and a 9-mm Sig Sauer. *But even the cheapest, crummiest gun can blow a hole in someone's head,* he remembered. Cardona controlled his temper as the man forced the muzzle against his skull and yanked the chain from his neck with brute force. But as soon as the robber turned to flee, Cardona instinctively gave chase. The thief fired, and the bullet caught Cardona in his right chest. But Cardona didn't feel a thing; he kept running while his cousin alerted the police.

Minutes later, the cops caught up to Cardona, who began recounting the story. He was wiping off sweat when he saw blood on his palm and discovered it streaming down his side. A clammy panic gripped him. "I don't know if I'm shot," he warbled. Whatever symptoms he hadn't yet felt suddenly throttled him. He began breathing too rapidly and sweating even more. Oddly, though, he felt no pain, just a peculiar discomfort.

One of the officers radioed for an ambulance, and University's Dispatch Center sent paramedics to the scene. While he waited, Cardona had time to think, *It was the stupidest thing I ever did, chasing this bum when I've got a baby son and a wife to take care of.*

The paramedics arrived and laid Cardona on a long board, which they used as a full-body splint. (Bullets can penetrate flesh with sufficient speed and force to continue tumbling inside the body, wreaking havoc with vital organs and tissues. The EMS workers don't have onboard X-ray equipment, much less the time, the tools, or the training to trace a bullet's path inside the body and correct the consequences. The long board minimized Cardona's mobility so the ride to the hospital wouldn't aggravate any internal damage the bullet might have done.) The medics tucked a cervical collar around his neck, cut off his shirt, slapped an oxygen mask on his face, pierced his arm with an intravenous line, and sped him to the ER.

"I'm not having any difficulty breathing," Cardona told the ambulance crew even as he wondered whether the bullet punctured his lung and whether his lung might collapse. "There's no tightness in my chest." They looked at him strangely before he remembered to explain that he works in the field, too. (At the time, Cardona worked as a trauma technician in another hospital's ER and provided basic life support—BLS—on the streets of Irvington, a neighboring city that some call Newark Lite.)

When they reached the hospital, the ER was packed. Cardona remembers that someone rolled him to X-ray. Soon after, a doctor visited and told him, "It was a really small hole, probably really small-caliber." The doctor injected a local anesthetic and then, using a clamp, extracted half a bullet from under Cardona's skin. He handed it to Cardona as a keepsake. The bullet looked like a gray pebble. The doctor stuck his finger in the hole and showed him where the bullet collided with his rib and bounced off. Cardona's rib, now chipped, stopped the bullet from doing further damage.

The doctor sewed up Cardona and sent him home the same night, with Tylenol for pain and antibiotics to ward off infection. As he healed, Cardona designed a crucifix with a skull and had it tattooed over the bullet hole. Now he carries the memory rather vividly wherever he goes.

As Cardona and Callahan pull up to 119 Broadway, they see a police car approaching from the other direction. Both drivers turn abruptly toward the curb, parking at angles in front of the pizzeria.

Sprawled on his back on the sidewalk by the pay phone, Aqeed lifts his head at the sound of the vehicles. He moans and clutches his knee. Blood, ink dark in the night, trails from him to the restaurant. Its security gate hangs a few feet above the ground, and a bright band of light glares through the gap. The Jamaican couple has retreated to their clapboard house. The wife watches from the second-story window. Her husband's dark silhouette stares from the front steps.

As Callahan and Cardona hop out of the bus, a uniformed cop rushes toward Aqeed. Still uncertain who he is, the cop kneels by Aqeed's side and almost topples into the pooling blood. "Oh, shit!" the cop shouts. "He's shot!"

"I don't know if these people go out or not," Aqeed warns the officer, who is still trying to piece the event together. "*Please*, go inside and see if my brother is alive," he pleads. But the cop declines to move until more units arrive.

Callahan and Cardona barely have a chance to bend down and examine Aqeed before more police cars screech around the corner, halting in a semicircle in front of the building. Officers scatter—some in uniform and others in street clothes with silver shields dangling from their necks. One strings yellow crime-scene tape to block off the restaurant and grocery from the rest of the neighborhood. Others, guns drawn, crouch under the security gate and push their way inside.

"Potential DOA here!" A cop's voice bellows from inside the pizzeria. "There's blood everywhere!"

Neither Cardona nor Callahan will take the cop's pronouncement for granted. Both have found patients others declare "dead" to be quite alive. Cardona wonders momentarily, *Is the shooter still inside?* Callahan, once carjacked at gunpoint, prays the cops will provide adequate protection. But neither Cardona nor Callahan hesitates to go to the second patient's side.

Callahan is twelve years older than Cardona. He is Baptist, and Cardona is Catholic. He is black, and Cardona is Hispanic. Callahan is six-foot-five, and Cardona is five-foot-seven. These differences disappear against backgrounds so similar they might be brothers. Both grew up in public housing rife with poverty and riddled with violence. As youngsters, both witnessed abuse and alcoholism in their daily lives. Both passed up opportunities to become thugs in favor of steady if grueling employment, college, marriage, and family. This is *their* city. This is *their* job. Aqeed is at least conscious and alert. They won't know about the other patient until they get a look. Here, EMS partners rarely split up; they do not leave each other's sight unless both feel comfortable. Assuring the weakened Aqeed that they'll return, they scramble under the gate to join the cops inside.

The pizzeria's harsh, white fluorescent lights and neon graphics blind them momentarily after the dark street's dim lamps. Poster-board menus hang on the wall. A cash register sits behind a cracked display case; its gray drawer dangles from ball bearings. Pennies and dimes shine on the scuffed linoleum floor, and Iyad's feet, clad in loafers, stick out from behind the counter.

Cardona and Callahan dart toward Iyad. But before they can fully absorb the sight of him lying there, they confront a blood slick as far as the eye can see. Jellied clots, the size of hamburgers, stretch back into the kitchen. *Man, it sure is a fuckin' bloodbath,* Cardona thinks. *This mofo is dead. I ain't never seen so much blood in my life. He must be shot in the head!*

"In the name of Allah!" Callahan exclaims, curling his long-limbed-frame over Iyad. Callahan puts his ear near Iyad's mouth to listen for the sound of breath or feel its warm gush. He looks to see if Iyad's chest rises and falls, and thankfully he sees Iyad's yellow button-down shirt move rhythmically. He signals Cardona, who is scanning Iyad's body for other signs of injury, such as pooling blood or deformities that might indicate broken bones.

"My man," Callahan urges Iyad, "wake up! Open your eyes."

Detectives enter the store waving their flashlights. "We don't know where the gun is," an officer calls to them from the kitchen. "*Anyone* could be the perp."

"That might be the suspect outside," another cop suggests.

Iyad lies on his back, breathing regularly. Although he has not yet opened his eyes, his lids flutter when Cardona flicks them, one of many techniques he employs to quickly determine who is faking. The partners suspect that Iyad is not truly unconscious; perhaps he is too scared to open his eyes. Iyad's skin is dry and his cheeks are blushed; he would be clammy and pale if he were in shock. Callahan measures Iyad's blood pressure; it's close enough to normal for him to relax just a bit. All this leads the partners, who have worked together for three years, to conclude that Iyad may have a concussion but that he's in no immediate danger.

Field supervisor Visoskas is just a street away when he overhears police confirm the shooting by radio. "401," he says, updating the Dispatch Center. "Radio car on the scene reporting a positive shooting."

"Received," says Smith, who has rotated from the call taker's station to the telemetry console. At University, telemetry monitors all radio communications between BLS, ALS, supervisors, dispatchers, and ER staff. Smith, Buzz, and many of their Dispatch colleagues have worked the streets when Newark was an even rougher town. They can well imagine what is happening on the street and wish their colleagues Godspeed.

Callahan and Cardona have assessed both patients and are ready to act. Cardona radios Dispatch: "1202, on the update." His voice comes across as one long squawk, and Smith can't make out the transmission.

"Last unit, say again," Smith requests, his voice raspy and raw from years of chain-smoking.

"1202, on the update."

"G'ahead, 1202."

"All right. Be advised, we may have two victims, stand by—one shot to the leg. It's an unsafe scene. I'm here with PD. There might be an actor inside the store, here," Cardona reports in one fast gush. *Actor* means "perpetrator" in law-enforcement jargon. "All right," he continues, breathing heavily. "You all stand by. Have units stay on Gouverneur, not Broadway."

"OK," Smith replies. "2202 and 401?" he calls, alerting the other responders. "Stay on Gouverneur. Stay on Gouverneur, *not* on Broadway when you arrive on the scene there." Hopefully, by avoiding the precise scene, no one will be caught in gunfire.

"2202, received," Drivet responds for his unit. "Jim, just let them know, we're still coming out of the south."

Instantly, everyone knows that means the paramedics are miles away.

Cardona and Callahan have to beat feet and get the bleeder to the trauma center. "I don't know if you can hear me, man, but help will be here soon," Callahan tells Iyad. The two partners scoot outside, but not before Cardona eyeballs the floor for shell casings.

Outside, a small crowd assembles behind the yellow crime tape. Visoskas arrives and will watch over Iyad until another unit catches up. Cardona hustles over to Aqeed and grasps his wrist for a quick pulse check. Aqeed's face is coated with perspiration. His heart is beating overly fast at 120 times per minute;

it's trying to keep pumping plasma throughout his circulatory system even though he's lost at least thirty percent of his blood volume. He needs a surgeon immediately. Cardona cuts Aqeed's jeans to expose the wound and put pressure on it.

Callahan hustles to the bus, yanks out the stretcher, hauls a long orange board (a full-body splint) from a side compartment, grabs the trauma kit, a bag of bandages, splints, sterile water, and tape, and wheels the supplies over.

Meanwhile, the police officer has not yet decided whether Aqeed is criminal, victim, or bystander. "What were you doing here?" he asks.

"Pizza. Delivery," Aqeed whispers. "They robbed me."

"Who robbed you?"

"Some men," he pants. Black curls stick to his head with sweat. Beneath his olive complexion, he is deathly pale.

"Did you know them?"

Wincing, Aqeed shakes his head.

"Where did they go?"

Supporting his weight on one arm, Aqeed lifts his wrist and points weakly down Broadway.

"Did you see the car?"

"White," he says, taking a breath. "BMW."

"Two or four doors?"

"Four."

As the officer murmurs into his radio, Aqeed clutches Cardona's arm. His almond brown eyes flicker with fear, pain, and confusion.

Callahan rips open a handful of five-by-nine-inch padded dressings and presses them against the bloodiest part of Aqeed's black jeans. Aqeed shrinks back with pain. The cop helps the EMTs roll Aqeed onto his right side so they can slide the long board along the wounded man's spine, scan for more wounds, and roll him back onto it.

Callahan and Cardona dispense with the spongy blocks that they usually place on either side of a patient's head to prevent lateral movement. They don't yet strap his head down or tie him to the board. The scene isn't safe; time isn't plentiful. Aqeed has lost buckets of blood and he has cooled on concrete too long. They hoist him onto the stretcher, tell the cop that they are going to University, and make for the shelter of their bus. Hopefully, the medics will catch them en route.

Having heard Drivet report his south Newark location, Visoskas gets an idea. "401," he says, announcing himself to the Dispatch Center. "MIC 1"—Mobile Intensive Care Unit 1—"has an ambulance." Usually, MIC 1 is just a truck with paramedics and equipment but no room for patient transport. However, as part of his supervisor duties Visoskas keeps a close eye on the equipment—so close some say he's anal. Yet, in a pinch, it's Visoskas who knows that MIC 1's everyday truck is in the shop and the two medics who use it are operating out of a fully stocked ambulance tonight—a nuance that neither Dispatch nor the GPS would pick up. "If they're available and you can use 'em, send 'em," he orders.

Visoskas is on top of his team's equipment and personnel, but he's still adjusting to another new policy. Just days ago, EMS administrators changed each unit's call numbers. MIC 1, during the graveyard shift, is now 2201. But in the excitement of the moment, Visoskas forgets. His error doesn't throw Smith, though.

"2201?" Smith announces over the system.

Paramedic Tracey Ann Fazio responds, "2201."

"2201, respond to 119 Broadway, 119 Broadway to the shooting."

And then Cardona calls Smith: "1202."

But Smith can't answer before verifying that Fazio is headed to the scene. "2201, received?"

"Received and responding from the General," Fazio replies, letting her colleagues know they're en route from a hospital in a neighboring town.

"And 2202?" Smith says, searching for Drivet. "You're canceled. Stand by for another one."

"All right," Drivet confirms.

Meanwhile, inside the ambulance, Cardona and Callahan begin to examine and treat Aqeed's injuries. Cardona loosens Aqeed's left sneaker and slides it off with a command: "Wiggle your toes."

"I can't do it," Aqeed cries breathlessly. That can mean nerve damage. It can mean broken bones. It can also mean Aqeed is plain terrified.

Using a pair of thirteen-dollar fishing shears he bought at The Sports Authority, Cardona cuts Aqeed's pant seam to expose the gunshot. He keeps the shears razor-sharp; more often than not, his patients wear several sets of clothes, sometimes all that they own. Purposefully, he avoids the bullet hole so he won't damage any evidence. He peels back the blood-soaked fabric to find a pulpy wound. A bullet has blown apart the fleshy part of Aqeed's left calf.

Blood flows from the wound. Blood soaks through the sheets. Blood drips on the floor. "There's too much blood here for one shot," Cardona says. *But where is it all coming from?* he wonders.

"My friend," Callahan says to Aqeed. "How old are you?" He wants to distract him from Cardona's comment and get Aqeed into a pattern of answering questions.

"Twenty-two."

"What city are you from?"

"Clifton."

"What's your name?"

"Aqeed."

"Aqeed, how many shots did you hear?"

"Five."

"There's a lot of fuckin' blood out there," Cardona notes, reflecting back on the scene, which resembled a slaughterhouse more than a pizzeria.

"Just lie still," Callahan instructs as he straps an oxygen mask over Aqeed's frightened face. Flushing the body with pure oxygen will help Aqeed's remaining blood carry as full a load of the nourishing gas as possible; cells throughout the body will die without it.

Cardona quickly pats Aqeed from head to toe, looking for more blood— gunshot wounds or injuries.

The back door of the ambulance creaks open and Visoskas sticks his head in. "Are you ready to roll?"

"We just got the fuckin' guy!" Cardona complains, exasperated. He and Callahan have been on-scene for barely four minutes. He tries explaining that they had to evaluate Iyad, too. "We coulda had a DOA."

"Get going," Visoskas grumbles. His raspy voice is one the team loves to hate. During downtime, they strain themselves imitating him, trying to capture the roughshod tones Burgess Meredith made famous playing the Penguin, Batman's archenemy.

Callahan and Cardona exchange discreet glances. They both feel they need a minute to get a clear picture of Aqeed's problems. Still, neither wants to argue. Callahan usually drives the first half of their twelve-hour shift, so he steps out of the box and takes the wheel. Seconds later, they are en route to Newark's University Hospital, one of the state's preeminent trauma centers.

Tonight, Billy "the Squirrel" Heber is running University's Rescue truck with a stand-in coworker. His regular partner, Eugene "Geno" O'Neill, is working with the Special Operations Group, monitoring the president's Independence Day visit and Operation Sail, a tall-ship parade on the Hudson River. The behemoth Rescue truck is a fully equipped, 275-horsepower turbocharged engine, packed with nearly every conceivable tool known to mankind. It is the EMS workers' best friend at crash extrications, on complex rescue missions, and at crime scenes. "3201," Heber says, calling Dispatch. "We're gonna take a ride down there and give them a hand." He and O'Neill have spent decades honing their skills and are accustomed to taking the initiative.

"Roger," Smith responds. "You're going over to Broadway, right?"

"Yeah."

"OK." Smith then redirects Drivet and his partner to a forty-seven-year-old female who fainted. He also deploys unit 1107 to West Bigelow for an assault and unit 1204 to Mount Pleasant Avenue for a man having difficulty breathing. Other crews call in to update Smith with their patients' conditions. And Visoskas checks in again, too: "401."

"401," Smith replies.

"All right, BLS is ready to leave. They got a gunshot wound to the leg. Lot of loss of blood, there. The second patient is not shot. He was just hit over the head. He may have blacked out. We're assessing him now. He's very upset; he's the brother of the other patient. You got another BLS coming for me?"

"Negative. I got 2201 coming," Smith says. "Do you need them?"

Visoskas reports that the gunshot patient needs the medics more and asks Smith about their ETA.

Smith calls: "2201?"

"2201," Fazio replies from her truck.

"You want to meet up with the gunshot wound," Smith says. Looking at the computer-aided map, which tracks the whereabouts of every EMS vehicle, he sees that the two trucks are just about to meet. "Let 'em come to you."

Callahan jumps on Channel 5, a secondary frequency, and the two units decide where to hook up.

Visoskas gets back on the radio: "401."

"401," Smith acknowledges.

"If MIC 1 doesn't work up the patient and there's nothing else available, I'll use them for the second patient. If not, get me another BLS."

Smith has a split second to process this before another bus calls in its availability. Jobs are holding now; there are just not enough buses to go around. Smith sends the free unit to an emotionally disturbed patient who is threatening people in a crowded lobby. Then he checks the job queue and the computer-aided citywide map and reassesses his strained resources.

Back on Broadway, Callahan stops his bus so Fazio and her partner can climb aboard, equipped with their intravenous tray, drug bag, and trauma kit.

"You didn't get to go inside?" Cardona asks.

"No time," Fazio says, shaking her head.

Without enough troops at his disposal, Visoskas ponders a solution. He wants Fazio and her partner to pull Aqeed out of Cardona and Callahan's bus and take him to the hospital in their ALS unit. And he wants Cardona and Callahan to come back and transport Iyad. He shouts the concept over the radio. The four EMS workers erupt in fury.

Ambulances, today, are mini emergency clinics. And University's teams have the expertise and the tools to get most situations under control given a minute to evaluate the situation. There are myriad options for deploying resources, but that is the Dispatch Center's domain. On monitors throughout the premises, Dispatch has the big picture, literally, displayed on computer-aided mapping programs. They also employ GPS, computer-enhanced triage systems, and almost thirty years of experience. Sometimes last-minute shuffling of resources is appropriate. But several B-teamers think Visoskas, whom they have nicknamed "Panic Paulie," can be too controlling.

The four rescuers argue with Visoskas that interrupting Aqeed's care and the time taken to effect the switch is time his stunned body cannot spare. He has lost a lot of blood; he is slipping deeper into shock. After some bluster, they all agree to stick with the plan. With everyone cursing under their breath, Fazio gets into her bus to drive to University, and her partner, Callahan, Cardona, and Aqeed get back on the road as well.

Visoskas, however, cannot sit still. Iyad is alert now and extremely agitated. "Where's my brother? Where's my brother?" he asks, his voice shrill with alarm.

"He's in the ambulance," Visoskas explains.

"I want to go see him."

"He's going to the hospital. You're going to follow him," Visoskas replies. But he can't help thinking, *Gee, you're really going through a lot for a little bump on the head*. Still, in an effort to hurry Iyad to the hospital, he radios Dispatch again: "401."

"401," Smith replies.

"MIC 1's gonna work up the gunshot," Visoskas reports. "Give me another bus."

Now he has called Dispatch one too many times. They've got sick and injured people all over the city. The Dispatch chief intercedes, grabbing the microphone to quash Visoskas. He promises the next available vehicle, and suggests that, if Visoskas can't wait, he have the rescue specialists, who are also EMTs, leave their truck at the scene and transport Iyad in 2201.

"All right, I will," Visoskas agrees. Looking down the street, he sees units 1103 and 2201 pull away. "Oh, it's too late. I'm gonna need another bus."

"You'll get the next available unit," Smith says for the umpteenth time.

Callahan radios again: "1202. Delta Zulu." Delta Zulu is a transport code that means the medics are treating their patient and BLS is assisting.

"Roger," Smith says, updating the computer yet again.

* * *

Inside the bus, the medic asks about Aqeed's injury. "Is the shot through-and-through?"

"No, I can only see an entrance wound," Cardona answers.

Aqeed struggles to lift his head. He stammers, but his words are unintelligible.

"Relax," the medic barks. "Put your head back. Enjoy the ride!"

To prevent him from lashing out in pain or panic, the medic ties Aqeed to the stretcher with strips of linen; then he ties a rubber tourniquet around Aqeed's lean upper arm. "We'll start an intravenous line," Cardona tells Aqeed as he takes hold of the man's other arm. The paramedic will infuse fluids, rich with electrolytes, to temporarily fill their patient's vascular container. That confuses the brain and heart so that they don't sense the blood loss and compensate by pumping so hard that the remaining blood gushes out through the wound. The medic takes Aqeed's forearm, swabs the tender part with an alcohol pad, and readies a catheter and a large-bore needle—nearly twice the size an ER nurse would use—to quickly infuse a bag of Ringer's lactate, a saline solution infused with electrolytes.

"He's gonna need two bags 'cause of all that loss of blood," Cardona suggests.

Deftly, the medic slides the catheter into Aqeed's left arm. The small flash of blood in the clear plastic chamber means the needle has found its mark. The medic draws blood for lab tests. Then he flips the IV tubing clamp, and the fluid flows into Aqeed.

"Open your eyes," the medic commands Aqeed, who has turned several shades paler and become totally still. Aqeed does not respond. The medic pokes him hard on the sternum, another technique to assess consciousness. People who do not respond to pain may be one step closer to needing more aggressive interventions.

"Open your eyes and let me know you are awake!" Cardona shouts.

Aqeed lifts his head slightly. His eyes wander, unfocused. He drops deeper into his daze.

Cardona hangs a second bag of fluids from one of several metal ceiling hooks. Certified in phlebotomy (blood drawing), Cardona ties a tourniquet around Aqeed's right upper arm. He won't pierce the patient, though, because state guidelines prohibit phlebotomists from working in the field.[1]

Newark's roads have their share of potholes, and although Callahan is a calm, careful, and efficient driver, everyone, except Aqeed, who is tied down, lurches to the left or right as if riding a nineteenth-century stagecoach. The working space inside the ambulance, which they call "the box," is roughly five by seven feet, and much of that is occupied by benches, cabinets, supply-filled shelves, the stretcher, and portable equipment. Three adult men and copious equipment crowded inside means scant room for movement.

Blood from Aqeed's wound permeates the dressings and spills onto the ambulance floor. "Put a sheet on that," the medic snaps. He lifts his leg to straddle Aqeed, crouches to lower his center of gravity, chooses a vein, and yells "Yee-ha!" as he slides the second catheter in place.

Aqeed's eyelids quiver briefly with pain.

"Hurts, don't it?" the medic asks.

Seconds later, Callahan turns in to University's driveway and radios Dispatch: "1202. We elect extra time." Customarily, they have ten minutes to transfer Aqeed to their hospital colleagues, report on his condition, wash their hands, remake the stretcher, clean up the bus, complete their paperwork, and get back on the road. Critical patients merit another five minutes. But all the blood has made the ambulance a biohazard, and they must now scrub the equipment clean.

"Roger," Smith replies, punching an additional fifteen minutes into the computer before it automatically makes them eligible for their next call. Seeing another BLS unit become available, Smith can finally send someone to Iyad. "1204?" he calls.

"1204," EMT Chuck Coles replies.

"Respond over to 119 Broadway—for the sickness. See the chief on the scene."

"OK."

At the pizzeria, rescue specialist Heber has already boarded, collared, and immobilized Iyad. Visoskas hates waiting idly. He bypasses Dispatch and radios 1204 directly: "Chuck, when you get on the scene we just need the stretcher. We got a patient with a head injury."

"Roger," Coles answers.

Having reached the hospital, Cardona and Callahan pull the stretcher out of the bus. They wheel the writhing Aqeed through the double glass doors, past the hospital police, beyond the crowded registration area, through a set of opaque sliding doors, and by the curtained ER bays with their assorted wounded. Finally, they reach the inner sanctum—the shock-trauma room, a special facility that the staff can convert into an instant operating room.

Lifting Aqeed by the bloody sheet beneath him, Cardona and Callahan transfer him onto a specialized bed designed to accommodate a portable X-ray machine. Nurses gather around to strip him of his brown-striped polo shirt, leather belt, rent jeans, socks, and remaining sneaker. They connect him to monitors that bleep and hiss as they measure his oxygen saturation, blood pressure, heart rate, and temperature.

But for a thin, gray pair of cotton boxer shorts, Aqeed is nude. He trembles with fear and chill. Still breathing through his oxygen mask, he looks anxiously down his nose only to see people in white lab coats slather his leg with molasses-colored Betadine, an all-purpose disinfectant. It mixes with his congealing blood and coats his curly black hairs.

It is the first week of July. Except for the attending physicians who supervise the staff, many of the residents have just graduated from medical school and arrived here for advanced training. The street-hardened paramedics call them "little boy and girl doctors" and pity the newly minted physicians' patients. They smirk as the residents converge hesitantly to poke, prod, and probe patients throughout the ER. But Aqeed will benefit from the trauma team's experience.[2] Except for the intern, the five residents have all been doctors for a year or more. The chief resident, who has been a physician for four or more years, supervises the team along with Dr. Sanjeev Kaul, the attending trauma surgeon and a professor at University.

"His rate is 120; his blood pressure is ninety systolic," the medic reports to the trauma team. "He has two lines in him and he's got palpable pulses." The fact that the medic can still feel blood pumping through Aqeed's foot means that oxygen is still reaching the tissue.

"Good," Dr. Kaul says as he cuts through the dressings to examine Aqeed's wound. Residents peer over his shoulder. No one should be standing by idly. "Let's get some fresh vitals!" Kaul commands. The residents scurry: one measures his pulse, another his blood pressure; a third assesses his skin temperature and condition; one checks his lung sounds; another looks at his pupils and how they respond to light. Comparing their findings, over time, with their baseline will tell them whether Aqeed is stabilizing or decompensating. EMS workers do this inside the ambulance, too.

"A *lot* of blood loss at the scene," Cardona reports. "He heard five shots, felt one."

"If he really lost all that blood, let's make sure he gets more fluid," Dr. Kaul instructs his residents.

One resident picks up Aqeed's shattered calf and twists it. "Oh, what's up, man?" Aqeed screams. His pale face winces, and although his eyes are squeezed shut, tears escape.

"They're just trying to mark the bullet hole," Cardona assures him. "Stay right there, boss. Don't move. We do everything."

The resident needs to mark the hole so the team can trace the bullet's path with a radio-opaque substance. That, in turn, gives them an idea of what muscle, tendon, bone, and nerves might be compromised. No one explains this to

Aqeed. And the docs won't even give him a shot of morphine until they are confident it won't mask any other problems. They do give him an amnesiac, though, so his memory of this fear and agony will be dim.

Dr. Kaul thinks that Aqeed may already be suffering from compartment syndrome. The lower leg has four compartments, each of which contains muscles, bone, vessels, and nerves covered by a protective sheath, or fascia. When one of the vessels is severed and leaks blood into the compartment, the muscles swell and pressure inside the compartment builds. The encompassing fascia is not expandable. Tissues compress and blood flow to the foot is compromised. If surgeons don't correct this, Aqeed might lose his foot.

Faint with pain, wet with the sweat of shock, Aqeed collapses on the bed and cries, "How is my brother, my brother?"

Everyone is engaged and no one answers. Aqeed weeps softly as a radiology technician enters. His mere presence clears the room. The faster the team gets an X-ray, the faster they will know what to do.

Callahan departs to scour blood from the equipment and put fresh linen on the stretcher. Fazio and Cardona pull chairs up to a nearby nursing desk to write their charts. Cardona prefers to write his on the bus and have them ready for the hospital staff to sign when he transfers patient care. But many jobs require several sets of hands to do everything necessary to get and keep a patient stable.

His paperwork on Aqeed is nearly complete, but Cardona still needs insurance data to avoid getting rebuked. (To prevent hospitals from turfing poor patients, the law prohibits EMS workers from soliciting such information until after they have treated *and* transported the patient *and* after the ER has examined the patient well enough to determine the course of treatment.) It's impractical, however, for Cardona to wriggle into the crowd surrounding Aqeed and ask him questions while the hospital staff is working on him. Theoretically, Cardona can get these data from the ER registration clerks who buzz around the patient's bed, too. In reality, though, it's the registration clerks who try and get the information from the EMS workers.

Spying Aqeed's wallet on the nurses' desk, Cardona flips through it for information. "He's from Jordan!" Cardona announces, surprised by the Hashemite Kingdom identification document he finds.

A doctor passing by gives him a withering look.

"Well, we got to get paid," Cardona says, somewhat sheepishly. "Governor!" he calls out. "We're trying to get you some money." Much of University's care is state-funded, and everyone is acutely aware of the medical center's financial crunch.

While the trauma team evaluates Aqeed, EMT Chuck Coles wheels Iyad into the ER. Strapped to a long board, his head securely protected by a cervical collar and spongy bookends, Iyad is still unsure what has happened to Aqeed. He imagines the worst and blames himself, wondering, *Why didn't it happen to me? I am older. Why my poor brother?*

Coles gives report, transfers care to the ER staff, and goes back on the street, where Callahan, Cardona, Fazio, and her partner are all off to their next calls.

But the chain of survival that got the Al-Atiyat brothers to the Trauma Center continues after the prehospital workers move on.

The Radiology Department makes quick work of shock-trauma patient X-rays, and Dr. Kaul and his team soon see where the bullet shattered Aqeed's tibia and fibula, too. Bullets or bone fragments nailed a significant blood vessel, possibly an artery, explaining the liters of blood on the floor and street, Dr. Kaul concludes.

Using a medieval-looking instrument called a Stryker needle, Kaul guides a resident through the process of puncturing Aqeed's calf to obtain a series of pressure readings. The resident preps the area with a local anesthetic then inserts the needle deep into his leg. "Push until you feel it pop," Kaul says, and urges the resident to keep going until she feels it a second time. Having penetrated the inner fascia, the instrument takes a reading. The resident repeats the procedure in the back of the calf, and the side as well. The findings confirm excessively high pressures; Aqeed will be going to the operating room.

Inside the creamy white shock-trauma room, he shivers on his stretcher, waiting to go to surgery. Beeping beige monitors, foreign-looking instruments, and surgical-steel shelves crammed with medical supplies loom over him. None of the bustling staff have time to hold his hand or cover him with a blanket.

Aqeed doesn't know that Iyad is secured down the hall, alive and complaining of pain in the left rear of his head and ankle. Dr. Will Gluckman, a paramedic turned emergency physician, examines Iyad and asks what happened.

"I was hit in the back of the head and I don't remember nothing," Iyad replies. "Please," he pleads. "What happened to my brother?"

Gluckman arranges for Iyad to have a CAT scan, routine protocol for head-trauma patients. Iyad asks about Aqeed again. Then their eldest brother arrives, brushing the curtain aside. With tears in his eyes, he embraces Iyad before striding down the hall to see Aqeed.

The trauma team sends Aqeed to an operating room, where an orthopedist opens his leg, cuts the fascia so the excess blood can drain, and repairs his broken bones.

Until their seven other brothers and their brother-in-law arrive from the party in Clifton, their eldest brother shuttles between Iyad and Aqeed, reassuring each that the other is, essentially, all right. Tall, powerfully built, and handsome, like his siblings, he looks like he could stand to lie down for a minute.

Tonight the B team and their Dispatch colleagues will handle several dozen other emergencies. It's not unusual for each two-person crew to respond to between twelve and twenty-five crises per twelve-hour shift, making it one of the busiest EMS centers per capita. There are no meal breaks, no sleeping is allowed, and one must get permission to go to the bathroom or risk being charged with delaying a response. Being part of such a busy, professional service is costly. Sometimes the price is burnout; sometimes skills boil down to cold efficiency. But friendships are rabidly tight. Laughter is cathartic and fierce. Challenges are frequent and furious. And, occasionally, the job is humbling, prompting even the most battle-hardened EMS workers to count their blessings.

The EMS workers have minutes to get to their assignment from anywhere in the city and to examine, treat, package, and transport their patient(s). The urgent pace leaves little time for learning what causes each patient's symptoms, much less their prognosis.

It can be maddening, but dumping patients off at the hospital without further thought can also be a blessing, they say. Many consciously avoid attachments to patients, convinced that the psychological consequence of seeing people in distress hour after hour, day after day, will undo them. They get only quick glimpses into their patients' distressed lives. Without closure, their professional memories are a vivid collage of half-stories.

Buzz, Cardona, Callahan, Visoskas, and the others will never know that Aqeed developed complications. The wound and subsequent surgery so traumatized his leg that his body kept shunting fluids to the area in an attempt to cushion and protect it. Such swelling meant the edges of skin where the scalpel cut couldn't meet, knit together, and heal. Aqeed underwent three surgeries and was one step away from a skin graft before he left the hospital, ten days later.

They'll never know that Aqeed had no insurance to pay for care, which cost forty thousand dollars. Or that he could not afford the extensive physical therapy he needed. Or that he knew nothing of the help he could get through the hospital's orthopedic clinic or the state's Violent Crimes Compensation Board. They'll never know that, five months after the incident, Aqeed still stumbles around in grotesque pain. He can't get up the stairs in his house without pausing between flights in agony. He can no longer drive for more than a few minutes. He and his teenage wife can no longer dance with wild abandon. He can't scramble on the floor in a free-for-all with his son, nieces, and nephews.

The B team won't see Aqeed's wife get weak in the knees when she and her sister-in-law go to the pizzeria to help clean up. They won't see her jaw drop when she first confronts the shattered glass, the overturned tables, and the crinkled black paper on the floor that turns out to be her husband's dehydrated blood. "It looks like a war went on here," she says, clutching her throat. She sees "Nike, Nike, Nike" on the floor. Blood from the bottom of her husband's sneaker stamped it there. The scene is appalling. But what strikes her as horrific is simply another B-team night on the job.

The B team will never know that the brothers carried barely enough liability insurance to replace the blood-soaked floor, smashed soda cases, burned grill, cracked counters, fractured lighting, and ruptured refrigerators. Or that upon their return, they say, fifteen hundred dollars in cash and cartons of Kool, Parliament, Marlboro, and Winston cigarettes had gone missing from Iyad's conjoined grocery. Police were the only ones with access, Iyad says. Aqeed thinks they helped themselves. The brothers are too disgusted and disheartened to file a complaint. They just want to repair what they must, sell the store, and get out of Newark.

That's not so easy.

Iyad stays out of work for nearly a month with a concussion and a sprained ankle. He has no workmen's compensation policy for himself or Aqeed. He has no income, either. He returns to work because he must pay his bills. But Iyad's wife says he is too depressed to talk. Iyad has nightmares. Iyad doesn't eat.

Aqeed stays out of work for five months. His brothers, grateful to have him alive, contribute cash to cover the cost of his family's rent and groceries. But that can't go on indefinitely.

Later, when the two do go to work it is with trepidation. Sometimes additional brothers accompany them to help protect the store from repeated assault. Every day they pray for a buyer.

The B team will never know that the Al-Atiyats' parents were robbed and shot in Jordan ten years ago. Their father, an Army detective, took three bullets in the leg. Rasmiah, their mother, was killed. In fact, she died in Iyad's arms. She was thirty-six. Iyad was fourteen. Aqeed was twelve.

3 THE SITUATION ROOM

People don't call 911 and say, "Two pies just
came out of the oven . . . come on by!"
Instead, they call and say, "Two pies just came
out of the oven and the chef is aflame!"

—CRAIG JACOBUS, PARAMEDIC AND CHIROPRACTIC
   PHYSICIAN

Just before 1830 hours one sweltering August night, emergency medical dispatcher Juan Ortiz punches his card into the time clock at the Regional Emergency Medical Communications System (REMCS). The EMS Department also runs the Dispatch Center for Newark and its environs. High aloft in the Martland building, which was once a 750-bed hospital itself, the burly, six-foot-two-inch man stares through wire-rimmed eyeglasses and panoramic, plate-glass windows at the darkening cityscape. Less than a half-mile from where he stands tonight, the city's infamous race riots erupted in 1967. Ortiz was five years old.

Residents, many impoverished, unemployed, and worried about displacement in the name of development projects, including the College of Medicine and Dentistry of New Jersey, were already on edge when an arrest went awry and rumors ignited one neighborhood after another until the city erupted into a full-fledged race riot. National Guard troops enforced a curfew to help restore order. Some University EMS workers were only children then but remember armored tanks rolling down Central Avenue. Armed troops made the Newark City schools' stadium their tactical headquarters and spread through the tangled web of streets. Five days later, twenty-six people had died; one thousand had sustained injuries; and authorities had arrested sixteen hundred more. Fear and suspicion lingered and etched psychological demoralization into the city's consciousness.

University Hospital is one of several institutions that emerged from the ashes. It sits squarely in the city's Central Ward, a section Ortiz calls "the dead zone" after its still-scarred streets, vacant overgrown lots, and torched buildings.

Ortiz was born and raised in Newark, a three-century-old city bookended by lush Frederick Law Olmsted parks. The South Ward sports Weequahic Park, an immense golf course, a racetrack dating back to the nineteenth century, an outdoor velodrome, and a sprawling industrial base. But there are high-crime areas there, too. In one neighborhood, which marks a transition between residential and industrial areas, windowless one-story warehouses dominate poorly lit blocks. Prostitutes slink in the shadows. Many blue-shirts believe the women are all HIV-infected. Nevertheless, they say, the hookers do a brisk business selling their wares to Newark businessmen and "regular guys" from nearby suburbs.

The East Ward incorporates neighborhoods as well as Newark International Airport and Port Newark. Many of the ward's narrow, one-way streets funnel into a slim stretch called Down Neck. A map of the area, turned on its side, resembles an animal's neck. Nineteenth-century train tracks encircle part of the area in iron, hence the nickname Ironbound. The Portuguese and Brazilian neighborhood's neatly kept streets bustle with seafood restaurants, trim storefronts that feature hand-painted porcelain, and small businesses, from tailors to dentists to the occasional go-go bar. Potted trees punctuate the sidewalks, and strands of tiny, white lightbulbs, draped between telephone poles like pearl necklaces, light up the streets. But there is drug trafficking and poverty here, too.

The West Ward is primarily residential, but many homes have been abandoned.

The North Ward, Ortiz says, is still the city's jewel. Massive, distinguished stone mansions dominate large, tree-lined streets. Indolent property owners have converted some once-grand properties into flophouses, but most are lovingly maintained. Branch Brook Park boasts an impressive spread of feathery pink cherry blossoms, and the Basilica of the Sacred Heart, a stunning religious icon, stands guard over the city. Hispanics now dominate what was, until recently, a predominantly Italian section.

Ortiz joined REMCS six years ago, after eleven years as a ground-pounder, which left him with a fractured ankle, a dislocated knee, other on-the-job injuries, and skyrocketing hypertension. He still takes pride in helping people, though experience has tarnished his view. A Catholic, he stares at the spectacular, illuminated cathedral with sorrow. Working EMS in Newark has sorely tested his beliefs, he says. If such a beautiful, vigorous, and sacred institution is powerless to stop the tragedies, the husky father of three asks, "can anything we do really make a difference?"

From the hushed, dim, cavernous communications suite, the glittering cityscape is draped in shadows. The streets sparkle—quiet, calm, and even serene. It's an illusion. "Time to wipe the ass of the city," he says. "Time to clean up its shit."

Ortiz and his colleagues spread out through the antiseptic technology suite, half of which sits on standby in case equipment fails or a major event occurs and Dispatch needs to double the staff. Each selects a console layered with up to nine flashing monitors and keypads. Shadows obscure the pale pink walls, which are studded with maps and memos. Slate blue carpet, flecked with color, mutes harsh street sounds. One can turn 360 degrees and never have a motionless view. A standing fan twirls and issues a perpetual breeze. Miniature lights vibrate across the surfaces of myriad machines. One emergency medical dispatcher (EMD) serves as primary call-taker. Another assigns jobs. A third supervises telemetry.[1]

For now, Ortiz will coordinate air medical dispatch and pick up any slack. The EMDs rotate jobs throughout the twelve-hour shift to enhance cross-training and quash boredom. A supervisor works with them, too, troubleshooting the inevitable calamities.

As the shift begins, they curl up in their cushy, high-backed chairs and steel themselves to guide the city through another rough ride.

DANGER, WILL ROBINSON!

The phones ring incessantly. At 2136 hours, the ringer sounds yet again, and a pale tangerine button flashes in tandem. William "Buzz" Busby takes instants to scout the three light boards in front of him; hundreds of ruby, emerald, and amber lights flicker, competing for his attention. Honing in on the latest 911 call, he presses it and taps into a fresh crisis. "Emergency medical?" he purrs into his headset microphone.

"Hello?" a woman's quavering voice inquires.

"Mmm-hmmmm."

She relays a Central Ward address.

"What floor and apartment?" he asks, typing a computer-generated report. The Dispatch Center has arrangements with the phone company which allow it to automatically capture the number, listing, and address, even from callers who block their caller ID intentionally. But still, dispatchers must confirm the listings. And so Buzz does.

"217B."

"What's the problem?"

"My husband," she says, her lush African accent emerging. "He's hurt."

"What happened?"

"We have—the lot of blood here."

"OK," Buzz replies. "He cut himself?"

"Yeah," she gushes breathlessly.

"All right, where at?"

"Uh, uh, for the leg!"

"On his leg?"

"Yeah!" she pants. "There has a lot of blood dripping."

"OK. Get a heavy towel and wrap it around the cut, and tell him to hold pressure on it," Buzz tells her. He calls on his own experience, fourteen years on the street and fifteen years as a dispatcher. And he consults a computerized database, which generates advice based on his input. He clacks away on his keyboard while conferring with the woman, so when the call is complete the computer will instantly shoot the crisis into the lineup, according to its priority and relationship to other emergencies. Some EMS dispatch centers operate similarly; others employ "system status management," a strategy that concentrates resources in high-call-volume areas to cut response times, reduce the frequency of no-holds-barred lights-and-sirens missions, and thus diminish the number of collisions.[2]

"A towel?" the woman asks, puzzled.

Buzz repeats the instructions. Many callers are just too emotional to focus on the conversation. "Get a heavy towel, wrap it around that cut, and just tell him to hold pressure as tight as he can."

"OK."

"All right. How old is he?"

"Uh, fifty."

Buzz verifies the address and reassures her: "All right, we'll get somebody there." He codes the call as a "hemorrhage/laceration," a condition the computer automatically classifies as "possibly dangerous." But because the patient is presumed conscious and breathing, the computer assigns it priority code B, Bravo, meaning emergent but manageable at the BLS level.

Ninety seconds later, a dispatcher assigns the job to Callahan and Cardona. They acknowledge, both via radio and by pressing a button on their onboard computer five seconds later. They arrive at the address within seven minutes, ride high up into the tower by elevator, and walk down a long stretch of hall to the very last apartment. A youthful, ebony-hued woman answers the door clad in braids, lustrous gold earrings, and a blue terry-cloth bath towel. Barefoot, she steps back to let the men inside. Cardona has barely one foot in the door when he turns to Callahan and whispers huskily, "I smell blood."

The air is thick with the sweet, metallic, nostril-curling aroma of the iron, carried by the viscous fluid's hemoglobin. "I smell blood, too," Callahan confirms with a deep sniff.

Cardona follows his nose down the hall and to the right. A man with a square-shaped head and skin that gleams obsidian sits upon a throne of a chair that is upholstered in pomegranate silk. His forearms flex as his muscular hands wrap around a thick white towel and squeeze his thigh. A large Pepsi bottle is overturned on the floor. Blood-soaked paper towels lie crumpled by his feet. A mattress is propped against a wall. A huge, glossy, burl-wood entertainment center dominates the room. Both EMTs can't help but admire it.

As he takes in his surroundings, something strikes Cardona as odd, but he can't pinpoint what. It might be the fear in the woman's eyes. It might be the tension in the man's jaw. Instinctively, he says, "I need to know what really happened."

The couple is silent. Many patients and their family members do not know what health-care options the law provides regardless of their economic, immigration, or criminal status. And not infrequently they attribute more power to EMS workers than the crews actually have.

"I'm not the police. I'm the ambulance guy," Cardona assures them.

"We were just talking," the patient's wife sobs into her long, delicate fingertips glossed with pearl polish. Her shoulders and heavy breasts, iridescent carbon silk, shake with emotion. "I take the knife and, I cut him."

"Let me see it," Cardona says. "I need to describe the knife to the doctors so they'll know how deep his cut is."

Tearfully, she turns and pads from the living room into the kitchen with Cardona close behind her. She reaches a slender arm into a sink full of dishes and extracts a ten-inch butcher knife covered with rice from their dinner and human blood.

"You need stitches, my man!" Cardona says, returning from the kitchen. "That's a deep cut."

The man gives a terse nod, and his wife timidly asks, "Excuse? I go, too?"

"Sure," Cardona replies. "If you want."

"Excuse, I go wake the baby," she says, turning toward a bedroom.

"Oh, if you have a baby, you should really stay here," Cardona advises.

"Yeah, you don't want to take a baby to an emergency room full of sick people," Callahan adds.

Uncertain what to do, she pivots, wringing her hands with frustration.

"He'll be fine," Cardona assures her. "They'll stitch him up and send him home."

Wincing with effort, the man pulls on a pair of sweatpants, slips on a pair of pink plastic sandals, and straightens up into a regal posture. He strides out the front door and to the ambulance, without assistance and without a good-bye.

The ride to the hospital is uneventful, but the ride back to quarters is strained. Cardona feels uncomfortable having left the man without some protection, at least a police report. "We have an obligation," Cardona says, considering domestic-violence law. "Let's say he goes home and she plunges that same knife into his chest?"

"Bottom line," Callahan agrees, "you got a fucking point."

"We probably would have treated this different if he had stabbed her, but he's all scratched the fuck up 'cause she was all over him."

"I'm just obsessed with men hitting women," Callahan says, recalling what he witnessed growing up and the wife abuse he sees regularly on the job.

"'Cause how do we know she won't lose her mind later, too?" Cardona asks. "Both seemed so adamant about not having the police involved." In the end, the two do not make a police report. But Cardona doesn't sleep easily for the next few days, and periodically he wonders how the man is faring.

When Buzz learns that the laceration was really a stab wound, he just shakes his head and chuckles. *Callers only give up enough information to keep themselves from being incriminated*, he thinks. It's his job to elicit the clearest possible picture in seconds. The software actually times how quickly he works. And the possibility of sending units into dangerous situations is always on a good dispatcher's mind, especially those who made their bones, i.e., earned their stripes on the street. But the interview is only a tool to give the EMS workers an idea of what's to come, Buzz explains. Their hands-on assessment is what counts, and there's no substitute.

Robert Resetar, a paramedic and the communication division's coordinator, concedes that the service can always improve. He's made sure each staff member has mastered a forty-hour EMD training course and spent six months training. He has appointed a quality-assurance specialist to evaluate transcripts and suggest possible improvements. He has required most of his staff to maintain their EMT and paramedic certifications. In the event of a wide-scale crisis, the department can send dispatchers to the street as certified caregivers. Several REMCS dispatchers graduated from Newark's school of hard knocks when resources were scarce, when the city was worn thin by corrupt government, when immense, widespread poverty enraged the community, when people were trapped in dilapidated high-rise housing projects, when modern EMS was in its virtual infancy.

Their experience, however, commands little respect from the men and women who work Newark's streets today. Many disparage the Dispatch Center, nicknaming it "the Land of the Lame."

EMD Judy Smith prefers to think of it as the Land of Broken Toys. "It's more of a forgotten place," she says, "like the rubber-gun squad where they send police who can no longer be trusted with a weapon, or firemen who sucked up too much smoke to climb the ladder." Her coworker Lorraine Murray likens Dispatch to a refuge for old soldiers who have done their tours on the street, but can still perform some valuable service.

Several colleagues who work the street scorn their Dispatch colleagues, even to the extent of proposing that they be replaced by "the handicapped." Conveniently, several EMS workers on the street ignore the fact that many of their REMCS colleagues are literally disabled and became so by working the streets. Murray, for example, was hired in the mid-1970s, before gloves and other personal protective equipment were required. She contracted hepatitis B. Judy Smith survived more than a dozen ambulance crashes; she was never the driver. She has a degenerative disc disorder that impinges her neck and spine. Jim Smith fractured vertebrae in his neck. Marion Shabazz broke her hand and her neck, too. Most EMDs say they were dragged upstairs to desk duty kicking and screaming. Some went with a grateful whimper. And several claim they would rush back to the street in a heartbeat, if only their old and broken bodies would allow.

On average, the warhorses upstairs at REMCS are older than their colleagues on the street, and that maturity helps them take the contempt in stride. They, too, remember hating dispatchers back when they worked the streets. It's tempting to forget that the jobs come in by way of the public and that the taxpayers throughout the state pay them to respond. "It's the nature of the business to get angry at the messenger," Resetar says. And he's honest enough to confess that he is guilty of dispatcher abuse, too, when he works as a paramedic, one or two shifts week in south Jersey. "As a provider, I have that same reaction to the dispatchers where I live," he admits. Dispatchers aren't malicious wizards who conjure up assignments to torture colleagues on the street, but when you are humping job after job, rushing from rathole to hellhole, carrying stinking, heavy, and combative patients hour after hour, it's natural to resent whoever is doling out the assignments, Resetar says.

To minimize conflict, Resetar insists that all new EMS workers spend one twelve-hour shift with REMCS to get a feel for the dispatchers' challenges. EMDs have seconds to wrest control of conversations, ferret out the nature and scope of the problem, determine the most appropriate type of response, juggle limited resources, and document, document, document. Every action is time-stamped, recorded on tamper-proof tape, and stored for years.

Still, it's a job the EMTs and paramedics demean as "easy." "REMCS," says one B-teamer, "is a haven for the weak, the lame, and the lazy." Compared with running up and down disintegrating, urine-soaked staircases, squeezing between roach-infested pipes and toilets to extract wedged-in patients, or scraping up body parts from industrial accidents, dispatchers work in relative comfort. The clean, spacious chamber is a protective bubble outfitted in institutional blue and gray. It shields dispatchers from the brain-fogged, waterlogged sensation of the street crews' utter exhaustion; the strain of endless flights of stairs; foul stenches; eyesores; visages of forlorn children; creeping, crawling vermin; violence; infectious disease; and grueling extremes of weather.

The department keeps the Dispatch Center cool and comfortable year-round, if only to preserve the computer equipment. Food, drink, and bathrooms are just steps away. EMDs can even ride up to their comfy chairs in an elevator instead of breaking their backs with hundreds of pounds of patient and "portable" equipment. "We sit at our desks, put our feet up, drink something cold from the fridge," Chief Thomas Austin Tryon jokes, "and one of us will say, 'Man, this job sucks!' Then we bust out laughing."

That Tryon and the others already invested years on the street doing what the B team does now is conveniently overlooked during griping sessions. Their hard work also yielded niceties that some present-day EMS workers take for granted. For example, Resetar improved the department's two-way, portable radios and developed panic buttons for the radios and buses. Previously, if partners got separated, everyone fended for himself or herself. One EMS worker still has his badge complete with the scratches and nicks it took the day it blocked a knife some thug used to stab at him. The palm-sized shield gave that blue-shirt the few seconds he needed to scramble and fight for his life. When his assailant attacked, his partner was outside near the truck—out of sight, beyond the call of his voice. The EMS worker had no way to signal him, or Dispatch for that matter. Now crews can summon help instantly. And Resetar has moved the department from phones, pads, and pegboards to a technologically sophisticated operation envied around the world.

The department's need to police itself motivated some improvements. Years ago, when thousands of impoverished families were crammed into decrepit high-rises, many blue-shirts were loath to respond. The projects were structurally convoluted, with the twists and turns of a maze and only one way out. There were times the EMS workers just couldn't face climbing another rank twenty-five floors up. "It would be nine hundred degrees outside and your feet would stick to the floor with all the urine and crap," Ortiz remembers. "If you're lucky enough to get an elevator that worked at all, you get in with a bunch of locals who just played a few hours of basketball. Now you're stuck in that box with the stink of urine and shit and garbage and body odor. By the time you get to the top you're literally crying to get out. But lots of times, the elevators wouldn't work. Or they wouldn't meet the floor, which means you'd have to touch that floor with your hands to push yourself up." He recoils at the memory.

Although management dismisses such tales as "folklore," veteran EMS workers claim that there were occasions, years ago, when some blue-shirts would do anything to avoid getting sent to the projects or to an out-of-town job where they would most likely get canceled before arriving on-scene. Some fabricated calls or claimed that people flagged them down from the street, diverting them from undesirable assignments. (In Newark, an empty ambulance cannot bypass a person in need, even if it is en route to a vetted emergency.) Since no alternative patient really existed, the crews would drive around for a bit and then show up at the ER with trumped-up paperwork. When the ER staff asked after the patient, the EMTs looked around, shrugged, and said "Oh! They musta walked."

Sometimes, the old-timers report, EMS workers stayed curled up in the Quonset hut that served as quarters before they took over the medical examiner's office twenty years ago. "Yeah, we're en route," they would radio in. "Yeah, we're on-scene." They faked entire calls, a veteran recalls. And since University EMS has never had an integrated facility for dispatch, BLS, ALS, supervisors, management, no one was the wiser—at least for a while.

Administrators added field supervisors, then GPS and automatic vehicle locators (AVLs), to discourage abuse and improve efficiency. Crews resent the scrutiny and allege that management has overreacted to the misdeeds of a few burned-out workers. (Many departmental policies result from punishing one person or another, they charge.) Despite their affection for Buzz and a few other EMDs, most see Dispatch as an obnoxious, bean-counting Big Brother.

Whether the conflict between the ground-pounders and the dispatchers is a fact of nature or a symptom of what is dysfunctional in this still-fragmented, still-youthful profession, it is ever-present.

Buzz may be the most successful at keeping himself smooth and unruffled. "Buzz could tell me I have to go to the eighteenth floor of a building where three people are dying and there's no elevator, and I'd say, 'OK,'" claims Vincent Francis Cisternino, veteran B-team paramedic. "But if some of the others even say, 'Seizure on the outside' "—a routine call with practically no lifting—"I just wanna kill them."

But even for the maestro it can be a Herculean effort. "Just the other day, a family called here," Buzz recalls. "The mother dropped dead of a cardiac arrest. I heard family members coming from all over the house, screaming and crying while I was telling them what to do. I got all choked up, putting myself in their place. What if it was *my* mother? What if it was *my* child?" A husband of many years, stepfather to three, and father to two, Buzz finds it easy to place himself in his patients' shoes.

"But I try to keep the emotions in, at least until after the call, because they're looking to me for help, man," Buzz says. "The last thing you want to do is break down. Sometimes, though, it brings me to tears."

Ortiz describes the weight of responsibility in the ambulance or behind the microphone as awesome. "To most people, callers are just a bunch of statistics, but they don't have to calm down the person who just smoked a half-inch dust bone"—a marijuana joint dusted with PCP (phencyclidine).

"We all live in terror for the one event that breaks the camel's back," Ortiz confesses. Shutting down emotions is just one way to forestall the flood. Coming upon decapitations, hemicorporectomies (bodies torn in half), suicides, child abuse, miscarriages, and other troubling scenes is stressful. But conversations with distraught callers can be trying, too. If even the slightest strain shows in a dispatcher's voice, the B-team blue-shirts smell blood and react viciously.

Even on their best days, EMDs have numerous strikes against them. Theoretically, when an EMS request comes into the city's primary public-safety center, the Newark police, calls are switched to REMCS at the touch of a button. When this works, REMCS can almost always automatically capture the address from which the call emanates and try, at least, to screen the caller. But many Newark residents lack phones and must resort to using pay phones, cell phones, and other means of accessing help. So interviewing callers to confirm the address and the nature of the emergency is crucial to getting the right help there promptly. For a variety of reasons, dispatchers can only interview callers a fraction of the time.

EMDs often get secondhand information or worse. Aqeed Al-Atiyat, for example, swears that he and the responding good Samaritans called 911 repeatedly—and that it took more than twenty minutes for help to arrive. REMCS received only one call from the police and sent an ambulance within one minute.

The hospital offered to build the EMS switching system at police headquarters so that software and hardware could be coordinated. But that offer was rejected, and it has neither the authority nor the technology to ensure that police route medical emergencies to REMCS properly. Each time a call is not transferred directly, however, a dispatcher notes it on a tally sheet, and the department submits this report to police.

Even when police operators do make the effort, callers sometimes hang up before the call is ever transferred.

The callers can be unreliable, too. Even with fifteen years' dispatching experience, Buzz can't explain why some people don't know their own address.

He often knows when people are wrong, partly from his years as a dispatcher, partly from riding the ambulance, and also from cruising the city with the fellas, something he did religiously as a younger man. One of Buzz's tricks is to ask people to read the address from a piece of mail.

Good Samaritans call to report car accidents but don't necessarily know where they occurred. So many of the street signs have been stolen or vandalized that it takes detective work and a historian's knowledge of the city to find them. One night, a caller phones 911 to report a car accident at Raymond Place and Jefferson. Buzz knows something is wrong. He checks the computerized street grid, and finds that both streets run through the city but they don't intersect. With a little bit of research, he determines that the caller means Raymond Plaza and Jersey Street. Buzz also calls on his mental database of popular landmarks such as parks, grocery shops, and ice-cream shops to locate emergency scenes.

Callers telephone from outside Newark, asking dispatchers to check on people who seem to have disappeared.

Some callers exaggerate, hoping to hurry the ambulance and leapfrog them straight to the back of the ER—beyond the registration area, past the double doors and nursing desks, back to where the medical staff gets hands-on with patients. Years ago, dispatchers had the discretion to prioritize calls and even to refuse to send an ambulance. But now society's propensity to litigate means that everybody who requests an ambulance in Newark gets one—it's just a question of when.

"The most we can do is downgrade a call," Buzz explains, "*if* we know the caller just wants to go to the hospital and get a meal and some heat because it's cold out." Currently, the department responds to at least a dozen "frequent fliers," from infamous drunks to a woman who snacks on talcum powder, frightening her neighbors and passersby on the street. Regulars might call five times a week, and, on a bad night, half a dozen times.

In parts of Washington State, one EMS system is experimenting with a program that allows EMS workers to triage patients on the scene and decide whether circumstances merit an ambulance trip. For those patients with less immediate needs, the EMS workers turn to nurses who help arrange appropriate alternative medical care.

University views ambulance requests from the callers' perspective. Chief Tryon defines medicine as "the alleviation of the pain as well as the healing of the illness." By that definition, he says, "even an abscessed tooth that is driving someone crazy with pain is considered legitimate."

People with toothaches and colds as well as those who have failed to fill prescriptions for chronic conditions (in spite of low-cost or free medicine) clamor for ambulances and compete for medical attention with victims of falls, appendicitis, strokes, and heart attacks. "I have a primary-care physician and I can't always see him when I want," a department manager says, throwing up her hands. "It can take people here three weeks to be seen. What are they supposed to do?" Experts estimate about one million people lack health insurance in New Jersey and thus have no regular physician, a problem echoed throughout the nation.

University Hospital's ER triages (sorts) patients by level of severity. Those with medically urgent needs go first. Everyone else waits. On a bad day, such as during a flu epidemic, delays can range between six and twelve hours. In a national Internet discussion group, EMDs from across the country share stories and query each other about how to handle frustrated patients and family members. Anxious and worn out by waiting, people are dialing 911 to ask for ambulance transfers from one hospital to another where they hope to get better service.[3]

Although municipalities have a responsibility to ensure their residents' well-being, the state of New Jersey does not legally mandate EMS access. Residents have cobbled together a patchwork of providers including volunteer first-aid squads, paid and volunteer fire departments, independent contractors, and hospitals. No one counts the number or analyzes the type of EMS requests EMDs log each year, here or nationally. Most EMDs admit that responses to some calls are seriously delayed. Resetar says he is not proud of the fact that it can sometimes take two hours to respond. There just are not enough ambulances to answer every call promptly. The lack of adequate EMS assets is unique neither to Newark nor to one type of system. And there are places in the U.S. where EMS cannot be accessed by dialing 911. Although there are laws that prevent emergency-care providers from turning patients away, there is no strategy, national or state, to coordinate and enforce EMS standards or fund EMS budgets.

A successful caller interview allows Dispatch to issue consistent, medically appropriate advice until the EMS crew arrives, determine which resources to send, and still keep the system staffed to address other crises. And it equips responding crews with enough information to begin thinking through scenarios before they arrive.

REMCS uses medical-priority software. Designed originally to help police, funeral directors, and other non-EMS professionals who once and still answer many 911 calls, the software features a database of medical emergencies, doctor-approved triage and assessment questions, and recommendations to classify and treat each threat. It standardizes the interview process, analysis, and advice.

Based on interview results, it determines each emergency's priority: A, B,

C, or D. A, or Alpha, is for nonemergent problems, such as eczema, wandering Alzheimer's patients, and rings caught on fingers. B, or Bravo, is for noncritical emergencies, such as lacerations and maternity calls. C, or Charlie, is for potential life threats, such as asthma. And D, or Delta, is for immediate life threats, such as unconscious patients.

Each priority is color-coded as well, in keeping with recognized triage standards. A calls automatically show up in Kelly green type, B calls in lemon yellow, C in hot-chile red, and D in skeletal white printed on a bloodred rectangle.

Dispatchers have some discretion in assigning jobs, but not much. They try to keep the paramedics free for more critical calls, but if a less urgent request waits twenty or thirty minutes and all the EMTs are still busy, they will assign it to ALS.

Once a dispatcher assigns the call, the computer updates the report. By activating their vehicle-based computers, the EMS workers record the time they receive the job, pinpoint when they arrive on-scene, and calculate the transport times. Based on their findings, EMS workers radio transport codes, which dispatchers use to adjust each job's status and augment their reports for billing. Depending on the nature of the emergency, crews may ask the telemetry operator to patch them through to medical control, i.e., supervising physicians at University Hospital who approve ALS treatment plans. The final product is a transcript, which, along with a corresponding tape, is preserved for years.

But there are obstacles. Lonely people clog the lines. One dispatcher posted a request for advice to an Internet listserv regarding a person who phoned 911 ninety-one times within seventeen hours.[4] Leading emotionally overwhelmed callers through interviews can be impossible. When information is sketchy, it impedes the EMS workers on the street. The blue-shirts have learned to be wary of everything that comes over the squawk box. Dispatch can announce that the world is ending, but even that won't provoke much reaction from seasoned B-team veterans. "You don't really get clear-cut information from the radio. They don't have both ends of the spectrum," Cardona explains. "So, you stay neutral because if you get too upset or think it's bullshit, you're not prepared. Just stay loose and get what you get."

CHIMERA

"Emergency medical?" Buzz answers at 2250 hours one close summer night.

"Hello? I need an ambulance," a woman gushes before rattling off a North Ward address. "My husband is having a heart attack."

"What floor and apartment?"

"B-1, basement," she says hurriedly.

"OK, how old is he?"

"He's thirty-six," she spurts.

"All right, what's going on with him now?"

"OK, he feels his arm is numb. His chest hurting. He's been complaining 'bout that fifteen or twenty minutes already, and he—Just get somebody while I'm talking to you!" she demands.

"Listen to me," Buzz says paternally. "The ambulance is on the way. Did this ever happen to him before?"

"No. He's felt his chest problems before but never like this."

"OK, all right. Just sit him down. Keep him comfortable. How's he breathing?"

"He's—Are you breathing good, honey?" she asks her husband. "Could you breathe good?" She tells Buzz to hold on, then reports, "He could breathe good, yeah."

"OK. All right. Just keep him sitting up. Keep him comfortable," Buzz instructs. "All right, and we'll get somebody over there." He completed the first phase of the report, within ninety seconds, while talking with her. The software classifies this as a C priority, a *potential* life threat, because the patient is young and has no cardiac history.

"He's numbing," the woman adds urgently. "Come on! It's numbing."

"All right, just listen to me. *Listen to me*," Buzz says, raising his voice a bit louder to get her attention. "The ambulance is on the way."

"OK."

"The best thing is for *you* to calm down so he doesn't get upset anymore. And you just keep him calm."

"OK."

"But you gotta stay calm also. The ambulance will be there shortly."

"OK, I'm putting my slippers on."

People tell Buzz all kinds of inanities. He doesn't laugh; however, he sometimes wishes he could. "OK, just keep him comfortable."

"Do you have your insurance card and your ID?" she asks her husband in the background, then mumbles, "I ain't even gonna think about it." Breathing into the phone, she tests Buzz: "Hello?"

"OK, I'm still here," he reassures her. "Just keep him comfortable and you stay calm."

"His face is getting numb!"

"All right, just keep him comfortable," Buzz instructs. "You can't get upset though."

"*You stay comfortable*; you stay comfortable!" the woman orders her husband.

"All right?" Buzz asks. "The ambulance is on the way. OK?"

"Yeah."

"All right. Look out for the ambulance."

"OK."

Within two and a half minutes, the Dispatch Center has interviewed and counseled the caller, chosen a paramedic unit, assigned the job, and received confirmation that the unit is headed to the man's home.

Buzz's phones ring fast and furiously. He can't get to them all. Ortiz, manning the air medical desk, helps out. He picks up a call without leaving his console: "Emergency Medical Service, 651. May I help you?"

"I got disconnected," a woman says. "Is this you again?"

"Who is me again?" Ortiz inquires.

"OK, I was just talking about my husband. My husband is having a seizure *and* a heart attack."

"OK, what's the address?"

She repeats her address, floor, and apartment number in one fast breath.

"You called already?" he asks, just before spotting it queued into the list of active jobs.

"Yeah, I did. But I just got disconnected!" she exclaims breathlessly. "But, I wanted to tell the dispatcher that he, we were smoking weed."

"OK," Ortiz says. *Pot can make a person paranoid*, he thinks. *And pot laced with PCP makes it worse*. He wonders where they bought the dope and if it was spiked. It's not uncommon for people to go to extreme lengths for a high, even dousing marijuana with roach spray or other household chemicals.

"And we was drinking."

"OK," he says. At least half the calls requesting medical assistance in the city have something to do with drugs and alcohol, he estimates. (Others say it's more.) Ortiz has even found people drinking antifreeze and sucking the contents out of hairspray cans.

"So, can someone hurry up, please?" she asks, urgently. "Make sure they're coming?"

"OK." He checks to see that the call has been assigned. "Yeah," assures her. "There is someone on their way now. What's wrong with him? What's he complaining of?"

"He's, his chest—his arms are numb. His mouth is numb. His face is numb."

"OK. How old is he?"

"He can't breathe. He's not breathing good."

"How old is he?"

"He's thirty-six."

"OK. We got someone on their way over there right now."

"Oh, God," she cries desperately. "*Hurry up.*"

"OK, calm down."

"Please, don't hang up," she begs.

"OK. Well, what do you want me to do?"

"I need to speak to somebody, just in case . . . I just need to stay on the phone, please."

"OK. Well, I'll be here, so if you need, if he changes just yell out. OK? But I'll have to probably answer another phone in the meantime. But if anything changes just yell out."

"OK," she replies quietly. Her husband mumbles something to her in the background. While she talks to him she also tries frantically to keep in touch with Ortiz. "Hello?"

"Yes?" Ortiz replies in a heartbeat.

"OK, I just want to make sure you're here," she sighs heavily. Then she resumes talking to herself. "Oh, goodness, where's his stuff?"

"Is he awake right now?" Ortiz asks.

"Yeah, I'm looking for his friggin' ID and stuff."

"All right, well, don't worry about that. Just take care of him."

"I don't want to leave him alone," she frets. "He's thirsty."

"Well, don't give him anything to eat or drink, OK?"

"I know."

"OK, just don't give him anything to eat or drink. OK?" Ortiz repeats, hoping something will penetrate through the caller's haze of panic. "I'm going to put down the phone again. I'll be with you in a minute."

"OK."

Then a man's voice murmurs, "Honey, get a spoon, quick!"

"Hello? HELLO? *HELLO?*" the woman shouts into the phone.

"Yes?" Ortiz replies.

"He just wants me to get a spoon for his tongue. What do I do?"

"For what?"

"Because he feels like his tongue is going to roll."

"No, don't put anything in his mouth, OK? You can't swallow your tongue, OK? Because it's impossible; it's attached to your mouth, OK? So just tell him to calm down. All right?"

"OK," she sighs.

"So, tell him to take some deep breaths and relax. You're getting all worked up for nothing."

"Take deep breaths," she tells her husband. "Oh, God," she moans. "Oh, where they at?"

"They're on their way."

"I don't hear nothing yet!"

"They're on their way."

"Hello? *You still there? Hello?*"

"OK."

"They're not here. Could you ask them where they are? Some way?"

"All right, just calm down, OK? You're getting all worked up over nothing."

"OK."

"So, just relax. They'll be there as soon as they can."

"OK," she says, huffing and puffing. He can hear her practically hyperventilating. "Can I put a cold rag on his head?"

"No, don't put anything on him."

"They're not here!" she cries to Ortiz. "Honey, how you breathin'?" she asks her husband. Then she yells to Ortiz, "His mouth is shaking!"

"OK," Ortiz replies calmly.

"Come on, *come on!*" she urges the ambulance. Then, to her husband, she says, "Take deep breaths, honey." She sighs deeply and repeatedly. "Come on! I don't hear them."

"All right."

"Oh, God," she says breathlessly. "My God! Sir, could you puh-lease? I don't hear anything."

"OK. Right away. Just relax. Right away. I promise. . . ."

"I don't hear anything! *Hello?*" she says to Ortiz. Then, with the next breath, she coaches her husband, "Take deep breaths, take deep breaths. Ohhhh, oohhh God! How you baby? Can you breathe?"

"I have to put you on hold for a sec," Ortiz says, and takes a minute to update the responding paramedics. Most callers withhold information regarding their recreational use of drugs for fear the police will come and lock them up. The police can and do listen to 911 calls, Resetar says. According to state law, there is no presumption of privacy.

ALS arrives, five minutes and forty-three seconds after the woman's initial request, to find that the man is not having a heart attack. Nor is he having a seizure. If anything, he reacted to the marijuana he smoked and the whiskey chaser. After an exam, including an ECG to monitor his heart, with his symptoms in remission and his vital signs stable, the man refuses to go to the hospital. He sends the medics on their way.

BEHIND THE SCENES

Dispatchers at University Hospital do more than play messenger. And keep the service's statistics. And run the computer systems. And coordinate resources for mass casualty events. They problem-solve. A constant stream of events occurs behind the scenes, hurling roadblocks into the fray and challenging system readiness.

One night, news broadcasters interrupted the program playing on the television that runs incessantly in the background. A huge condominium complex on the banks of the Hudson River is ablaze eighteen miles away, in Edgewater, New Jersey. As news helicopters fly over sizzling flames hundreds of feet high, images flicker on the Dispatch Center's TV. Soon, a call comes from the state's First Aid Council, an umbrella organization that unites 430 volunteer first-aid squads and uses REMCS for mobilization dispatch.

Chief Tryon, one of the state's first paramedics, is on duty tonight. "Frank?" Tryon says, looking at the caller ID on his screen. Frank Goodstein is the First Aid Council's mobilization coordinator. "What's up, man?"

"Two things. Anybody keeping you aware of the situation up in Edgewater?"

"No. MICOM"—the regional dispatcher for Bergen County, north of Newark—"sounded way too busy. So I said, 'We're just here, you know. Call us if you need us.' I haven't heard from them."

"All right. They're going to activate statewide in just a few minutes because they need to communicate a couple things and I just wanted to let you know."

"OK."

"And number two—is the mass-casualty response unit working?" (The department's Special Operations Group (SOG) staffs the MCRU, a special vehicle capable of treating dozens of patients simultaneously. SOG members are EMS workers proficient in incident command, hazardous materials mitigation, confined space rescue, and other specialty facets of EMS.)

"As far as I know, yeah."

"All right. Can you do me a favor?" Goodstein asks. "Can you verify that it is in working order? I heard it was out of service."

"I'll do that while you are on the phone. Hold on." Tryon switches to Channel 5, a secondary frequency, and pages Mario Piumelli, the field supervisor on duty tonight. "408," he says. (BLS units begin with 100, 200 for ALS designations, 300 for the rescue specialists, 400 for supervisors, and 500 for managers.) A minute goes by—an eternity in EMS time. "C'mon Mar," he mumbles before getting back to Goodstein: "I'm waiting for him to get on the radio."

Another minute passes. Piumelli returns the call from the field, and the telemetry EMD patches him through. "That fire in Edgewater," Piumelli says, "you know anything about it?"

"They may need the MCRU," Tryon reports. "I got Frank Goodstein on the other line inquiring."

"Yeah, we're OK with that."

"Thank you very much," Tryon says, promising to keep Piumelli informed. All the while, he types.

Tryon creates a report to track the event, readies his paging system, and alerts SOG that they might need to mobilize the MCRU. (Earlier this year, the department helped direct rescue operations at Seton Hall University's dormitory fire in the neighboring town of South Orange. In the wee hours, some students perished, others sustained life-threatening burns, and several students jumped from the windows to avoid the flames. Approximately six hundred spilled onto the snowy campus, quickly overwhelming the small volunteer squad that serves the town. The year before, a plane crashed into one of Newark's residential neighborhoods. A candle factory went up in flames. For these and other calamities, the department activates SOG.)

Tryon also briefs department higher-ups, hospital officials, elected representatives, and other VIPs.

He's about to get back to Goodstein when one of his bosses calls to inquire about the fire. Tryon updates him. Then another field supervisor phones. He, too, wants to know about the fire, because in addition to his EMS duties at University he helps run a volunteer squad that has been summoned to help out. Tryon fills him in as well. Then Resetar checks in. The conversation is more of the same, except that Resetar adds that the apartment complex is located next to a gasoline refinery. He authorizes Tryon to summon another dispatcher if necessary.

An overly eager EMT calls. He doesn't have any relevant training, but he offers to help man the phones. Tryon, an aging hippie with an uncommonly relaxed demeanor, just laughs. "It's always the same cast of characters," he muses, "the ones who don't know any better than to call the chief while a crisis is under way. They'll start calling now and want me to pull them off their trucks so they can go to the 'Big One.'"

Sure enough, another EMT calls from the road. "If they happen to need anyone to go to that Edgewater thing," the EMT offers, "being that I'm a Bergen County resident and very familiar with the Bergen County area, my partner and I would be very willing to go over there, if needed, sir."

"Understood," Tryon replies, rolling his eyes.

"Just keep that in mind, OK?"

"OK."

"That's *my* area," the EMT says proprietarily.

"I really don't think anything's going to come of this, but you know me," Tryon laughs, downplaying the commotion. "I have to follow procedures."

"And *you* know *me*," the EMT says, still trying to wedge his way into the action. "I'm here to help people. Whether it's Essex County, Bergen County. If they need my help I'm willing to help."

"You're an inspiration."

"You *know* me."

"OK, buddy," Tryon says. His warm, easygoing style means that most everyone earns an endearment: "buddy," "bro," or "pal."

Piumelli calls back wanting the latest. If news had occurred, Tryon would have sent out a bulletin. But Tryon tells his old friend what he's learned. Piumelli wants to know what frequency the state officials are broadcasting on to see if he can pick up their transmissions.

"I got the statewide band up here, and I'm not hearing anything," Tryon reports.

Next, Piumelli asks if the "whoopee pager," the alert system for volunteer EMTs, is going crazy. Tryon taps into it. "The whoopee pager is going nuts," he reports, reading Edgewater's call to arms: "Clifton, Edgewater. General alarm. River Road between Russell and Underhill are burning or exposed to fire. Fire has extended to brush and numerous cars are burning." Tryon also discovers a slew of other crises unraveling throughout the state. Tonight EMS volunteers are spread far and wide.

Goodstein calls Tryon back. "Hey. It looks like the fire is burning itself out."

"Uh-huh," Tryon grunts, clacking away at his keyboard, freshening the report.

"Most of the firemen are refusing medical assistance. They made a quickie evaluation and don't think they're gonna need the MCRU at this time. But they'll make a final decision as soon as they can. But definitely within fifteen minutes so we don't keep anybody on hold, OK?"

"All right, good enough," Tryon says. "We're here all night, man. You know the deal."

"All right, thanks a lot."

A BLS worker calls in on Channel 5 so that his colleagues won't hear him admit that he left the ambulance unlocked while assessing his patient and someone stole the equipment he now needs. He asks Tryon to have a supervisor bring a replacement to the patient's house.

A private ambulance company, which subcontracts nonemergency patient transportation from University Hospital, calls with a request. They have a 500-pound patient whom they need to move, but they don't have a stretcher strong enough to take the weight. They want to borrow a Stokes basket, a reinforced plastic container, from Rescue. By aiding a number of morbidly obese patients in Newark, Rescue has developed an expertise in safely extracting them from and returning them to their homes, be it through the rapid construction of ramps and rope riggings, the removal and reattachment of doors and windows, or even more exotic techniques.

Tryon relays the request to Piumelli, but Piumelli won't authorize the loan. The subcontractors are not trained to use the equipment, and if they drop the ball, or the patient, the hospital will be liable. He refers Tryon to EMS management, which always leaves an administrator on call. Tryon informs the subcontractor but holds him off while he consults the schedule and pages the EMS manager on call.

When the manager responds, Tryon rehashes the request. It could be straightforward, but it's not. The manager wants to help the subcontractor, but not at Rescue's expense. "First, it's Rescue's equipment. What if they need it?" the manager asks. He worries about what might happen if Rescue gets pressed into service while their equipment is in someone else's hands. "Second, there is the liability issue." Third, he assumes the subcontractor is going to need hand-holding, if not more. "What if they pull up with Ken-and-Barbie EMT who collectively weigh 110 pounds?"

"Yeah, well my goal with these things is to make sure the folks getting paid to do this job have enough people to do it without our guys busting their chops. And if our guys are there in an advisory capacity—I kind of sound like it's Vietnam or something." Tryon laughs at his own melodrama. "You know, then they can be in an advisory capacity. In other words, the bottom line is, from my point of view, they're getting paid to provide a service. They're not going to have us provide half of that service and our guys just get a thank-you and they get a fat check, you know?"

"Yeah," the manager chortles. The department's Rescue service is a one-of-a-kind asset, and although it has gotten the community out of tens of thousands of jams since it was created, in the early 1980s, no one has yet figured out how to pay for it.

Tryon waits patiently, letting his boss du jour think through the decision. When silence follows, he gently encourages him. "So, when I talk to the sub-contractor, I'm going to tell them make sure they have enough people there."

"And tell them we want to work with them," the manager adds.

"Oh, absolutely," Tryon assures him.

"We're warm and fuzzy and all that stuff."

"Uh-huh."

"And, regardless, we should make some kind of documentation of what they're doing even if it's just loaning the equipment out and we're standing by."

"We're fine," Tryon says, subtly trying to wrap it up. Then he reports on the fire's status, which is starting to look like a nonissue.

"You know the right thing to do," the manager tells Tryon. "You're not doing anything different now than you were when you called me."

"Exactly," Tryon chuckles.

"That's usually the way it is ninety-eight percent of the time," the manager laughs.

Tryon hangs up and dials the subcontractor. "Here's what we are able to do," he explains, "and here's what we are not able to do. I can't outright loan you equipment; it's a liability thing. But, if you guys want, I could have our Rescue meet you at the house, put the guy from your stretcher onto the Stokes, get him into the house, and then they'll take off."

"Oh, OK."

"All right. Bottom line is because of the payment, nonpayment, nonemergency versus emergency and all that, if I've got to pull our guys, I've got to pull them, and you'll just have to live with it until they can get back to you."

"OK."

"And, secondly, you got enough people that you can handle this without our men?"

"Yeah, I got about six people going."

"All right, good."

They agree to touch base when the patient is ready. Ten minutes later, the subcontractor calls back.

"REMCS, Chief Tryon, good evening."

"Hi, this is us again," the subcontractor says. "My crew's going to be able to do it after all."

"OK. Glad you could, brother. Thanks very much."

Then, Tryon phones Piumelli. "Hey, the subcontractor just called. They don't need us after all. So, you need not concern yourself about any liabilities or anything."

"All right," Piumelli says. "Thanks."

"If Rescue is wondering why I told them to call me, tell them don't bother."

Piumelli agrees and signs off moments before a fresh crisis erupts.

University's ER requests a two-hour BLS bypass, meaning that EMTs should transport noncritical patients to other hospitals. *They must be getting swamped*, Tryon imagines as he sends an alert to everyone. Soon a problem flies up from the truck to the telemetry EMD and then to his desk. Paramedic Tracey Ann Fazio is en route with a cardiac patient whose internal defibrillator keeps shocking him. She wants to bring the patient to University and muster the cardiac response team, a group of heart specialists. But the charge nurse warns her not to come, claiming the whole ER is on bypass.

The telemetry EMD tries informing the charge nurse that the bypass only pertains to BLS patients, but he is having none of it. Rather than argue, the EMD refers it to Tryon. He pages Dr. Gluckman, and the two talk the situation through. Within seconds, they agree to admit the patient to University. But five minutes later, another problem threatens the chain of survival that links this patient's prehospital and hospital-based care. Tryon discovers that the cardiac response team pager has malfunctioned. Unless he can correct it, he can't notify the specialists to meet the patient in the ER. That takes a few mechanical diagnostics and another round of phone calls to solve. Ultimately, he clears the board of crises and asks, under his breath, "Where's the Valium?"

The laid-back, self-deprecating joker with hippie-length hair really does need some kind of stress relief. Although he has a cardiac catheterization scheduled shortly, the forty-seven-year-old goes outside for a smoke. He takes deep drags, drawing the tar and nicotine way back into his lungs.

4   *THE COAST IS CLEAR*

It's not a good day at work until you are at home.

—University Hospital paramedic Chuck Coles

*B*ecause the job is inherently dangerous, EMS curricula warn workers about on-the-job hazards, from blundering into scenes with patients felled by invisible, odorless, and sometimes lethal chemicals to encountering downed power lines—still live and capable of frying them in seconds. Careless drivers follow emergency vehicles' strobe lights like a beacon only to mow down roadside rescuers. In spite of the advisories, EMS workers die every year.[1]

Although crime is down, the city is still a dangerous place. According to the Uniform Crime Report, in 1999 Newark suffered 70 murders, 114 rapes, 2,497 robberies, 2,303 aggravated assaults, 3,117 burglaries, 8,984 thefts, and 5,365 auto thefts.[2] Blue-shirts here have been stabbed, bitten, attacked with two-by-fours and chairs, spit at, cursed at, and hit with fists and hurled objects. Once a bullet sailed right through an ambulance windshield with the crew inside.

People who attack EMS workers in the line of duty in New Jersey earn enhanced charges under the law. At the time of sentencing, judges consider mitigating factors and aggravating circumstances, and assaults on rescuers are incendiary. If a prosecutor argues a case in which a blue-shirt was murdered on the job, attacks on a rescuer may be a factor in seeking the death penalty. Such protection offers the blue-shirts some comfort, but that is only if police catch the assailant and only if the EMS workers want to press charges, which, though they were hurt on duty, they must do on their own time.

Some EMS workers here wear bulletproof vests and others do not; they are not standard issue and cost hundreds of dollars. Anyone who wants a vest must buy it with his or her own funds. "My wife bought me this," one blue-shirt says proudly. He wears it every day. Walter Drivet, who has worked urban EMS for two decades, used to wear one, but he says it was heavy and it made him hot: "I'd be nauseous by the time I climbed my fifth flight." Another figures, "The vests give a false sense of security. If you didn't have it, you might not put yourself in situations. You're either gonna catch a bullet or you're not. Besides, it does nothing for your head, and some of my most valuable real estate is below my waist."

The department teaches EMS workers to avoid or remove themselves from dangerous settings and summon help from Dispatch, which will alert superiors, and police and firefighting colleagues. If a paramedic spies firearms in a patient's residence, for example, he may tap his partner on the shoulder, call him or her by a false name, and ask if they have a particular piece of equipment. Fashioning an excuse for them to go back to the truck allows them to alert Dispatch and request police assistance. Avoiding conflict is paramount—theoretically—but evasion is not always possible. EMS workers value their law-enforcement colleagues, but experience has taught the team that police are often otherwise engaged and sometimes unwilling to take the responsibility.

Confronted by dynamic threats, the action-oriented problem-solvers find it hard to stand by idly. More often than not, they follow their calling and intervene. That can mean spotting a conflagration, alerting firefighters, running into a burning building, and waking and escorting out seven people on three floors (and their pets) before a fire truck ever arrives, as paramedic Henry Cortacans did.

EMS workers learn what works from veterans they respect; ever resourceful, they invent tactics on the fly, and each brings life experience to the task, which colors perceptions and confidence levels. Callahan and Cardona have had the odd advantage of having grown up around crime, poverty, and myriad social ills. Life has taught them to take suffering in stride. They choose to meet challenges head-on, and proactively involve themselves in the community to make their faces known. Drivet uses skill and humor to negotiate his journey. O'Neill has trained so extensively with law enforcement at local, state, and federal levels that he might as well be a soldier. Fazio cracks wise with her teammates but rarely stints on sharing the milk of human kindness. Others try and out-tough the toughest people on-scene. Like paramedic Vincent Francis Cisternino, most seek to achieve a balance of toughness and tenderness.

IT'S A BEAUTIFUL DAY IN THE NEIGHBORHOOD

At 1900 hours, Callahan is already behind the wheel when Cardona hoists himself into the bus. The sun, a ripe orange hanging low in the sky, vibrates and showers the city with oppressive summer heat. Baked tar sends hot air shimmering upward. Caught in the middle, the men feel like a roast-meat sand-wich. But Cardona is fairly quivering with excitement. "Look what my boy made," he boasts, handing Callahan a piece of paper festooned with crayoned stick figures, balloons, and the words *Happy Father's Day*. "When I picked him up from school, he ran into the car waving it and shouting 'Here! Here! Here!'" Beaming, he says, "I'm going to hang this inside my locker so I see it every day!"

Callahan smiles as he holds the drawing. "My son called me for Father's Day, too," he volunteers. Shaking his head sadly, he reports, "He said, 'Dad, I hope you don't have a headache on Father's Day.' Man, I miss my boy." When Callahan and his wife celebrated the birth of their son, after a fifteen-year effort to conceive, they uprooted themselves and moved to Maryland, where their boy could enjoy a bucolic lifestyle and attend private school. So Callahan commutes to the job, at least three hours each way, and bunks with relatives between his shifts.

Besides the heartache, Callahan has had dull, thudding pain in his head for days. His frequent headaches are inevitable. No matter how strenuous a shift, Callahan can't just drift off to sleep. He's had six hours' rest in the past three days; between last night and tonight he has slept only ninety minutes. Perpetual sleep deprivation hurts. Tonight he woke up behind schedule. He hasn't eaten yet. Cardona has the hots for a cooling lemon ice. Dreaming of refreshment, the two go instead to a succession of emergencies and stumble onto the first of two domestic-violence calls.

First, they meet a petite and angry woman who concedes that her nose is probably broken. Her boyfriend rained down blow after blow, she says. She is injured and aggravated, but her condition is not life-threatening. A slave to the paperwork that eats up several hours per shift, when Cardona knows a patient is stable, he tends to keep the bus on-scene an extra minute or two to organize his thoughts and work his way through the chart. A self-confessed "neat freak," his handwriting surpasses even the precision print of engineers and architects. But this, too, comes at a price. "If I have to cross something out, I'll just start a new sheet," he explains. Meanwhile, his patients lie on the stretcher and wait.

This woman, however, won't lie down or sit down. Restless, she studies her misshapen reflection in the ambulance's smoke-colored supply cabinets as Cardona interviews her. She is irritated that the police have not arrived. The crew's pace is too sluggish for her taste. So she tugs up a pair of jeans she just happens to have on hand over her tight turquoise shorts and grumbles, "Forget all that! I'm outta here." She lets herself out of the ambulance and waves off Callahan's attempt to tell her that the police will either meet them on the way or speak to her at the hospital. With fury in her eyes, she explodes, "*This man, he's going to kill me!* And he's got a warrant. And he's on probation. If a nigger says he's gonna kill you, he's gonna motherfuckin' do it." As she slams the ambulance door in Callahan's startled face, she vows, "He's not going to take me away from my three kids. I'm gonna kill that motherfucker first!"

As she stalks off, he tries telling her that the city's housing police have a trailer right across the courtyard, but she disappears into the darkness.

Well after midnight, the two pull up to a deserted section of the West Ward where a young, thick-waisted woman in a glossy tangerine wig waits for them under a street lamp. Her lower jaw, clearly deformed, thrusts left. Sighing, she accepts help, clambering into the bus.

"What's bothering you tonight, ma'am?" Cardona asks.

"My boyfrien' hid me," the twenty-two-year-old mumbles through a stiff, unmoving mouth. Incongruously, her perfect white teeth gleam unblemished.

"Did he knock you out?"

"Nah. But he bid me on my chest."

"Did he break the skin?"

Lifting her striped T-shirt, she shows him two enormous breasts that jiggle in her bra cups like pudding. One wears an angry purple bite mark. "I had him in a headlock," she explains.

"So that's when he bit you?"

"Uh-huh." She sits on the gray vinyl bench, her jeans partly unzipped, homage to a current fashion statement. Her belly flesh, laced with stretch marks, spills over the waistband.

As Callahan takes her blood pressure, Cardona asks about her last period. It's not a routine question per se, but he tries to let the ER know which patients are pregnant or might be.

"I'm five months pregnan'," she mouths.

At 158/90, the woman's blood pressure is a bit elevated. Callahan asks about prenatal care when the hushed, almost intimate environment inside the ambulance is interrupted. Someone pounds on the bus's back window so hard it rattles. Everything and everyone trembles.

"Open this door motherfucker!" a man's irate voice demands.

"Do you know this guy?" Callahan asks.

"No."

"Are you sure you don't know him?" The streets are dark and empty. Police are nowhere to be found. Callahan has to size up the risk this man poses.

"Tha's him," she sighs, thickly. "My boyfrien'."

"That's the mother of my motherfuckin' baby!" the man roars. "Let me in."

Callahan knows not to let abusers near his patients. But he takes pains to avoid getting tough. He asks the woman, "Does he carry a weapon?"

"No."

Callahan feels a rapport with his patient and decides to take her word. "All right, I'll talk to him." Turning patient care over to Cardona, who has been writing the chart, he steps outside the bus. The air is a sponge soaked with humidity. Streetlights are sparse on this block. The buildings blend in a dull montage of burnished browns. Callahan senses that the man is drunk, and possibly stoned as well. Rather than confront or chastise the angry male, Callahan tries to defuse him. With his tall, 250-pound frame, hoop earring, and street smarts, Callahan is an imposing presence. But, surprisingly, his deep voice is warm and gentle. And that helps calm the man, too. One can't hear even the muffled sound of voices outside the ambulance.

"For your own sake, bro," Callahan advises, "you better take off, because the police are coming."

"But she's getting high, smoking all kinds of shit, with my baby in her," he protests.

"I do understand you're upset, man, but you just can't justify hitting a woman," Callahan says. "Let us take her to the hospital and get her checked out, and you can both use the time to cool off."

The man wants to accompany them. "My man, they're going to lock you up if you come to the hospital," Callahan says, shaking his head no. "You can count on getting arrested."

The man seems to appreciate the advice and slaps Callahan's hand before taking off. Callahan steps into the driver's seat and points the bus to University.

Inside the bus, the woman tells Cardona she is tired of the violence. To save herself she has had to "cut him up" in the past. But she hesitates to leave, she says, "because it will cause a lot of trauma to the families."

When the EMTs arrive at the hospital, they try to transfer care. A nurse delays them, unsure which pregnant patients should be admitted to the ER and which she should direct to Labor and Delivery. A doctor pauses to examine the woman, and Cardona reports, "Her boyfriend bit her tit." He has barely gotten the sentence out when shouts and scuffles erupt in the hall.

The woman's boyfriend chose to come to the hospital despite Callahan's recommendation. Tall, wiry, and clothed in jeans, which he snaps and belts below his buttocks in exaggerated jailhouse fashion, he tries forcing his way in, but hospital police march him outside. Minutes later, Newark police officers lean him face-first against a concrete wall, cuff him, search his pockets, and take him into custody.

"I told him if he came to the ER the police would get him," Callahan says, distressed. He really tries to help most everyone, and it hurts him to see people who find no alternative to drowning in self-made misery.

A graduate of the city's Prince Street housing project, Callahan says he grew up around violence, and it simply doesn't faze him. "On my way to school, I used to step over bodies in the hallway," he recalls with a shrug and a such-is-life view of reality. "In fifth grade, I saw someone beaten to death."

He might have become a thug himself and admits that as a youngster he "wasn't too nice" when he "got with the fellas." In junior high, he set up a makeshift tollbooth and charged other kids ten cents to get to class.

Fortunately, he says, he had the opportunity to get out of Newark on occasion. During summers, he visited his grandmother's farm in Virginia. After high school, he joined the Army Reserve, moved to Colorado, and saw people of color succeed as he had never imagined. And then he met "a girl from the suburbs" who, Callahan says, changed him for the better with her consistent love, affection, and kindness. He married her.

Callahan sees most every patient as an opportunity to heal the city's wounds. He believes his EMS work makes a difference, and he revels in the good feeling it generates. It's no surprise, then, that he has few safety concerns. But at age forty-two, sometimes he wonders how much longer he can do the work and provide for his family on $370 a week.[3]

Money is always an issue. So Callahan and Cardona prefer to eat cheap. "A lot of guys say there's no place to eat," Callahan reports. And some EMS workers who swear they can't get a fast, clean meal in Newark will visit eateries in nearby towns. *Well, maybe there's no place they wanna eat,* Callahan thinks. *But there are plenty of places for me to eat.* He and Cardona find nourishment inside city limits.

Tonight the partners agree on hot, made-to-order steak sandwiches with grilled onions and melted cheese. Lucy's Mini Market on the corner of Eighteenth Street and Eighteenth Avenue is the best place for that, they say. Some dub the area "Dodge City" owing to the prolific shootings. Callahan admits it's a rough area: "A lotta guys would say, 'You got what? Where?' But a steak is a steak." And he swears by the popular bodega. Here they can fill their bellies deliciously for an economical $2.50.

Besides eating well for less, the two enjoy eating locally for its opportunities to polish the hospital's image. As they strut toward the storefront, grinning, boys rush up to them, hands raised in search of high fives. More heavily muscled youths glance up, nod, and step aside respectfully to let them through.

Inside Lucy's, a wide product assortment fills the shelves, from Happy Boy margarine to deck mops and cigarettes. The meat counter is in the back. Smoked neck bones, pigs' feet, ribs, an astonishing assortment of hot dogs and sausages, ham hocks, beef bacon, smoked turkey wings, and more squat in glass cases, issuing heady aromas. The proprietress chats with them as she cooks their steaks on the griddle. She seasons Cardona's with a medley of Spanish spices. When they pay, the cashier greets them warmly from his bulletproof booth.

Later, in a rare moment of free time, they park their bus, buy some smokes, and hang out on South Tenth Street. The two enjoy "going into the community and getting to know people." Their proactive strategy harks back to the days when Callahan brought his bus to block parties, let people explore it, and gave free blood-pressure checks. EMS workers used to hand out lollipops, one says, make a point of patronizing local vendors, and otherwise be outwardly friendly and accessible. Callahan and Cardona are two who still make the effort. Sometimes, between calls, Callahan will visit young shooting victims. Just "hanging" is a way to see and be seen, making EMS a little more familiar, a little more approachable. Leaning against a brick wall, smoking in the summer night, they smile and wave at most passersby.

The two are popular. Females especially flock to Cardona, a dark-haired Ricky Martin look-alike. A fourteen-year-old approaches and shyly asks if he remembers taking care of her. He does, and the girl is pleased. Then, rather less shyly, she asks for his phone number. "I'm married!" Cardona laughs. She shrugs. "I'm old enough to be your father!" he protests.

"I like older men," she persists.

Eventually, Cardona charms her on her way, and the partners chuckle over his many admirers.

Another night, the two still pine for cool, citrus Italian ices from Rita's and are heading toward their goal when they see a Toyota Corolla weaving down Lyons Avenue. A child's plastic swimming pool slips off the car's roof, where it had clung by a poorly tied piece of string. As the pool rolls into the middle of the busy roadway, the Toyota shrieks to a halt in front of a White Castle hamburger restaurant and a boarded-up brick warehouse. A woman opens the driver's door, shields her eyes from the sun, and squints into the glare to see what has become of her children's new toy.

Callahan and Cardona look at each other. Then Callahan flips on the light bar and carefully parks the bus so as shunt the traffic away. Cardona dives into the roadway, grabs the pool, and dashes back to the curb.

Inside the car, two children are strapped into car seats. A girl clutches a white teddy bear and stares wide-eyed at the EMTs. The youngest, an infant, sucks on a pacifier and breathes oxygen through a nasal cannula, a double-pronged, green plastic tube. A fuzz-covered plastic Dalmatian bobs its head in the rear window.

Ever resourceful, the EMTs fashion a brace for the pool on top of the car with bungee cord and gauze. It won't endure hurricane-force winds, but it's secure enough to get the woman home without further mishap.

Cardona and Callahan do more than extend common courtesy during jobs. Between calls and on their own time, they regularly make efforts to help people, which gives them enhanced standing in the community. Callahan even has a rapport with the drug dealers and thugs, whom he has passed on street corners and in hallways countless times. To those who think that puts him in a questionable light, Callahan shrugs and points to the many cops and state police who are his friends also.

The dealers are a fact of life; they do brisk business in Newark. Callahan is a realist who has learned how to survive in the most ruthless sections of town and go about his job unmolested. "I'm like the Switzerland of Newark," he explains. "I try to stay neutral." But that doesn't mean he is sympathetic to dealers. Drugs claimed his brother's life. He strives to shelter his son. He counsels his patients against using drugs. For the sake of his patients and his own safety, he has learned to coexist.

Years ago, he noticed an eleven-year-old boy from the neighborhood had begun selling drugs. Callahan, who hadn't had any luck yet becoming a father, made a point of befriending him. Frequently he would pull his bus over to chat casually with the boy and try pointing him in a more constructive direction. "He told me he was going to North Carolina," Callahan remembers. But one day Callahan found him shot, the result of a soured drug transaction. He rushed him to the hospital but was so broken up by the event that his supervisor told him to go home. Instead he waited outside the operating room with the boy's family. When the boy died, a piece of Callahan did, too.

When Dispatch later sends them to care for a "thirty-five-year-old male, sick," they calmly drive to a run-down brick building in the South Word and march, unafraid, several flights up a narrow staircase. The pungent stench of cat urine greets them before the animals appear themselves, patrolling en masse on a sixth-floor landing.

Straddling an apartment doorjamb a weathered black woman stands, arms folded across her chest, waiting. When she sees the EMTs, she waves them in.

They literally have to twist, squeeze, and almost hold their breath to get inside the tiny space. The front room is nearly wall-to-wall mattresses. Two large beds are shoved together. Several bodies huddle on mismatched sheets under blankets despite the June night's heat. Children sleep head to foot in the beds, packed like sardines. The patient, a twig-thin black man in a stained checkered shirt, lies on the edge under a scarlet cover.

Callahan sidles up the foot-wide alley of stained, tobacco-colored carpet between the bed and the only other furniture in the room, a bureau. The frame of its mirror is crammed with photographs. He smiles before beginning to measure the man's vital signs. Cardona, keeper of the charts, takes up residence in the doorway. He can't see ahead into the next room, which is utterly dark. *In case anyone comes flying out of there, I gotta make sure we get out of here*, he thinks. Keeping the exit accessible, he begins the interview.

"What's wrong?" Cardona asks.

"His kidney," the older woman, the patient's cousin, answers. "He's supposed to go on dialysis. He's suffering."

"My head's hurting because I ain't got no pills," the man croaks from his bed. He has lost several teeth and his gums shine an obscene pink. Drool cakes in his wispy beard. "It's just, my head hurts."

"Did they give you something at the hospital?" Cardona asks, noting that the man wears three hospital identification bracelets on his wrists.

"Once they gave me some pills," the man says, scratching at a hairy birthmark. "Last time I didn't get anything."

"What other medical problems do you have?"

"None," the man answers. His sallow skin clings loosely to his bony, birdlike face. His fuzzy hair is one giant six-inch cowlick.

"How much do you weigh?"

"One twenty-eight."

Callahan's blood pressure cuff reads 180/140. The dim room is lit only by a one-bulb lamp. He doesn't trust the finding and wants to try again. "Sit up, my man, I got to get a better reading."

Light from the hallway is thin. Cardona pulls a black flashlight out of his equipment belt for Callahan, who wears a tool belt, too, albeit empty. Cardona, always prepared, takes pride in his arsenal of equipment, even decorating it with discreet Puerto Rican flag stickers. His cell phone and protective helmet are similarly festooned.

With a flashlight pointed on the gauge, Callahan reads 200/140. "Bro, if your BP is what I just took, you need to go to the hospital, now," he tells the man. Still incredulous, he suggests, "Let's do it on the other arm. Don't talk for just one minute. Lie still."

As he reapplies the blood-pressure cuff, a small young woman pushes her way into the apartment, her arms full of packages. "He's not going anywhere," she states, defiantly.

As she struts into the darkness of the other room, her chin in the air, Callahan asks the older woman, "Who's that?"

"That's his lady."

Cardona is unsettled by the newcomer's attitude and considers what and who might be inside the hollow. *Is there a threat?* he wonders.

The young woman reappears and stamps her foot. She looks directly at Cardona and announces, "He's not going."

"Yes he is," the older woman says. "He's not going to lay here and die."

"He don't want to go," the young woman replies. The two women square off. The girlfriend stares so intently at the sick man that he lies back down in his bed.

This time Callahan's blood-pressure reading is 210/110. The man's pulse is humming along at 92 beats per minute. Callahan sets up the oxygen tank and tells the man, "You're messing around with a stroke." As he positions the oxygen mask over the man's face, he cautions him again, "You don't want to bust a vein in your head."

Cardona knows that the paramedics can use medicine to lower the man's pressure, so he radios for assistance. And, sensing that the woman is going to cause a problem, he requests a supervisor, too. Pugnacious, she stands at the foot of the bed, arms crossed in front of her chest, shaking her head no and taking occasional drags of her cigarette.

"Listen, do me a favor," Cardona asks the woman. "Before we all blow up—put that cigarette out." She glares at him, perhaps unaware that oxygen speeds combustion. But she steps into the hallway to grind it out with her foot. Cardona uses this as a reason to keep her from escalating the argument. He follows her out as if he wants to talk privately. She tells Cardona, "I've got five kids that's on him." Her voice is loud and grating. Apartment doors in the building open and people collect in the stairwells. Other EMS workers would have the patient in the bus by now, but Cardona still feels the situation is under control.

Meanwhile, Callahan continues persuading the patient to go to the hospital. Unless the man is unconscious or otherwise incapable of making a competent decision about his health, Callahan can't force him. Glancing at the lumps under the covers, he asks, "This is your family?"

The man nods.

"Do it for them. You gotta understand something. You're only in your mid-thirties. They don't want to put you on a whole bunch of medicines for the rest of your life, because you are a young man. They want to get you well."

"Every time I go to the hospital I have to wait," the patient complains. "They told me to wait for a doctor. I waited six hours."

"You are going straight to the back, man," Callahan assures him. *The back* is the actual treatment area. Going *straight to the back* does not mean no waiting, but it does mean less waiting than those stranded in the front, that is, the purgatory known as triage, where less urgently sick people check in and wait their turn.

The man's girlfriend snatches jeans and sneakers from a pile of clothes and shoves them at the patient. Callahan helps him dress. "Partner, you won't regret this."

"Thanks, lady, for everything," Callahan whispers to the man's worn cousin.

The man tries to stand up but Callahan tells him, "Just sit there. We're not going to let you walk." He sets up the collapsible stair chair near the end of the bed, and the half-dozen people who have collected outside the apartment step back to make room.

As Cardona and Callahan carry him out, they see that the other room is also full of unmoving bodies crammed together on the floor.

Having arrived at the building entrance, Visoskas hears them on the way down and begins clearing away milk crates, cushions, tires, and other miscellany cluttering the vestibule so they can pass.

The man's pressure rises to 212/160, then 220/160. The man denies using drugs. *Bullshit*, Cardona thinks. No angel himself, Cardona admits that as an adolescent he "smoked a little bush" and experimented with "a little bit of this and a little bit of that." And he is by no means the only one on the team. Most are refreshingly candid about their youthful use of alcohol and recreational drugs. Having done it, having grown up around it, the EMS workers are not easily fooled. Experience coupled with exceptional interviewing skills can persuade even the most clandestine users to fess up. Minutes later, the man concedes that he smoked cocaine, although he swears it was days ago. After transferring care to the ER staff, Cardona whispers to Callahan, "Shit. The old fucking lady that was talking to us—it's fucking nighttime and her pupils were like darts. Everybody in the house was high. I think it's a smoke den."

MIDGETS AND MONSTERS

Cardona and Callahan drive toward a brick tenement in the North Ward for an EDP (emotionally disturbed person). "There he is," Callahan says, spotting a youth huddled against the autumn chill in a hooded Bulls sweatshirt, a leather jacket, and voluminously baggy jeans. Other people are on the corner, but Callahan senses that this is the patient. As he slows the bus, he and Cardona watch the young man pace, stepping in and out of the building doorway, his eyes flashing furtively. "That's gotta be him, you see his eyes, man?" Callahan asks. *He's got that EDP glare: he just looks right through things*, he thinks. *He's just asking for help.*

Cardona nods. They park and both climb out.

"What's up?" Cardona asks a pale, auburn-haired woman who starts toward the bus, clutching herself for warmth.

"My brother," she says, nodding her head at the young man, "he's got some problems. If he stays out here, he's gonna get killed or someone's gonna kill him." Then she whispers conspiratorially, "He wants to hurt me and my son." At her side, a boy about ten years of age nods; his eyes bulge with fear.

On cue, the patient panics and yells at Cardona, "They're after me!"

The woman shrugs her shoulders, shakes her head no, and rolls her eyes upward. As far as she is concerned, it's all in her brother's head.

"Well, how about if we take you somewhere where they can't hurt you, man?" Cardona asks politely. He stands a few feet away from the patient, at an angle, which is less of a threat.

The patient wants to believe Cardona will protect him. He nods and walks toward the bus with Cardona on one side and Callahan on the other.

Climbing up on the runner, the patient sticks his head in first to check it out. He's dazzled. "Wow," he exclaims enthusiastically. "It's like a room in here!" He takes a seat on the bench and swivels about, scouting the cabinets, overhead lights, stretcher, and various dials and switches for oxygen, suction, and temperature control. "You got your own little room here."

His chiseled face has fine sculpted features, an ivory complexion, and a downy mocha mustache. Only a missing front tooth, a few angry-looking pimples, and the mad look in his dark eyes mar his striking good looks.

"Let me fasten this belt around you, man," Callahan says, moving toward the patient and reaching for the safety belt. The patient eyes him suspiciously, but Callahan just keeps talking softly. "Yeah, so you don't go flying if I hit a pothole or something." Casually unwrapping his blood-pressure cuff, he asks, "Can you take that jacket off, bro, so I can get a pressure?"

The patient shrugs off his thick leather jacket and bundles it next to him, within arm's reach. "Is it gonna hurt?"

"No, man. It's like a balloon in here. I squeeze this pump and it gets a little tight on your arm, but it won't hurt." Callahan shows him the cuff. "Nothing to worry about."

The patient acquiesces. His sister has been sticking her head in the ambulance the whole time. Now she asks, "Can you take my pressure, too? I had cancer."

Not infrequently, family members and bystanders will horn in on a situation and try to obtain care for themselves. Callahan figures an extra minute on-scene will give Cardona time to shore up his bond with the patient, so he obliges.

"This your address?" Cardona asks the patient.

"No, this is my house," the patient's sister interjects. "He visits me sometimes."

"Where you live?" Cardona asks the patient again.

The man tilts his head slightly and screws up his face in confusion.

"You staying on the streets?"

"Nah. I got friends," he says. "I been up in Annandale for four years," he volunteers. Annandale is home to a state youth correctional facility.

"What for?" Cardona asks. Each month, police arrest more than forty Newark juveniles for violent crime and about 230 others for lesser offenses.[4]

"Drugs," the patient replies, unabashedly. Shifting restlessly in his seat, he confesses anxiously, "They're coming for me!" It's unclear whether he's actually hallucinating or misinterpreting the reflections in the bus's back window. Either way, his agitation soars. "They're coming for me! *Get the fuck away!*"

"You do any drugs today, bro?"

"Two bags of heroin," he says with a shrug. Then he looks sharply over his left shoulder and tosses his head at a hallucination. "*They* told me to do the drugs. If I did, they said, they would leave me alone. But they haven't. They're liars. *You're liars!*" he screams at the air.

This kid obviously has a psych history, Cardona thinks, *but the drugs don't help; they aggravate the situation.* "You take any medication?"

"Yeah, but I don't have any."

"What do you take, Haldol?"

"Nah, I hate that. It makes me sick."

"What do you mean?"

"It makes my jaw like, all stuck," he says, distorting his face and sticking his tongue outside his lips. An antipsychotic, Haldol can cause an extra pyramidal reaction, prolonged muscle contractions, which can leave patients with twisted, abnormal appearances.

"When's the last time you had your medication?"

"I don't know, man," he answers. "Two days? They gave me a thousand milligrams of Thorazine at Greystone. I don't have to go there now, do I?" Greystone Psychiatric Park is a state-run psychiatric hospital that houses some criminally insane patients. "I don't want that again."

"Oh, they're having a party," he informs Cardona, snorting contemptuously at the hallucination. *"You think it's funny that I'm going to the hospital?!"* he screams at the delusion. Then he delves into a pocket of his jacket on the bench and extracts a heavy-duty pair of wire-cutters. He brandishes the twelve-inch makeshift weapon at his imaginary nemesis. "There's this little guy here; he's two feet tall!"

"Yeah man, I believe you," Cardona says. "Do me a favor though, will you?"

The patient looks at him searchingly.

"Put those wire-cutters back in your jacket. You won't need them here," Cardona assures him. "I won't let anyone hurt you."

The patient sizes up Cardona and sees a clean-cut, soft-voiced, muscular professional looking him straight in the eye. "I won't need them?" he asks in a childlike voice.

Cardona shakes his head no and adds a genuine smile.

The man slides the wire-cutters into the jacket sleeve and folds his hands in his lap. Cardona jots a note to Callahan and hands it to him through the small opening between the back of the box and the cab. It says, "Notify Dispatch to tell the hospital police that he has a possible weapon." And Callahan does.

For years Cardona did special transports, ferrying the country's most deranged patients to asylums, an experience that still gives him nightmares. And just days ago Cardona watched a 130-pound patient exercise a mammoth tantrum. It took nine correctional officers in full tactical gear to get the self-abusing patient out of a jail cell, and six inside the bus to accompany the man to the hospital. Still, the enraged man thrashed about so violently he ruptured the stretcher. *This guy could go either way*, Cardona thinks.

When Callahan arrives at the hospital, he deliberately parks next to a concrete wall. Outside the bus, a half-dozen armed hospital police are waiting. Callahan climbs inside and Cardona asks the man, "Why don't you let my friend here hold those wire-cutters for you?"

The patient looks carefully at Callahan.

"You won't need them in the hospital," Cardona adds. "It's safe here."

"You wanna hold them?" the patient asks Callahan in a childlike manner.

"Sure." Callahan nods. He smiles sweetly as he takes the cutters. "I'll watch them for you." Then he opens the door and steps out. The patient follows, but as soon as he sees the police, he freezes and grabs the ambulance door, afraid to step down. *"WHOA, whoa, whoa!"* he shouts. "What are *they* doin' here?"

"They're here to protect you, man," Cardona assures him. "No one's gonna hurt you with those guys around."

The patient looks back in the ambulance, then at the concrete wall. His forehead wrinkles with anxiety.

"You don't worry about nothin', man," Cardona says, throwing his arm protectively around the man's shoulders. "You're here with *us*!" And the three walk in to the ER together, the best of friends. Three armed officers precede them. Three follow just feet behind.

They walk through the corridors toward University's psychiatric ER, a separate division, as are its pediatric ER and domestic-violence center. Along the way, the patient stops several times, unsure whether to proceed or to tear and run. Each time, Cardona and Callahan coax him forward with quiet, friendly reassurances. By the time they reach the psychiatric ER, however, the patient is feeling altogether boxed in. Reluctantly, he takes a seat beside a desk, but glares at the staff from under his brow.

Cardona shares information with a clerk who checks to see whether the man has been admitted before. The computer confirms that the patient has been a frequent visitor, and the clerk retrieves his file.

Callahan tries to keep the patient's attention focused. "This here's the man!" he tells him, pointing to a psychiatric resident who is hurriedly flipping through paperwork for clues to the patient's problem. "He's gonna take good care of you."

The patient isn't buying it. "He's the man?" he asks uncertainly. He calms down considerably, however, when a female staff member approaches authoritatively. She recognizes him and engages him in calming conversation.

One of officers recognizes the patient, too. "He always comes here and has no idea he was here before," he says, shaking his head sadly. "He's always seeing these imaginary midgets." No one laughs. None of the security measures are lifted. The man has become explosive in the past, and they have to be alert until he is safely sedated.

"I can't stand seeing that little man," the patient says, rolling his eyes back into his head as he points to the empty air in front of him. "Why he has to be here?"

"How about if I give you some medicine so you won't see him anymore?" the resident offers.

But the patient is still suspicious. "What are you going to give me? They gave me a thousand milligrams of Thorazine up at Greystone."

"Oh, no, nothing like that," the doctor assures him.

Eager to bring the man more under control, the woman asks, "How about if we move you into that room where there won't be so many people and you'll be safe?"

The patient agrees. Inside the room, if he erupts, restraints are waiting. As he enters, the police cluster by the door in case they are needed. Callahan turns over the wire-cutters to one, who tosses them into a biohazard container.

The doctor signs off on their chart and Cardona and Callahan go on to their next call, but not before they give each other a friendly punch on the arm. "Man, that went well!" Cardona says. Callahan agrees wholeheartedly. "It takes a real professional to walk a violent patient in."

Callahan and Cardona take pride in their unsung talent, grateful that their skills and personalities permit them to deescalate most situations. The two rarely manhandle their charges. Some on the team are too fast to throw a punch, they say. But sometimes it seems there is no other way.

ROADWORK

EMS workers in Newark are not astonished to see people on the street all night. Newark's 8.1 percent unemployment rate is more than double the state's average.[5] Drivet and Cisternino are unfazed if not blasé when they turn a corner one night to find a crowd of males playing football in the road by the weak light of a single street lamp. Players spy the ambulance. Unimpressed, they continue the game. Neither team feels inclined to stop the action and let the ambulance pass. Drivet sits patiently until one of the teams scores. "Touchdown!" he cheers through the loudspeaker with genuine enthusiasm. The players freeze and stare at the ambulance. Then they applaud and wave their fists in celebration. And they part so it can pass.

When Cisternino and Fazio are partners and when they're not exhausted from moonlighting, parenting, schoolwork, and their myriad other responsibilities, when they're not engaged in a heady discussion on the theology of ancient cultures, the two can be downright giddy. Sometimes, they take a can of Cheese-Whiz and a box of Triscuits and drive about town handing out appetizers with cheesy smiley faces or a caduceus, the snake and staff that has come to symbolize medicine. Like Callahan and Cardona, they find ways to spread cheer throughout the community. Fazio is driving very late one night when they pull up to Bloomfield Place. Both partners look to see if they can safely make a right turn. The white sedan next to them threatens to overflow with young adults.

"How many people are in that car?" Fazio asks dumbfounded. "Can you see?"

"I can't count," Cisternino chuckles. "It's stuffed." A proud Tau Delta Phi brother, Cisternino loves high jinks and perhaps wishes he could sandwich himself in there, too. Leaning out his window, he grins and shouts, "How many people you got in there?"

"A lot," one young woman laughs. "How about you?"

"We got *lots* of room."

"Well, you should give us a ride home then!"

"Yeah!" Cisternino snorts amicably.

"Hey, we got a guy back here whose leg is broke."

"No wonder!" Fazio chimes in.

When the light changes, a second later, the two vehicles speed off, occupants all agiggle.

LIONS AND TIGERS AND BEARS, OH, MY!

Dispatch is charged with instructing callers to confine family pets, but not all EMDs do and not all patients comply. Dogs are naturally protective of their human companions, but the threats are orders of magnitude more severe when people use their pit bulls and Rottweilers as bodyguards, street-tough fashion accessories, and betting devices.

Callahan and Cardona march into the Prince Street projects unafraid. The buildings, now emptied of seventy percent of the residents, have the abandoned look of empty egg cartons. Window after window is boarded up, and those that aren't are gaping black holes. Inside, the two step around snoring bodies and willingly box themselves into cramped metal elevators, but they can't get to their patient on the thirteenth floor until Callahan throws his weight behind the door to make it close. Contorting themselves to avoid puddles of urine and scum-covered walls besmirched by felt-pen phallus sketches and misspellings such as "FUUCK," Cardona jokes, "Someone should take a culture of this floor."

But a menacing bark behind a patient's front door is enough to make Cardona want to cut and run. "We ain't going in there!" he says, backing away from the door and off to the side. Fortunately for the patient, Callahan does not retreat but barks right back: *"Put that dog away!"* It's not unheard-of in some cities for police to come in and tranquilize threatening pets, but law enforcement has no time for that here.

Except for dogs, Cardona has few worries on the job. Callahan's weakness is rats. Naturally, then, Cardona takes perverse delight in spotting respectably sized rats, which make Callahan shiver. Scaring each other silly is one way to deflate anxiety. Sometimes, though, anxiety has just the sting EMS workers need to stay attentive while they negotiate what one calls "the ragged, jagged edge."

DRUGS, GUNS, AND UGLY WOMEN

Gene O'Neill sits in the peony pink concrete square that the Rescue unit uses as an office. He hums a Led Zeppelin tune and tweaks his new personal digital assistant. He keeps an ear tuned to his EMS radio's chatter. He also listens and laughs along with *Opie and Anthony*, his favorite radio talk show, and takes in a BLS pal's "foolproof" secrets to better sex, which the EMT promotes to everyone within earshot. Walter Drivet, who welcomed O'Neill to the Rescue truck in 1991 with the words "May God have mercy on your soul," sits catty-corner to O'Neill, listening to a Rescue wanna-be and twirling and tightening the minuscule screw that holds his glasses together.

Heber and O'Neill can hear one another through the window they keep open to air out the tiny office, although after seven years as partners they don't have all that much to say to each other. The notion of fresh air is a curious delusion, since it's mostly thick diesel fumes—from the perpetually running trucks—that float in and cover their desks and computers in a thin, slick film.

The ambient noise also includes a cross section of rumbling motors, beeping pagers, snippets of hallway conversations, an assortment of technomechanical sounds, knocks on doors, swinging doors, and change-of-shift prattle. Amazingly, the dissonance doesn't distract them. Without straining a muscle they can screen out miscellany and, when called upon, hone in on the softest sound or translate the most opaque mumble into a clear call to action.

A fresh coat of New Year's Day snow makes the Newark night sparkle. Cars huddle under snowy crusts, which have encased them for more than two days. Most sidewalks go unshoveled, forcing pedestrians to take their chances walking along the edges of the eight-foot-wide paths that traffic has carved. Rescue's first call brings them to Bergen Street, just blocks from the hospital, where police arrest an unlicensed, uninsured, drunken driver whose car spun out of control and hit several others. A vocal crowd is on hand to make certain police take the right man into custody; the driver and his passenger tried swapping places before the law showed up. "People always lie to the cops," O'Neill says, bored. "They expect it."

This crowd is having none of it. Someone shouts he got the whole thing on tape. The community is edgy. Stolen cars whiz down their streets maiming and killing people all too routinely. Since no one is hurt, O'Neill and Heber can't do much at the scene. Both are hungry for rat burgers, their nickname for the small but delectable steamed hamburgers and onions available at White Castle, so they drive north. O'Neill washes his eight burgers down with a Coke. Heber matches him burger for burger but slurps a vanilla shake.

They have barely bolted down their meal when their police scanner alerts them to a possible gunshot victim with an active shooter still at the scene. "We listen to every channel on God's green earth," O'Neill explains. Although the department prohibits "self-dispatching," the partners are initiative-takers. They reach out to Dispatch, tell them they are near the incident and free to ride over to see how they might help.

Pulling the leviathan vehicle up to an intersection, they find a hulking and dilapidated old home squatting on an otherwise barren corner. It appears deserted. No lights glow in the windows. Squad cars have already blocked access by cordoning off area streets, but they wave the Rescue truck into their circle.

So accustomed are they to working together, the cops don't shoo O'Neill and Heber away. A founding member of the city's tactical medical support group, which supports Newark's SWAT team, O'Neill has joined police on more than 150 missions, from high-risk warrant service and hostage rescue to quelling civil disorder. He's taken some of their toughest courses and taught some as well.

One of the cops briefs the two EMTs. Nearby, a black woman sits in the back of a patrol car crying hysterically; she flagged down the police as she ran up the street screaming that someone was shot in the head. The cops are still trying to sort out what the woman is saying and what type of threat they might find if they enter the building to investigate.

Four officers scout the building's icy perimeter from a distance of thirty feet. In dark of night, they search for signs of life, a viable entrance, and risks that might trip them up. A crowd coalesces behind police lines. When the police decide to go in, Rescue goes, too, with equipment essentials on their backs. If a victim turns up, if a cop goes down, they'll be on-scene instantly.

The cops lead an exploratory patrol, sticking close to the home's soiled siding. They move with stealth; the pathway is solid if lumpy ice. Sharp, massive icicles suspended from a rickety fire escape dangle over their heads.

Man by man they enter the home through a back door. It's a terrifying black chasm—so dark they can't see their hands in front of their faces. Everything is still, silent but for one incongruous sound. Somewhere, up on a higher floor, Gloria Gaynor's voice belts disco tunes. The cops' flashlights flicker just long enough for the party to get its bearings and spot a wooden staircase that winds up several stories. Long-neglected plaster walls, marred by graffiti and peeling paint, crumble at their feet. Spiderwebs as thick as nets sprawl across the ceilings where each flight meets the next on coarse wooden landings. The men can hear themselves breathe. When the group nears the third floor, a scuffle occurs. One cop's voice whispers urgently, "You got a victim?"

"I got a man bleeding!" another answers.

The small group crushes together inside one large, dark room off the landing. A silver-haired black man sits in the dark on a bare mattress, which lies on the floor. He looks up at the company that just stormed his hovel. Silent, he appears bewildered. The radio next to him pumps music out at a deafening blast. A paper plate of fried chicken sits in his lap. It's peppery aroma scents the air.

A tall, thin, and much younger man emerges from the shadows into the flashlights' glow. "She cut me 'cause—" he says, holding his arm forward, showing a wet, red slice of flesh.

"That looks self-inflicted if you ask me," a cop replies, training his light on the laceration.

"Turn that goddamn radio down!" someone shouts. But the music continues full force. It's disorienting. The silver-haired man makes no move.

"Turn it off!" another commands. Finally Heber reaches around and lowers the volume.

"This is *his* apartment," the tall, thin man argues, pointing to the older man. "I kicked his door in running from y'all."

The smell of gas wafts through the air. *He was not in his own apartment because he knew the cops were coming,* O'Neill figures. *So he crashed the other guy's place so the cops could only do a plain-sight search.* There are lots of gray areas when it comes to search-and-seizure in multidwelling units, O'Neill explains. *I bet he's got something in his apartment that he doesn't want police to find—drugs, guns, or ugly women.*

"Me and her had a fight," the thin man says of the woman inside the police car. "She hit me and I fell on the floor."

"Fan out and search for bodies shot to the head," one cop orders. The group thins, spreading in all directions.

"I don't know what the hell—" the tall thin man interjects. But the cop holds his hand up, signaling the man to shut up.

More flashlights flicker, and in their light a can of mixed nuts appears, as do blankets tacked over the windows, a box of cookies, used tissues, and eyeglasses. Someone flips a switch, but there is no electricity in the apartment or in the building.

"You take it down. Relax, man," the tall, thin man urges the cop. "You take a little DNA, and you'll find it's all my blood."

"Yeah," one of the cops grumbles. He handcuffs the thin man's wrists by flashlight and nudges him out the door.

"You guys brought the Sixty-Second DNA Kit, right?" O'Neill interjects. "If not, you can borrow mine. I've got it downstairs in my Dick Tracy Kit."

As the posse heads downstairs, a dog barks somewhere down the street. There's little conversation as they troop through the building, which might well be condemned, and gingerly retrace their steps over the icy path.

"We had this fight, over this gun. Two shots went off—" the man in custody ventures, seeing if a different version of his story will sell. As they parade past the crowd toward a waiting ambulance, some in the crowd seem frozen in place. Perhaps they are. Despite the subfreezing temperature, one man stands in shirtsleeves and open-toed sandals.

"My guys will sit on him until you say," an EMS worker assures the cop, who returns to confer with his colleagues while the crew treats the man. Ultimately he refuses their care and sails off to jail in a cruiser.

FINISHING SCHOOL

If common sense were common, everyone would have it.

—VINCENT FRANCIS CISTERNINO, B-TEAM PARAMEDIC, 1999

Summer is skel season. *Skel*, a corruption of the Scottish word *skellum*, means rascal, rogue, or plague-infested corpse.[6] But in EMS circles *skel* stands for the unwashed, malnourished, infested, infected, self-abusing people who clutter the planet. The frank expression is one of many coping mechanisms some EMS workers use to fight their way through the ugliest sides of the job. It may be pejorative, but it is no more so than GOMER—Get Out of My Emergency Room,[7] a term a physician-novelist coined in his book *House of God* to mean "a human being who has lost—often through age—what goes into being a human being." *Gomer* is one of several such blunt terms that has become ubiquitous in certain medical circles. Although it is uncomfortable for the uninitiated to hear "healers" make jokes at their patients' expense, it is one way those confronted with constant illness and grotesque physical deterioration and tragedy cope with the total and frequent assault on their sensibilities.

Skels make people uneasy, especially when they collapse in public. Skels are those whom people call the police to "do something with." The police, at least in Newark, call EMS. "The city has ordinances that prohibit public drinking," a police spokesman explains, "but being drunk is not a crime; it's a medical condition."

Skels are the patients many EMS workers dread most. Some EMS workers have alcoholics, drug abusers, and criminal lowlifes in their families who have left them hurt and bitter. Others resent having to practice their craft on people intent on self-destruction. (Overeating, which can cause diabetes and heart disease, and smoking, which can lead to congestive heart failure and cancer, are two habits EMS workers indulge in that might also be considered self-destructive. Certainly, enough such patients end up in ambulances. And EMS workers sometimes turn excessively to drugs and alcohol, too, especially in times of stress.)

Every night, skels personify massive human and social failings. Society abandons many of its weakest and most intransigent people to EMS. After brief hospitalizations (often a matter of hours), health-care workers and policy-makers turf them back to the streets, where they tumble into trouble again, because they can't manage to correct themselves or simply don't care to. Skels are part of the job.

At times, Cisternino and Fazio are as fed up with this aspect of the job as anyone. After all, they are smart and exceptionally skilled ALS providers. They do their best work, they say, on people who die in front of them, patients who pose complex challenges in which their skills and drugs and tools make a difference. But EMS Utopia is elusive, and when tasked with helping stinking, marinated drunks, psychotics, or taffy-brained users, they try to set a good example for those who look up to them.

Spring is in the air when Fazio and Cisternino and two EMTs hump their equipment into a homeless shelter to revive a semiconscious woman who trebled her methadone dose and has aspirated her own fluids to the point of near drowning. Cramped in a concrete-block corner by the woman's dirty bare feet, her hands full of IV equipment, Fazio makes time to help sensitize one of the EMTs.

She knows he is grossed out from having to hop over vomit chunks and blood clots that resemble leeches, which the woman hacked up onto the cheap linoleum. She noticed that he took the easiest way to squeeze into the cubbyhole this woman calls home: instead of rearranging her sparse furnishings, he stepped on the patient's clothing, which is piled into dresser drawers stacked on a margin of floor. Fazio sees his horrified grimace as he wipes seven shades of mucus, blood, and vomit from the woman's cheeks and chin. Besides holding a sheet up as a shield against the flow of infectious fluids, the EMT can do more, and Fazio challenges him.

"Fix her bra!" Fazio orders; she would do it herself if she could reach. The simple act of adjusting the woman's underwear so her breast doesn't flop around as she spews all over herself might remind the disgusted EMT that this skel, despite her weaknesses and self-destructive habits, may still have the sense to be embarrassed by her nakedness and her condition. And onlookers who peer through the door will see their neighbor treated respectfully.

Some EMS workers can compromise scene safety and require more straightforward taking in hand. Fazio is not the only one who regrets that some people come to the job poorly schooled in manners and common courtesy. She's willing to coach the ignorant. It improves customer service and makes for a better impression on observers, which reduces the chance that the next EMS workers who visit will be greeted with disdain and distrust. It's one thing to gripe about job conditions and be comfortable spiking one's speech with cusses, which Fazio does, but when patients or family members open their door to her, she becomes as a veritable "game-show host."

"You need to show more respect," she tutors newcomers when they carry cups of hot chocolate or edibles into people's homes. "Who the fuck are you to say their emergency isn't important?"

"I didn't say that," they retort.

"Yes, you did, with your demeanor," she explains. Fazio, affectionately called "the Redheaded Bitch from Hell," "Ma Barker," and "Bella Faccia" (beautiful face), is also nicknamed "Sister Mary Fucking Fazio" for the gentle way she tends to her patients.

She is intolerant of coworkers who jab the air while talking to a patient or pound their clipboards for emphasis when they talk. God forbid someone fails to keep patients warm and dry because they forgot to stock their ambulances with sheets and blankets. Other cretinous behaviors the B team despises include failing to wipe one's feet before entering a home, flipping off a TV without asking permission, putting one's foot up on a table in order to write on one's thigh, or whining, "You called the ambulance *for this?*" Fazio says everyone is allowed to "fuck up" and "everyone does." But neither she nor her colleagues will tolerate much.

Veteran B-team paramedic Daniel R. Gerard, Sr., also chairs the paramedic division of the National Association of Emergency Medical Technicians. On the job for decades, he thinks it's miraculous that "people pick up the phone and call for help when they don't know your qualifications."

"There's that faith—dial 911 and get help. They don't know me from a hole in the wall," he marvels, "but they let me in their house, give me their medicines, let me open their wallet, let me put my hands on their body and give them needles and drugs. It's a sacred trust."

Another Newark native, Gerard is street-smart and sufficiently rough-and-tumble to protect himself. He is also a registered nurse, with a master's degree in hospital administration, an international consulting practice, and occasional overseas medical rescue missions. Yet Gerard, Fazio, Cisternino, Drivet, Callahan, and Cardona share the streets with others whose approach to patient care is considerably more crude.

One former team member supplemented his uniform with a pair of metal welder's gloves. "He'd hold people like this," a veteran remembers, extending his arm and forming a pincher claw. "He'd say to the patient from arm's length, 'OK, ready to go?' "

Another bragged about having her patients self-bandage. She says she'd climb on top of her bus, dangle a strip of gauze, and instruct patients to hold it to their head and twirl.

A third turned away from a patient who had been discharged from an area hospital. She had been picked up earlier from a street corner, where she lay in a fetal position, holding her ribs, barely able to breathe. She should have been able to file a complaint against her assailant, a former boyfriend. But no one at that hospital reached out to the police, or let her use the phone. And no one felt compelled to help the woman find her way safely home, although she lived outside city limits, far beyond walking distance. A University EMT witnessed this and shrugged. "The city is a hard, hard place," he remarked. "It's about survival. You just can't feel sorry for everybody, because that's when you get taken advantage of. Besides," he added, "maybe she deserved the beating."

Field supervisors, such as Visoskas and Piumelli, cannot be at every call; the crews respond to hundreds of emergencies per day. And when B-teamers discover socially retarded colleagues, including well-intentioned but ignorant FNGs, they find ingenious ways of disarming them. For example, chumps might be sent from the scene to the truck in search of the "orange" Kendrick Extrication Device (KED) or the "left-handed" bag-valve mask (BVM). There is no orange KED (only a green one) and no "left-handed" BVM either (the handle swivels to accommodate the user). But the ruses get troublemakers out of the way.

HIGH-WIRE ACT

Paramedics Fazio and Cisternino have worked Newark's streets for over ten years apiece. Like Callahan and Cardona, neither had an idyllic childhood. Unlike Callahan and Cardona, neither Fazio nor Cisternino grew up in Newark. Therefore, their perception of what makes a scene safe is different. They prefer to actively mitigate risks.

At 2230 hours one warm night, Dispatch sends Cisternino and Fazio to an unconscious patient at an address where the two have been before. "It's a shit-hole, courtyard building," Cisternino says, concerned about a vocal crowd of onlookers who may surround and hassle them. Fazio just bangs her head on the steering wheel.

When they arrive, Fazio backs the truck up to a flight of concrete stairs and the partners hop out. From the back of the bus they remove their airway kit and defibrillator, stretcher, long board, and Reeves, a sturdy sheet of flexible plastic reinforced with wooden slats that functions as a carrying device. They pile everything on to the stretcher and wheel it toward the stairs. Because public-housing residents have rained bricks, metal doors, glass bottles, and even refrigerators down on crews, few are cavalier when they approach the buildings.

"Ambulance people coming through," some have learned to holler up stairwells, so their uniforms and shields won't take drug dealers, users, prostitutes, and others by surprise. Others still scan the windows before approaching buildings to see what if anything might be hurled at them. Tonight, however, the building seems still. Each shoulders a few of the heavy items and, stationing the stretcher on the ground, begins to climb. Under the weak golden light cast by a few bare bulbs, they plod up flight after flight. Choking humidity sends sweat down Cisternino's back. Fazio wears a turquoise bandanna around her neck to soak up the perspiration. "The most important piece of equipment in *The Hitchhiker's Guide to the Galaxy* is a towel," Fazio says. "For us, it's a bandanna." She has tied her copper-colored hair back before it fully frizzes and donned a baseball cap—two tactics to avoid getting tangled in the ubiquitous curly adhesive strips used to trap flies.

They scale several flights before coming upon a small crowd of children and adults gathered around an ashen-skinned man propped up against a cinderblock wall. His eyes are closed.

"He all right?" a woman asks, before the partners can get near the man.

"The neighbors say he's been drinking. He fell down and hit his head," a Newark police officer reports. Having an officer on the scene helps, but it's no panacea. Many people in the city are armed, including some of the patients.

"He fell here?" Cisternino asks.

"No, we dragged him upstairs from outside," an elderly man volunteers.

Another nods and reports, "We put a cold rag on his face."

Cisternino takes a quick look over a balcony and sees the ocher glare of broken brown beer bottles below.

"He had some beer with him when we found him," a woman adds.

Fazio stands at the man's feet, counting his breaths. Cisternino squats at the man's head to begin the exam. Such positioning allows them to watch one another's backs and do their jobs. The man's dark skin is glazed with sweat. The medic taps him on the shoulder and asks, "Sir?" He gets no answer.

The man breathes regularly but only four times a minute—three to five times slower than normal. Besides overdose patients, the only people who might breathe as slowly as this man are those with head injuries, and their breathing is irregular. Fazio whispers, "I think I know what this is."

"I'll almost bet you are right," Cisternino replies. Taking out his flashlight, he pushes up one of the man's eyelids to inspect his pupils. The size of pencil points, they don't react to the bright light. "Well, he's unconscious now."

The medics suspect that the man overdosed and passed out. But since bystanders said he fell and then reported dragging him, Cisternino and Fazio must also treat him as a trauma patient.

The patient needs oxygen, a narcotics antidote, and fluids. Rather than treat him in the hot, dingy, open-air stairwell, with people drawn to the commotion, they elect to get him into their ambulance. It's the closest thing to a controlled environment. Still squatting, Cisternino stabilizes the man's cervical spine by fastening a rigid collar around his neck. He grasps the sides of the man's head as Fazio grips his lower legs. They slide the man flat on his back and roll him onto his side. The officer helps hold the man steady as Fazio slides the long board into place, and they rotate him onto his back.

Cisternino continues holding the man's head in position while Fazio spreads the orange Reeves flat, forcing the crowd to step back. Gripping the long board at each end, the partners heave the patient onto the Reeves, wrap it around him, and secure its Velcro straps. They both hoist several pieces of equipment over their shoulders before lifting the man waist-high and beginning the hot hike down the twisting stairs. The full package is just plain heavy. But no one makes an effort to help or even to open a door.

As they load him into the ambulance, Cisternino whispers to Fazio about the man's pupils, "Way constricted." She nods knowingly, starts up the truck, and radios the ER.

Inside the box, Cisternino growls, "I could say you shouldn't be fucking getting high," but he knows his words are wasted on the unconscious man. *Society says he's entitled to waste my time using illegal drugs*, Cisternino fumes. He turns on the oxygen and straps a mask to the man's face. If the patient vomits suddenly, the clear plastic mask offers some protection from HIV, hepatitis, tuberculosis, and the other communicable diseases with which this drug user might be infected.

Cisternino must start an IV for the antidote and fluids. When pricked, the patient does not wince or show any sign of distress. Cisternino draws five tubes of blood in less than one minute for labs. He blots a stray drop of blood off the sheets. He wipes drool from the man's mouth. The unconscious can't swallow. Saliva and blood are just two of several potentially contaminated fluids to which this patient exposes his rescuers.

This is their second overdose in an hour—still nothing compared with the February 1991 weekend when crews treated 180 overdoses. Two-person EMS crews arrived to find three or four people clustered together—all dead or near death. The crews soon discovered that Narcan, their traditional antidote, did not work as expected. Normally, an injection or two would send the medicine to the patient's narcotic-receptor cells, where it would bump the opiate out of place, abruptly ending the drug-induced high. On this particular weekend, though, crews had to quintuple or sextuple the Narcan doses to get any effect. When roused from their deathlike stupors, patients became exceptionally combative. Very shortly, the EMS units were overtaxed physically and emotionally, and their medication reserves were depleted. Managers and supervisors drove to area hospitals, borrowed whole cases of Narcan, and chased ambulances from call to call to resupply them. The ER was "sheer bedlam," one remembers. All this from one innovative street chemist's blend of heroin and fentanyl, a hybrid nicknamed "Tango and Cash."

Because such events, which occur every few years, are so memorable, the crews do not take chances. Even the average heroin user can react violently to Narcan. Accordingly, before Cisternino injects the antidote he tucks the patient's hands and wrists inside the man's waistband. If the man responds aggressively, he'll first have to extricate his hands from his pants and the constricting Reeves strap before putting up a fight. And the mask will constrain him from biting, spitting, or puking . . . at least long enough for Cisternino to protect himself.

Fazio pulls into the hospital driveway just as Cisternino pushes the Narcan. A moment passes and nothing happens, so he shoots a second dose. Even that does little to rouse their patient.

Cisternino drops the needle in the protective sharps container, gathers bits of paper, plastic, glass, and blood- and drool-covered gauze in his hand, and peels his glove off in reverse. When he chucks the medical waste, it's encased in the latex packet and falls neatly into a biohazard container.

As the partners wheel their patient into the trauma ER, a tired nurse greets them: "Why did you bring him here?"

That's a question Cisternino loves to hate. *Because my toy box at home is full,* he thinks. *I would have taken him to 7-Eleven but he needed a doctor, not a Slurpee.* Finally, he chooses a retort: "Because you were closer than Chicago Memorial."

By now the man has opened his eyes. He looks around, dazed.

"Hello! Welcome to University Hospital," the nurse says, her voice dripping with false cheer. "How much heroin did you take tonight?" She receives no reply. Rather than cut his clothes off in preparation for a CAT scan, she unbuttons, unzips, and unties his garments. But she doesn't conserve his wardrobe out of sympathy. "I don't want to cut your clothes off because I want you to go home."

As she yanks off the man's jeans, a box cutter, a cheap and popular street weapon, falls from his pocket and clatters on the floor. "I'm going to keep your blade until you leave," she tells the man. Unless he develops some signs or symptoms suggesting a serious medical condition, he will go home in four to six hours or as soon as the drugs wear off. Overdoses are so prolific here that the ER does not consider them automatic grounds for admission. There are no compulsory rehabilitation programs, so patients are free to dance on the edge of life repeatedly, calling on EMS again and again and again.

DUEL

In the dark, poorly lit city it is easy to miss an address. One night when Drivet and Cisternino are paired together, Drivet slows down as he approaches a location, taking a few seconds to size up the scene's safety.

As soon as they near their destination, the medics see two tall black men stumbling erratically on a chipped sidewalk outside a sagging white-clapboard house. One is lean and wiry. His tan pants have footprints on them. His denim jacket is askew and his hair is wild. The other man is chubby, wall-eyed with fear, and wearing a bloodied, torn white T-shirt and jeans.

Pulling on their latex gloves, Drivet and Cisternino hop down from the ambulance cab. Drivet approaches the bleeding man with slow, steady strides and says, "Sir, we are the paramedics. Are you hurt?"

"I'm stabbed," the man says, his eyes wide open with surprise. "What happened?"

Drivet moves toward the man from the side, holding his attention with a gentle series of questions and guiding him toward the back of the bus, whose doors Cisternino has opened. The white light from the ambulance is so bright in contrast to the dark road that both street fighters gawk and shield their eyes.

Meanwhile, Cisternino deflects the other man, who may be the victim's friend or assailant. No police are on hand to help. He refuses to answer any of Cisternino's questions and is getting too close for comfort. "Hey, buddy, back up," Cisternino says. "Back up, I tell ya."

"What you doin' to him?" the man asks in an alcohol-soaked haze.

"We're taking him to the hospital. You need to back up, man."

"What's going on in there? I got a right to know, damn it."

Cisternino looks over his shoulder quickly to check on his partner's progress. Drivet has the patient inside the back of the ambulance and is about to step up there himself. Cisternino mumbles under his breath, "No you don't. I'm a card-carrying member of the International Association of the Brotherhood of It's None of Your Fucking Business, and I say butt out."

Not wanting to risk a stab wound in the back, he retreats to the bus's runner and steps up into the ambulance, never taking his eyes off the other man. Once inside, he pulls both doors shut and locks them. He is still stooping when he turns around and deftly negotiates the tiny space between Drivet, the patient, and the green, translucent tubing that is already shuttling oxygen to the patient. Because he and Drivet anticipated several traumas, Cisternino only needs to reach up to the radiator and pull down preassembled fluids and blood tubing, which he quickly sets up to treat the man.

"Let's get your shirt off, sir, so I can see what is happening," Drivet says to the man.

"Whoa man, what's happening? I didn't see nothing. My man just gave me a hug," the patient says, his breath pungent with alcohol.

"Don't talk," Drivet instructs. He takes a pair of shears out of his holster belt and starts to cut the man's T-shirt. To save the hospital staff time, EMS workers usually make badly injured people "trauma naked." But medics here generally avoid cutting their patients' attire, because they know from experience that many Newark residents have precious few clothes. This man's shirt, however, is irreparably torn, sopping with blood, and masking the stabs.

"Hey, man, don't—"

"Don't worry about your shirt. You are hurt. Don't talk for a minute. Let me see what's going on here." Drivet places his hand on the man's collarbone and asks him to sit forward for a minute so he can inspect the injuries.

The patient slumps forward on the paramedic's gloved hand as Drivet scans his back. "I see four wounds," Drivet says to Cisternino, who is now taking notes. "One to the right axilla, one to the left kidney, two under the left shoulder blade." Penny-sized openings of pink wet tissue glisten beneath the man's caramel-colored surface skin. The stabs are all life-threatening.

Cisternino takes a handful of four-by-four gauze pads from one of the built-in cabinets, tears them from their sterile wrappings, and hands them to Drivet, who presses several against each wound and helps the man sit back. Cisternino hoists the LIFEPAK 10 heart monitor/defibrillator off its shelf; unzips a pouch; peels the paper off three round electrodes; snaps them to red, black, and white wires; and, holding the strands like a bouquet, hands the bunch to Drivet, who places them at strategic locations on the patient's chest. The two partners work quickly, efficiently, and without a word.

With the wounds padded and the heart monitor on, Drivet completes the patient's vital signs. "His heart rate is 100. His pressure is 162/104. Lung sounds are equal and bilateral. He's not diaphoretic," he calls out to Cisternino, who writes the data on the chart. "How old are you, sir?"

"I'm twenty-three."

Without his shirt for cover, the man's rubbery stomach, scarred with stretch marks, spills over his pants. His eyes are bloodshot. His hair is unkempt. He looks fifty, at least.

"You want to go to University, Sir?"

The man nods.

"OK, I'm gonna drive. My partner here is going to take good care of you," Drivet says, rising to take a few steps and crawl through an opening to the cab. He urges the bus along at 40 mph.

Cisternino turns the man's forearm upside down and is about to insert the IV when the patient starts crying, "Someone hit me in the back. I don't know where it came from."

"Yeah, it's fucked up," Cisternino sympathizes. "Now hold still, bro, because I don't want to have to do this twice."

"Am I hurt bad?"

"I got to be honest with you," he says, locking his aqua eyes into the man's soft brown ones. "We can't tell how deep the cuts are, but they are in bad spots." Then he slides the needle into the man's arm like a candle into birthday cake.

"You got a steady hand."

"Yeah, bro, I try."

"I think I got hit here, too," the patient says, touching his thigh.

"Hold on a minute, my brother," Cisternino says as he fills the blood tubes and tapes the catheter to the man's arm. "Let me see what you got." He helps the man unzip his jeans and pull them down over his jockey shorts, which are soaked with urine. A ruby-colored, four-inch gash disfigures the man's thigh.

As the ambulance pulls up to the ER, the patient points to his feet and says, "I think I got more down there."

Cisternino jerks the man's pants down to his ankles. Two more wounds appear—one slice to the knee and one cut to the calf. He grabs more pads and dresses the wounds. "They are going to do a chest X-ray to see how deep the cuts are," he tells the man, preparing him for the hospital staff. Then Cisternino takes one more blood-pressure reading.

"It hurts when you be putting this on me. It's cold."

"Sorry, bro."

Cisternino covers the patient with a sheet and blanket. He transfers the oxygen from the ambulance's main tank to a portable cylinder, buckles it onto the stretcher, unhooks the heart-monitor wires, grabs the paperwork, and holds the IV solutions up as Drivet opens the door and pulls the patient and stretcher outside.

"Cisternino is a tough guy. But he's gentle. He's not a punk," Cardona summarizes. "The people in the street can sense that. And that bald head is intimidating. But he's a nice guy and they can sense that, too."

Cisternino is strong, but he is not bulletproof and he knows it. Called to resuscitate a youth whose chest was blasted apart by a gunshot wound, he refuses to acknowledge the people surrounding the ambulance as he steps inside. They want information. He already knows the man inside is dead but he doesn't yet know if all is lost. Men try to catch his attention and shoulder their way behind him into the truck. He won't talk to the crowd while they pound fists on the truck and scream at him from all four directions. He looks straight ahead, climbs inside, and locks the door behind him. Ignoring the throng leaves him free to focus on the problem and how to fix it. The dead man's injury is complex and probably irreversible, but the anxious crowd doesn't know that. And as long as they're unaware, they won't fix the blame for their friend's death on Cisternino and his colleagues. Unfettered by that concern, he puts his all into it.

The injuries are fatal, however, and doctors pronounce the boy dead on arrival. Before the hospital informs the victim's loved ones of his death and lets them in to see his corpse, nurses wipe away blood, close his eyes, cover his nakedness, and gather his possessions into a neat pile. The law, however, requires them to leave the endotracheal tube, chest tubes, intravenous lines, and other evidence of lifesaving effort in place for the medical examiner. Even in a city where it is not uncommon for young men to die before their time, often as a result of crime, death still comes as a shock to friends and family.

It's routine, even sadly predictable, for the EMS workers, though. They see it most every shift—several times a shift, some nights. Cisternino does not grieve for the boy. He does not know what circumstances led to the death. He did what he could, and now his part in the drama is over. Back on his bus, he swabs blood from the ambulance floor with a sheet and wipes down his equipment with phenol, an industrial cleaning agent. A cigarette dangling from his lips, he jokes with his buddies that the man died from "acute lead poisoning." In spite of the posturing, Cisternino spies the man's friends and family emerging from the ER. A compactly built man who was at the shooting, followed to the hospital, and then waited for nearly an hour before getting the news, shouts, "No, no, no!" He yells at the heavens, "Man! Oh, man," and pounds his fists against the hood of a car in the parking lot. *"Shit!"*

A smooth-faced young woman trails after him, weeping into cupped hands. The right thigh of her blue jeans is still smeared with the patient's blood. From the corner of his eye, Cisternino watches her lean her head against the concrete wall, sink to her knees, and sob in uncontrolled grief. He lumbers out of the bus and over to the woman. He hands her a wad of tissues. He means well and she knows it, but her sobbing only increases. Finally, her friends interrupt their own mourning to console her.

One asks Cisternino if he can buy a cigarette from him and extends a $10 bill. Cisternino and his fellow EMS workers are accustomed to being asked for cigarettes, money, bandages, aspirin, medical advice, rides, directions, food, change for a hundred or a single dollar bill. Those who don't want to get something usually want to sell something: jewelry, perfume, a bus ticket. Cisternino usually rebuffs the "get-overs," local slang for low-level con artists. This time, however, he takes out his Marlboro Lights, packs them against his curled hand, and gives one to the man. He pulls out his lighter and ignites it for him, too. "Sheesh, I wish I had ten bucks on me, bro," he says, declining the money.

ALL FOR ONE AND ONE FOR ALL

Partners choose each other for lots of reasons. The ability to trust one another is the top of the list. Separations, schisms, and splits occur, but for the most part teaming up twelve tough hours a day inside the box makes for sturdy relationships.

Sometimes it's the little things that make a partner a friend. "I always have to carry gloves for him," Cardona says, chuckling about Callahan's trademark forgetfulness. "He'll wear that big ol' tool belt with nothing in it." Callahan does forget his gloves, loses his magnetic access card, and constantly misplaces his cell phone. Once he drove home to Maryland with Cardona's keys in his pocket.

Each EMS worker has a repertoire of tactics for making and keeping scenes safe. But there is one rule that is not subordinate to individual styles or preferences. Every B-team member rushes to another's aid when a true threat arises.

One tender spring evening, Fazio and Cisternino take a breather in the headquarters parking lot. The dashboard radio is tuned to *Saturday Night with the Eighties*, and the partners immerse themselves in a passionate sing-along. EMT Pat Vogt's voice cuts in over the dispatch radio: "We need assistance, please." Instantly, everything changes.

Fazio guns the engine and quickly turns the bus on a dime, shouting "*Where are they?!*" at the radio. Cisternino's face freezes. He turns off the tunes and sweeps their customary clutter from the dashboard. Fazio's journal, a Nora Roberts novel, a package of Celestial Seasonings Vitamin C drops, two-liter bottles of Fiji water, a copy of *New Jersey Monthly*, a pay stub, assorted hair-restraining devices, an inhaler, a hairbrush, a glasses case, textbooks, crumpled tissues and napkins, a cosmetics case, Quality Assurance sheets, and baseball caps tumble to the floor.

A stream of people streak from quarters and jump into emergency vehicles; a cavalry of ambulances, supervisor sport utility vehicles, and the behemoth Rescue truck assemble. Lights flash. Sirens blare. It's enough to cause a seizure. Despite the crush of activity, none of the trucks collide as they rumble toward the narrow exit.

A B-team member asking for help is akin to the call that scrambles the fighters for rapid deployment. Some very tough, very competent people are in trouble. And when the EMS workers hear that, a switch flips. They run full force toward the danger.[8] They don't take time to acknowledge their fear. "It's not that we don't have it," Cisternino explains. "It's just that it doesn't stop us. Until I am standing next to the person in trouble, I'll do anything and everything to get across and worry about the liability later."

Vogt's patient, a petite, pregnant woman who suffers from epilepsy, is exploding with rage. With superhuman strength, she's thrown Vogt across the ambulance. *For a little thing, she's very powerful*, Vogt marvels. *She probably weighs as much as one of my legs!* Now Vogt has a smattering of contusions, and her arm is scraped and bleeding. Fortunately, she and her partner are just blocks from quarters. Still, nearly every bus in the city barrels there. The convoy screeches down the avenue, but no accidents occur. No rescuers can afford to get hurt.

As Fazio parks the bus, Cisternino jumps down and hustles to the troubled ambulance.

Guttural screams rupture inside the ambulance. People on the sidewalk stare at each other in alarm, but Callahan is already on hand to reassure them. Cisternino climbs inside the bus to help subdue the patient. Fazio coaxes the family members away from Vogt's ambulance.

"She's irrational!" a cousin of the patient exclaims. "Why is she acting like that?"

Several medics are there to answer questions. In short, the patient is undergoing successive seizures. She hasn't time to recover fully before the disability strikes again. Unaware who she is, where she is, or what is happening, she can't process information and knows only that strangers are grabbing at her. Naturally, she resists. Unable to harness her full mental capacities, the woman reacts at a primitive level. She lashes out, bringing all her adrenaline to bear, much like someone who finds it possible to lift a car when a child is trapped.

A tall male relative listening to the explanation decides the EMS workers make sense. Raising his hands above his head, he pushes the crowd to retreat, shouting, "Step back and let them do their job!" The man is an EMS worker's dream. One scene-safety technique is to take the biggest mouth in the crowd and distract him by putting him to work.

The medics let the family know when the patient is ready to go and ask if anyone wants to accompany them. They all decline but promise to come to the hospital later. "Do me a favor and make sure she's all right before they let her out," the male relative asks. "She go in and out of the hospital all the time. They don't fix nothin'."[9]

The bus takes off. Cardona drives. Vogt, her partner, Cisternino, and rescue specialist Gene O'Neill stay inside the box with the patient.

Everyone else leaves, too. "You don't want to hang around while the crowd gathers," Fazio says, of one of the consequences of working EMS in an urban setting. "Luckily, they were pretty reasonable. But it's not uncommon for them to react poorly to that." How many people can feel comfortable hearing a woman shriek and scream while others coerce her into submission? How are outsiders who happen on a scene supposed to know the woman is utterly out of control, a genuine danger to herself and everyone around her?

Callahan, Fazio, and others drive their buses to the ER, where they meet up with their partners and quickly debrief. "Even though the job just happened, everybody gets together, real animated," Fazio explains. Such events "make your adrenaline spike. You need to bounce that off with people who know what you just went through. It's a way of coming down, defusing. It'll go on a few minutes then everyone will go about their way."

"Never, never touch the ambulance driver," Cisternino says ominously, and he is not joking. Vogt is a popular if quiet member of the team. A fifty-year-old, chain-smoking EMT, she's known to pull her weight and keep her mouth shut. And that has earned her the team's respect, even when she sits in the box between calls doing something as sentimental as knitting for her grandchildren. When Vogt called for help, her coworkers were only too happy to answer.

But even if a rescuer is less popular, an attack upon one is considered an attack upon all. Since ambulance crews often go about their business unaided by police, they have learned to defend themselves. Strictly speaking, weapons are prohibited. But almost anything can become a weapon when threats loom. In some places, EMS workers carry "instant anesthetic" in the form of heavy-duty flashlights. Others carry knives, ostensibly for cutting seat belts, and cravats. Even a radio can be pressed into action. To hit a combative patient or bystander with a radio is to "Motorolaize" them. Even empty-handed, EMS workers will defend themselves. "There's always brutacaine," one says, inventing a pharmaceutical name for what might otherwise be called brute force.

Outside the ER, team members are still cooling down. "People on the block won't ever forget that," Callahan chuckles.

"At least no one was hurt," someone else says thankfully. That everyone on the patient's bus was either punched, slapped, scratched, kicked, shoved, or worse does not count. Sometimes the job is rough. Although they'll wash their scratches off to discourage disease, they'll wear no Band-Aids.

Inside the ER, the patient, in four-point restraints, has comported herself well for several minutes. So the nurses plan to release her, a decision that infuriates the B team.

"It took a lot of big and trained folks to tie her down, just minutes ago," Fazio protests. "But then, they're the *higher* medical authority."

It irks the paramedics when their assessments are so casually ignored. Paramedic training varies throughout the country, but in New Jersey, candidates follow the Department of Transportation's nationally accredited program.

Paramedics spend at least two college semesters mastering anatomy and physiology; respiratory emergencies and management; cardiac arrhythmias; electrocardiograms; advanced cardiac life support; trauma; infectious disease; burns; math and pharmacology; the digestive, lymphatic, endocrine, immune, renal, respiratory, reproductive and musculo-skeletal systems; body fluids and electrolytes; sterile intravenous techniques; triage; caring for patients at crime scenes, hazardous materials incidents, and rapes; sudden infant death syndrome; pediatrics; obstetrics; geriatrics; death and dying; the legal implications of care, charting, and more. And, they invest eight hundred or more hours of clinical time before they can test for certification and become eligible for employment. It's not the *Arthur Murray School of Paramedicine and Dance*, as Cisternino likes to say. As a paramedic student in Massachusetts, he stayed late when he worked in the ER. As the staffing levels decreased, he got to see more action. A decade later, he still vacuums up knowledge in the ER, at University's many libraries, in the labs, and virtually everywhere he goes. Unlike nurses, paramedics recertify throughout the course of their careers. Depending on the state, paramedics can perform many nursing skills and several specialty skills that many nurses cannot. Yet when they report this woman's consecutive, violent seizures in the field, the ER staff can virtually ignore the information and usher her out the door and back into the care of her chagrined and perplexed family—who may well chastise the next EMS worker to appear at their door.

The medics are concerned that they will have to treat her and transport her for free if she becomes ill again within twenty-four hours. They don't begrudge the woman her right to care or the cost of it. They just resent expensive, otherwise preventable trips that keep the department operating in the red, unable to invest significantly in salaries, equipment, training, research, and initiatives that can make EMS a more proactive community-health asset.

There is no program to ensure that patients follow up on the care and instructions they receive at the hospital—measures that can get many insurance, free medicine, and free transportation to neighborhood clinics. "You can't have the medicine police," Cisternino says (although there are places where police accompany social workers to make sure patients take medicine to combat infectious diseases such as tuberculosis). Some patients are too poor to comply. Some are incompetent. Some are irresponsible. Regardless, when they need care EMS, the community safety net, provides it. But even a safety net has costs.

The team is still decompressing when someone comes outside with an update. Before the nurses could complete the discharge papers, the patient seized again and earned an overnight stay. Hurray!

5 RESCUE ME

It's our toolbox on wheels. It slices. It dices. It
juliennes. It really does!

—WILLIAM HEBER, UNIVERSITY HOSPITAL EMT AND RESCUE
SPECIALIST

GOOD SAMARITAN

At 0250 hours, Dispatch sends Rescue Specialists Eugene "Geno" O'Neill and
Billy "the Squirrel" Heber to one of the busy highways that loops around the
city for a motor-vehicle accident. Heber and O'Neill are in the truck and out
of the compound in thirty seconds, per usual. Conscious of stolen cars that
speed unchecked throughout the city, Heber pushes his truck as fast as he dares;
he swings his head both ways at each intersection and waits for his partner's all-
clear sign. It is all too common for drivers here to disobey speed limits, stop
signs, and red lights; tailgate; create their own lanes; fail to use turn signals; and
otherwise motor along recklessly. Satisfied, O'Neill cocks his finger like a gun
going off, and Heber rolls on through.

The truck pounds the road like an angry battleship at full throttle. The six-
inch-tall hula dancer with the plastic grass skirt who lives on a perch in the cab
shakes as if she is having a seizure. Heber leans on the horn. The earsplitting
blast mimics a freight train; it's loud enough to make people cringe, and so
deafening that the uninitiated might be tempted to grab one of the protective
headsets that gather dust in the cab.

The city is soiled with four-foot mounds of soot-encrusted snow; piles of rubble studded with chunks of concrete and wood; and crushed, rusting barbed-wire fences. But for a few people clustered outside liquor stores and phone booths, the streets are empty. One B-teamer claims that "snow and rain are the best policemen," because they keep people off the streets. "It's no fun stealing a car if you can't drive it around."

By habit, Heber chooses the fastest route, steering the truck through the congested streets and convoluted thoroughfares that they visit night after night.

Adrenaline surges through his veins. His brow knits with concentration, his mind already engaged in the problem that he has yet to see. *How do I get to the patient? How many patients do I have? How am I going to get them out? How fast can I do it? What tools will I need? How many more ambulances and personnel might be necessary? What type of personnel—BLS, ALS, cops, firefighters? How many hospitals do I need and what types of hospitals? Do I need trauma or burn-care centers or can they go to the local cat-and-dog hospital?*

Meanwhile, O'Neill dons his protective gear so he can thrust himself into the action the instant they arrive. Even after ten years on Rescue, the slowest part of the job for him is adding these twenty-five pounds of turnout gear. He's learned to save time by first shedding his pager, wallet, cell phone, keys, and portable radio. An avowed agnostic, O'Neill nevertheless takes care to tuck his Celtic cross beneath his collar. As the truck slams and bounces, he wriggles into mustard-colored, fire-retardant pants that zip down the sides and cover his leather boots. He stuffs himself into a flame-resistant coat. It's February and it's freezing, so he tugs on a navy watch cap and favorite pair of wool gloves, the ones with nubbed palms that enhance his grip but no fingertips to impair his dexterity. He stuffs a pair of heavy-duty work gloves in his pocket and a few latex gloves, too. His hates the safety goggles, which tend to fog up, but he can't forgo the egg-yolk yellow helmet.

O'Neill likes to pop a smoke to blow off excess tension, but Heber hates the stench. In between butts O'Neill always fidgets with something. Tonight he twirls an oral airway he found in his pocket. The rigid plastic tube, which is shaped like a question mark, helps prop open patients' throats and prevent their tongues from falling back to block the vital exchange of oxygen and carbon dioxide.

The two don't speak much inside the truck. Longtime partners who compare their relationship to a bad marriage, they're pretty much talked out. Besides, it's too noisy. Their cab sits above a turbocharged engine, and an exhaust pipe rises up right behind them, spitting diesel fumes up toward the sky. They designed the unusual ventilation system so the stinking, noxious fumes wouldn't smother them when they work at ground level, which is most of the time. (They can't shut off the truck while they work. Its motor powers the generators, which in turn drive their exhaustive collection of tools.) They blare classic rock from one radio and set another to surf; it pipes in a constant stream of police and firefighting activity, and other municipal nightmares.

Approaching the designated mile marker, they see no wreck. Two sedans have pulled to the left; a taxi and a glossy black four-door are parked on the right-hand sliver of shoulder. They can also make out the pale lemon color of a Newark engine company up ahead. A body lies facedown in the express lane. On O'Neill and Heber's watch, the first guy out of the truck identifies possible hazards and assesses the patient(s). O'Neill leaps down first. When he squats near the man he spies a three-inch-wide, eight-foot-long stream of blood flowing from the patient's head. The ice-cold asphalt is freezing it into a ruddy slush. *That's gotta be 2,000 cc's of blood*, O'Neill figures. The body only has 5,000. "He's down! He's hurt! He's bleeding real bad, Billy," O'Neill shouts as he changes into latex gloves. "Get me a collar and a board. Get me an MIC unit!"

Heber updates Dispatch at 0257 hours and yanks equipment from the truck. In addition to several hundred tools and various rescue supplies, it has all the first-aid basics they need, except the means to transport the man.

O'Neill's top priority is to ensure that the man's mouth, nose, and throat are clear so he can breathe, but first he must turn the patient over. Scanning the roadside for somebody, anybody to help him reposition the man, he sees that Heber's hands are full and the firefighter and bystanders are too shaken. With one hand on the back of the man's head and another reaching across his torso, O'Neill rolls him over.

The man's eyes stare up at the night sky, unseeing. He's unconscious. His neatly trimmed mustache and goatee are saturated with blood. It leaks from his ears, nose, and lips. His breaths are few and irregular; between them blood gurgles in his throat. *If this guy's gonna make it, he's gotta get tubed*, O'Neill thinks. He needs to address the airway, but he also needs to splint the man and get him out of the express lane before they all get pancaked.

Heber hustles with the equipment as O'Neill presses the man's wrist, searching for a sign of life; he finds none. Moving his fingers to the man's neck, O'Neill feels the pulse bound. Blood is leaking out of the man's vessels and his heart is beating faster to keep his circulatory system from shutting down. As O'Neill works, the firefighter tells him that the man witnessed a fender bender between two other cars and got out to help. A minivan came flying down the highway at "a high rate of speed," which O'Neill estimates was at least 50 mph, and whacked him. "I saw him get launched," the firefighter claims, pointing to his turnout coat, which is spattered with body fluids.

Heber hands O'Neill a cervical collar and reports, "They're sending MIC 5"—paramedics stationed at the airport. As the crow flies, the crews are a few hundred yards apart.

O'Neill glares up in frustration, and Heber cuts him off with "I know, I know." O'Neill hoped Dispatch would send a city MIC unit—they might be farther away, but they would probably arrive before MIC 5. Leaving the airport, the ALS crew is forced north, while the accident is in the southbound lanes. High-speed traffic, cement dividers, and guardrails will force the truck miles out of the way and impede a fast turnaround.

O'Neill slides the collar behind the man's neck, wraps it around, and fastens it under his bloody chin. He and Heber logroll the motionless man onto their long board. Heber secures him in place as O'Neill searches for other signs of injury by cutting through the man's coat, his brown argyle vest, his spotless white shirt and dark tie.

Dispatch also sent a BLS bus, which arrives with an EMT and his paramedic partner. In New Jersey, paramedics can work BLS because they must also maintain their basic skills. When paramedics work with BLS partners, however, they have to leave their advanced lifesaving skills and equipment behind. State administrative code limits paramedics to practicing with partners trained to their level or beyond, always under an authorized physician's command, and only in a licensed MICU or ER.

The law harks back to the 1970s, when New Jersey was first piloting advanced-life-support programs. The State Department of Health and Senior Services found that ALS caregivers working with nonparamedics "could not perform all the critical tasks fast enough" and "excessively delayed patient care."[1] It issued certificates of need to qualified hospitals and restricted paramedic resources to them.

"He's ALS!" O'Neill roars when he spots the BLS unit. "The guy is agonal already, for Christ's sake," which means the man is taking his dying breaths. *New Jersey prehospital medicine is so archaic, it's pathetic,* O'Neill thinks.

Although the man needs ALS in the field, the crews know he needs trauma surgeons more. They can't wait until MIC 5 figures out how to find them. Hoisting their patient onto the BLS stretcher, they rush him to the bus. The man's hands are bloodied. He wears white socks but no shoes; it's not uncommon for high-speed accident victims to be literally thrown from their footgear.

O'Neill drives the BLS bus, leaving the EMS workers two sets of hands in the box to do as much as they can. He pushes the speed up to 50 mph, alerts the trauma team by radio, and hopes to hell the guy doesn't code.[2]

The patient's olive skin is cool, pale, and damp, classic signs of shock. He doesn't respond to voice or touch. Blood pools in his throat and bubbles in mouth. *This is heinous,* the paramedic fumes, frustrated that that he, by law, has no intubation or intravenous equipment. He connects a football-shaped pumping device called a bag-valve mask to an oxygen tank, cranks the liter flow up to fifteen liters of oxygen per minute, and squeezes the vital gas into the man's chest through a mask over the man's face. Because it's 100 percent oxygen, whatever gas gets through is almost five times as concentrated as the man would receive from room air.

The bloody mouth doesn't offer much resistance, although the onboard suction unit might help clear the airway. Tilting the long board on its side would be cumbersome but it could encourage secretions to drain from the man's mouth. Since the air is going into the man's lungs, however, the paramedic keeps bagging. He lays his hand on the man's shoulder in a comforting gesture, and says, "You're gonna be OK, buddy." EMS workers choose whether and when to tell patients they are dying. The medic believes the man will die before sunrise, but he doesn't say so.

The EMT works the man's torso, cutting off his shirt to check his body for additional signs of injury. He sees none, but before he continues his exam he rechecks the patient's circulation. "I can't get a pulse, man," the EMT reports after carefully palpating the man's wrist. The medic bags with one hand, and digs for a pulse in the man's neck and finds one, albeit thin, with the other.

"I can't get a pressure either!" the EMT states just as O'Neill pulls into University's parking lot. The men haul their patient out of the truck, roll him briskly inside, and turn him over to the trauma team. By the time they scrub up and finish their paperwork, it's 0327 hours. The medic shrugs his shoulders and walks outside. The EMT writes the chart.

"It's what we signed on for," O'Neill surmises, long accustomed to going from one horrible situation to another. "If I took the time to dwell on it, I'd be outta my mind." He pauses for a cigarette and gets his first drag down when Dispatch sends them to the next wreck, a Taurus with four passengers and a stolen silver Porsche.

POETRY IN MOTION

B-team Rescue is part art, part science, and part sweat equity. In their combined thirty years, doing many hundreds of auto extrications each year, O'Neill and Heber have learned to read wrecks before they ever step out of the truck. "If we think the situation is critical, we go slam-bang fast and pull the doors off the fucking car," O'Neill explains. They stare at crushed metal and glass, estimate the vehicles' mass and velocity, and figure in the effects of probable rotational spins and successive impacts. Applying these rough calculations to their knowledge of anatomy and physiology, the rescue specialists do a fair job of predicting what damage their patients may have sustained as well as how best to get them out of the ruins without further injury. When their patients don't survive, it's not for lack of trying; it's not for lack of expertise. Sometimes it's not meant to be—an outcome they have come to accept.

Called to a two-car collision at Park Avenue and North Fifth, they rush their nineteen-ton truck to the busy North Ward intersection. Cherry-colored neon flares light up the night and warns traffic away from the chunks of shiny car parts. A cop contends with traffic, bystanders, and a hazardous debris field. A dull beige Cavalier sits in the crossroads, having completed half of its right turn before crashing into a gleaming black Honda. The Cavalier's front end is crumpled. The driver's door hangs open; he dashed down the street before police or EMS arrived, leaving it empty, except for the screwdriver he probably used to bust the steering column and jiggle the starter. (The B team has cut several thugs out of stolen cars, which Fazio calls "instant karma.")

The Honda, however, has what O'Neill calls "Spam in the can." The driver is still inside; her door absorbed the impact and now intrudes, pinning her between it and the console. Her husband climbed out only to pace frantically. The windshield is cracked, but there's no spiderweb pattern to indicate unrestrained heads smacked against it.

A BLS crew beats O'Neill and Heber to the scene by a few seconds. It's time enough for one to climb into the car and hold the patient's head steady, in line with her spine, while the other takes out a few windows with his center punch. The EMT inside the car quickly assesses his female patient. "No head injury," he shouts to Rescue. "She's only complaining of hip pain." He helps his partner apply the protective neck collar. His partner stays inside the car with the patient. The noise and vibrations, the sight of shattered glass and razor-edged metal, is frightening for trapped patients. It's soothing to have someone explain what is happening and offer assurance. When patients are calm, they are less liable to panic and exacerbate injuries. And their EMS workers can alert colleagues to any change in the patient's status.

Before either rescue specialist takes a tool to the car, they make their scene safe. Heber calls for engine-company backup in case an electrical fire ignites. As he gets dressed, he powers up the quartz light tower, which rises forty feet in the air to illuminate the intersection. When the bright lights go on, the scene smacks of a major-league ballpark. Whole fields of Coke-bottle green and obsidian glass glitter.

Heber draws two fire extinguishers from the truck. The red one sprays a dry chemical powder, which denies oxygen to fire and flammable liquids and solids. The silver one mixes aqueous film-forming foam to dilute and coat burning fluids, retard vapors, and starve the flame.

"It's nice and stable so we can take our time," O'Neill explains, training his steel blue eyes beneath both cars in search of leaking fluids. Finding none, he walks to the Honda and pops its hood. "We're slow and deliberate; we stick to procedure and still we beat the national average. The national average is thirty minutes, and we habitually never go longer than twenty minutes." O'Neill uses a cable cutter to disconnect the car's battery from its electrical system, reducing the chance of fire or the sudden deployment of airbags.

Meanwhile, Heber pulls out wheel and step chocks. The EMT grabs a few wheel chocks and stuffs them in front of and behind the tires to help stabilize the car. O'Neill shoves wooden step chocks underneath the vehicle frame, behind the two front wheel wells. He wedges two more in front of the rear wheel wells. As he deflates the tires, the frame comes to rest solidly on the four supports instead of the springy suspension. Now the car won't shake, rattle, or roll, much less collapse and cause additional injury to the patient or her rescuers.

Both rescuers say they witnessed another town's rescue service work on a wreck without securely stabilizing it. The car collapsed on a patient and crushed her. Fortunately, the woman was already dead. Another time, when Heber worked Rescue and O'Neill worked BLS, they reached an auto accident just after an engine company and just after the car exploded. "The car was blazing," Heber recalls, mesmerized by memories of firefighters attacking the inferno. "Little did we know there was a person in the passenger seat." But as soon as that became clear, and as soon as they "screamed like little girls," they called for medics and immediately plunged in—despite the fact that the car was still burning and each time firefighters knocked down the flame it reignited.

"He was melted to the dashboard and seat of his car," Heber says, remembering the patient. "We had to literally peel his skin off. His knees were stuck under the dashboard—it melted over his legs, arms, even his back had melted to the seat. When they ripped the dashboard out his hand skin came off, but it was the only way." This was one of several dreadful calls where O'Neill and Heber's actions earned them the rarely issued Class A medals equivalent to the Medal of Valor.

Exposure to such horrific incidents only reaffirms their overriding strategy. "We let the patient's condition, and best interest, determine our action," Heber explains. Their unique approach and training distinguish them. No other hospital that they have been able to find dispatches heavy rescue, much less in teams of two who are as qualified in extrication and other rescue disciplines as they are in patient care.

O'Neill, for example, is a nationally registered EMT-B, which means he has passed a rigorous test designed to bring caregivers up to Department of Transportation standards. O'Neill is also certified in at least eighteen other emergency-response specialties. And he is an expert instructor in fourteen key areas such as confined space, hazardous materials, and natural and man-made disaster management, including several types of terrorism. He earned his credentials from hands-on work with the state police, the Federal Bureau of Investigation, the

Federal Emergency Management Agency, the National Fire Academy, and the U.S. Air Force as well as other law-enforcement agencies and military divisions. And Heber has racked up extensive firefighting and disaster-management credentials of his own. All that training might make a simple extrication seem tame, even boring, but the two never tire of polishing their craft.

To shield the entrapped woman against shards of glass, slivers of metal, and sparks to come, O'Neill tosses a thick, flash-proof blanket to the EMT, who drapes it over his partner and the patient. O'Neill peels back sheets of fractured window glass from their metal rims; most of the cracked glass hangs together by dint of illegal tinting film.

The bright lights, sparkling glass, buzzing tools, super-sized truck, and twisted metal are sheer spectacle, although crashes due to car theft happen frequently here. In 1990, nearly 15,000 cars were stolen in Newark, which helped earn the city its reputation as car-theft capital of the world. Last year, 5,365 cars were stolen here (not counting cars snatched from affluent suburbs and brought to Newark for parts or joy rides). O'Neill compares car theft in Newark to a fatty tumor. "It's not attractive," he says, "but it's there."

As if the circus has come to town, crowds gather and camp on all four corner properties: a Hess station, a Kentucky Fried Chicken restaurant, a car wash, and an industrial building. It's night, it's dark, it's winter—nevertheless, boys wander and ride their bicycles through the surreal scene. A man in sweatpants and open-toed sandals takes it all in. Someone in open-toed sandals is always in the crowd of onlookers no matter what time of year. The cop is beside himself keeping onlookers at a safe distance and directing traffic around the colorful mess. He leans on his cruiser and honks, and he points, and he shouts.

Heber and O'Neill prepare for the demolition by lugging the tools they will use from compartments on the truck's right side. The entire truck is geared for a two-man operation. They designed it so that each side is the mirror image of the other. The duplication of tools and power supplies is intentional. Whichever way they approach a scene, they have quick, convenient access to their power and their rich bank of equipment. Both men have their favorite tools, and both insist on "the right tool for the right job." Sometimes it's a metal-cutting Slicepak, a torch that burns pure oxygen and runs at 10,000°F, and sometimes it's simply a pair of pliers. "I can't tell you how many times we've been called to an entrapment to find the people on scene just didn't unlock the door!" Heber chuckles.

Rescue rides under the theory of "preconnection," which means that its tools are stored set up and ready to go, which saves them five minutes a job, O'Neill says. Colored tubes connect each device to its air compressor, generator, or other power source; this minimizes confusion if a hose blows or they need to shut down a single machine. Heber extracts several hydraulic contrivances: a standard O cutter, which weighs about thirty pounds, and its dull red hose; a forty-six-pound spreader connected to a mustard yellow hose; the thirty-five-pound Combo tool, fed by a royal blue hose; and their Speedway cutters, which also weigh thirty-five pounds and are hooked up to a smudged-black hose. By the time he has everything lined up, perspiration shines on his ruddy, freckled face. Four minutes have passed since they arrived.

Heber lowers his safety goggles over his eyes and uses the spreader to nudge the driver's crushed door out the way it would naturally open. "We take advantage of physics," Heber clarifies. "It's easier and it saves time."

He takes the whole door off, walks a few feet away, and tosses it aside as if it's a soda can. O'Neill uses the O cutters to sever the hinge between the door and the kick panel while Heber uses the spreader to defeat the locking mechanism, then press the door down and rotate it off its Nader pin. When he tugs, it comes off as easily as paper towel torn from its roll. *This is emergency-service poetry in motion*, O'Neill thinks. *It's so clean, logical, and linear, it's almost science.* "Usually in rescue a single act is performed at any given time," he explains. "With us, we've been together so long, I'm comfortable working right next to him while he's using a hydraulic tool that can take my head clean off."

With the front and the rear doors gone, Heber needs only to use the customized Sawzall to cut the B-post, the vertical column between the doors. The pine-scented air freshener that hangs from the mirror barely twitches. Their technique yields an opening, roughly six feet wide by three feet high, for patient extrication. "A lot of other rescuers do door pops, pulling it back a little for patient caregivers to work their way inside. After a door pop, though, it's only another two cuts and a wire snip to make a much bigger opening," Heber explains. "We remove the vehicle from the patient, not the patient from the vehicle."

O'Neill wraps a ballistic nylon pad around the roof edge to protect everyone when they reach in for their patient. "OK to take her out!" he announces.

Heber kneels and slides the long board beneath the woman's behind. With one EMS worker still holding the woman's head and back in line, the other reclines the seat, then takes control of her skull and spine, leaving his partner free to guide the woman's shoulders. The EMT at the patient's head controls the count, and on three they glide her upper torso in one smooth movement over the long board in line with her hips. Heber and an EMT slide the woman slowly onto the board as the other lifts her calves from the floor and rests them on the body splint, too. As they pull her out, her head, spine, and legs are aligned. O'Neill braces the stretcher, where they rest the boarded woman down and buckle her in.

This technique, called "rapid takedown," is accomplished in moments, and usually reserved for patients whose vital signs signify distress. If a patient's condition is sufficiently stable to tolerate a slightly longer procedure, EMS workers suit up patients in KEDs (Kendrick Extrication Devices) before removing them from wrecks. A KED is a short, cushioned board with straps and padding to secure and protect the abdomen, legs, chest, and head. Patients end up resembling overturned turtles that have been stuffed into hockey or parachuting getups. But the device goes a bit further in protecting their spines and backs. KEDs are a national standard of care for stable patients. But things move fast and furious in Newark, and sometimes they seem like an excessive impediment to care, and they are ignored.

"Get a blanket on her!" O'Neill barks at the EMS workers as they roll her to their bus. "It's fucking freezing." Despite the cold, he's now down to his shirtsleeves, and Heber's rosy cheeks and curly brown hair are wet with sweat. The job, a simple one by their standards, took all of eleven minutes.

A police-approved towing service hauls the wrecks away; it leaves a car seat and a stuffed Bugs Bunny on the ground. O'Neill gathers information for his report and the billing form he helped design. Heber shuts off the hydraulic pumps, breaks down the equipment, and switches his mental checklist back on. Inevitably the hoses get tangled, so he disconnects the tools, puts everything back in its place, and then reconnects everything. Methodically, he examines each blade to see if it has dulled. Heber is nothing if not fastidious and also checks the remaining gas, the hydraulic fluids, and whether he needs to replenish the compressed air.

Most of the blue-shirts think Rescue has a posh deal, working anywhere from zero to ten jobs, sometimes more, a night. O'Neill says it used to be "slam-bang, bing-boom, crisis-to-crisis" when Newark was drowning in violent crime and chockablock with high-rise projects that crammed thousands of poor people into a few tall acres. At three thousand to six thousand jobs per year, the Pros from Dover are content to let their work speak for itself.

NINJAS-CUM-JACKS-OF-ALL-TRADES

During one of its economic crunches about twenty years ago, Newark slashed fire-rescue and police emergency budgets. The money-saving tactic did not prevent people from falling into construction pits, wrecking their cars, and becoming otherwise imperiled and in need of EMS. Back then, the EMS director padded the schedule with two extra EMTs who ran hospital errands, such as transporting blood to an off-site lab and retrieving results. Mario Piumelli and Artie Hayducka, both of whom are now field supervisors, served as those float EMTs. Of their own volition, they obtained rescue training and volunteered to start up a departmental rescue service. It seemed pointless to send EMS to calamitous scenes without access to ensnared patients, they argued. Spotting a novel opportunity to combine technical rescue with EMS, the former department director seized it.

At first, they self-limited their practice to mini-rescues, strictly auto, Piumelli recalls. Over time, the unit invested in the training and equipment needed to handle diverse challenges. Rescue tackles elevator mishaps and accidents in the city's myriad industrial parks; for example, when a worker gets entrapped in a conveyor belt, Dispatch sends Rescue. Sheets of metal crushed a lone after-hours worker once. He used his cell phone to dial 911 before falling unconscious. Dispatch tasked Rescue to lift the load, but first it had to locate the man, who lay somewhere on an acres-large property. By emitting shrill blasts from their near-deafening horn, Rescue sent signals through the open channel on the patient's phone. Dispatch used the noise to discern Rescue's distance from the patient. Taking this cooler-versus-warmer game to a new level of import, Dispatch guided the truck to the patient.

Rescue manages water incidents, too—for example, the person who jumped from the Bridge Street Bridge into the mighty Passaic River, or the car that sped out of control and into Branch Brook Park's lake, or the many occasions cars careen off area roadways to sink into swampy marshes.

Rescue addresses structural incidents, also. Once, for instance, a man plunged through the floorboards on a decrepit home's front porch. Rescue cut away the porch support beams and planking and shored up the remaining structure so they could extricate the man without further mishap.

Rescue executes special lifts and lowerings, too, such as the time when Newark's $187 million performing arts center was built. A construction worker high up on the iron framework injured himself. Rescue brought him down using their ropes and Stokes (a rigid plastic container).

With police participation, Rescue handles forcible entries so emergency workers can help trapped patients or access those who have barricaded themselves. It also participates in Federal Aviation Administration drills and weapons-of-mass-destruction exercises.

Besides making it safe for coworkers to treat patients in otherwise hostile environments and get out of jams, Rescue opens car doors for colleagues who lock their keys inside and makes it possible for broken trucks to limp back to quarters. These all-purpose, go-to guys have a female team member, too. They are ninjas-cum-jacks-of-all-trades.

Most of those who work Rescue have other certifications, too, which they exercise staffing the MCRU, the Urban Search and Rescue Team, the Special Operations Group, and the Emergency Response Team, which backs up police SWAT missions.

Occasionally, the ER calls them for help. Rescue has used its Dremel drill to cut rings and other objects (including a trumpet) off patients' limbs. Rescue has also removed patients from large machines; loaned a three-eighths-inch drill to an orthopedic surgeon; and used its generators to provide power during blackouts for essential hospital equipment such as ventilators.

Even the medical examiner's office sometimes needs Rescue's assistance. People burned in car fires, for example, are considered crime-scene fatalities until proven otherwise, Heber explains. "The medical examiner does a lot of investigation while bodies are still in the vehicle. Sometimes the ME has the entire vehicle flat-bedded to his office in Newark and calls us to extricate it."

Of the burned corpses, Heber says matter-of-factly, "Their faces shrivel in the heat. A lot of them burn right down to the bone or they blow out from the inside—their brain matter and organs. Sometimes you can't make out if their mouth is opened or closed. A lot of people think the extrication of dead bodies is difficult, but to us it's not. I find it interesting. We do things other people cannot, be it because of the type of call, the knowledge, or the use of equipment."

Rescue and their EMS colleagues "do things" because they are passionate about disaster management. Except for auto extrication, which helps recoup a small portion of costs, all of Rescue's services are gratis. Management has not found a way to convince recipients to pay for the help they receive. The department has billed auto insurers for cutting people out of car wrecks for only two years, although EMS workers say they lobbied this point for more than a decade after reading about other states who set precedent.

Last night, Heber and O'Neill spent three frosty hours lighting up a dark street so detectives could investigate and a police photographer could piece together the scene of a triple shooting. Police had the equipment and manpower to do the work, but their truck was broken. Heber and O'Neill not only lit the scene but also did the better half of diagnosing and fixing the police emergency-response truck. "Tell the City of Newark to pay its bill and put lighting in our contract," Heber growls under his breath. Like his colleagues, he's become bored with what seems to be perpetual payment delays and a permanent budget crunch. "Police are always considered the first service. Fire comes second. EMS is the bastard stepchild. Nobody wants to pay for it. It's a pain in the ass to run. But everybody wants it when they need it." In 1999, law-enforcement expenses in the city were approximately $92 million. Firefighting cost just over $48 million. The city paid EMS $1.3 million.

The department's contract with the city expired this year. Like those of many EMS services, the department's revenue stream is largely tied to the number of patients transported, which is almost like paying police for the number of crimes solved or compensating firefighters for the number of fires extinguished. The flawed model does not cover the expenses of maintaining a state of readiness.

Some forty percent of EMS calls here turn out to be false alarms or people who ultimately refuse aid and don't pay a penny for summoning the medical cavalry. Many patients are uninsured. Some have insurance companies who refuse to pay, arguing that transport by EMS was not medically necessary or that the patient had not obtained advanced approval. The city's contributions to EMS's costs are limited to Newark residents who take no more than one trip to the hospital per day. It issues payment only after an annual audit and after hospital administrators have proven that no other payer can be tapped.

Policymakers and the public expect the department to maintain its fleet of emergency vehicles and equipment, keep a sufficient stock of supplies, employ crews, and provide a timely response as well as medicine for everyone who calls 911, regardless of their ability to pay. This year, those costs have left the department several million dollars in the red. University EMS isn't the only system confronting such problems.

The director is following NHTSA's lead and renegotiating on the basis of cost preparedness as opposed to reimbursement for a fraction of patients transported.[3] She wants to establish a predictable budget. She wants the city to distribute its payments monthly instead of as its annual, postaudit sum. She wants land on which to build an integrated EMS facility, for blue-shirts, dispatchers, supervisors, managers, and vehicles. She wants money for capital renewal.

If she can't achieve her objective, there are other tactics to cut costs and increase productivity, she says. The fire department can take on the role of first responder. "Firefighters are located in every neighborhood. They would be getting to calls first, validating the need, and letting us know whether to keep coming or cancel. It would reduce our unproductive-response rate."

She may have to cut programs that everyone has come to value, from dispatch and fire standbys to dignitary protection. "It's all on the table," she says ominously.

BASIC TRAINING

The Rescue unit is small and tight, operating with eight full-time members. Six more have earned Rescue status as well as three part-timers, aka "per diems." (Per diems have the same certifications as full-timers but only work occasionally.) In addition to O'Neill and Heber, Drivet, Callahan, Opperman, Piumelli, Mendez, and Hayducka, the unit's chief, have worked Rescue. Hayducka even competes internationally in extrication championships on his own time. This fall, Rescue lost four members. Two left to work for the union, and two were injured. Per diems can fill in the holes temporarily, but O'Neill wants a firmer plan. Over homemade spaghetti and sauce, which he prepared with a touch of molasses and brought in to share with Heber, the two wrestle with obstacles that have made it nearly impossible to hold a new Rescue-class and identify qualified recruits.

Prerequisites for the Rescue training course are daunting. To ensure that everyone who joins is steeped in patient protection and care, Rescue requires at least three years' experience on University ambulances and a top-notch record—no warnings or other disciplinary actions for at least two years. Candidates must also have mastered courses such as Confined Space Rescue and Incident Command, which teach EMS workers how to organize complex incidents that may also involve military, elected officials, bureaucrats, media, other emergency-response agencies, etc.

The Rescue class is not offered frequently. Competition is fierce. Some think of Rescue as a step up the EMS ladder for BLS workers; they get off the insanely busy trucks and into an interesting niche.[4] With hundreds of tools and machines, even one that can boil a sidewalk and slice through iron reinforcement bars, the job demands mechanical aptitude and the ability to grasp fluid mechanics, physics, and other applied sciences for real-time problem solving.

When management posts a sign-up sheet for the next Rescue course, more than thirty-five applicants volunteer.

The first phase, ninety-six hours, is a far cry from the first classes. "In 1983, Rescue class was two days and some practice cutting up cars on a Sunday afternoon," Piumelli recalls. Now candidates must master Basic and Advanced Vehicle Extrication, Knot Craft, Basic and Advanced Rope Rescue, Rescue Vehicle Operations, and High Angle Rescue, followed by a written and hands-on skill test. High scores are not enough; no one gets rubber-stamped.

To progress to phase two—a grueling 120- to 180-hour internship—candidates must pass a prequalifying test. "To work on the truck, you have to have knowledge, applicable skills, and the physical attribute of being able to carry two-thirds of your own body weight," O'Neill says. "It's intensely physical. You gotta have enough upper-body strength or you're going to fail at a critical juncture. You gotta be able to pick up the tools, or you'll have nothing left, and the time for that not to happen is when two critical patients are trapped in a car." He also looks for applicants who have continually added skills throughout their careers.

Learning the tools, where they are located, how they are powered, handled, cleaned, and maintained is no small accomplishment. "From the time they get here until the time they leave, they go over the tools, learn knots, rub our feet, and clean the truck," one Rescue specialist says, laughing now that he's survived the ordeal. "They made me wash the truck at the beginning and end of each shift," he remembers. But he doesn't begrudge them. "It's the best damn job in the University. They give us a $375,000 truck with a million dollars' worth of equipment and they give us the keys. The city is our playground and we come to play!"

The internship, like the prerequisites and the time invested in taking the classes, is at the candidates' expense and on their own time. Contenders must test out of the internship by working through challenging scenarios. For example, O'Neill may order them to execute a rope rescue technique called the "incline pickoff." Hopefuls will set up and rappel down ropes, find an "unconscious victim" in a precarious position, free the patient from any entanglements, attach him to their own equipment, and either haul the injured party back up or lower him to safe ground.

The six-hour driving class that follows teaches candidates how to handle their gargantuan vehicle with professional truck-driving skills. "It's an average-sized truck about the size of a school bus," Heber explains, "but it can pull a semi." He compares its power to that of six cars or five sport-utility vehicles. Candidates must take and pass the same test as those seeking commercial driving licenses.

Their final exam is pure hands-on problem solving.

The last hurdles are a six-month probation, a course in hazardous-materials operations, and training to become a technician on the department's MCRU. It's a bit of an uphill sprint to the finish. O'Neill admits that when he first joined the truck "it was fucking bedlam." Between him and his partner, "neither one of us could get soup out of a can."

Once appointed to Rescue, specialists get a patch for their uniform and the ability to safely do with two people what the rest of the Rescue world usually does with five. "That's what makes it fun," Heber says. "We could use a third person definitely, to do the driving, set up, get us additional equipment, act as our safety officer. Yeah, a third person would be nice." But for twenty years now they have made do without.

Rescue specialists spend their own time, money, and muscle mass to earn their positions, but they earn no extra pay.

CRUSADES

O'Neill is the chief shop steward for the blue-shirts' union, Teamsters Local 97. Among his duties, he advises employees as to their rights, suggests what action to take or not to take, advocates for them, and files formal grievances, too. He devotes about twenty-four hours per week to this, for which he is paid $75 per year.

Each week, O'Neill deals with eight or nine cases. He just finished helping an EMT who wanted to change shifts. "Except for a couple of smudges, this guy is a model employee," O'Neill says, leaning forward in his seat. "He's worked here two years, and whenever they"—management—"needed someone to fill in, he always came. When they needed people to work Newark high-school games, he came. He even volunteered his time to work on the bike team.

He was given custody of his kid. Well, he's been working 2:00 P.M. to 2:00 A.M., and he asks for a transfer to the 7:00 A.M. to 7:00 P.M. shift because it's easier for him to arrange day care. He was basically told the 2:00 P.M. to 2:00 A.M. truck is hard to fill, and that we put new hires in the 7:00 A.M. to 7:00 P.M. slot, 'cause new hires won't wanna take the 2:00 P.M. to 2:00 A.M. I seriously think they don't give a fuck." KinderCare, where employees can safely stash their children, is a hundred yards from the EMS compound. But O'Neill notes, "There's no KinderCare here at night. And the night-shift differential is only ninety cents per hour"—the extra pay overnight workers earn to compensate them for arranging their lives according to vampire hours.

To argue his charge's case, O'Neill subjected management to "warfare."

"We hounded them—calling seventeen or eighteen times a day, leaving as many voice mails. We E-mailed them thirty times a day. 'I need to know why we're not transferring him. Why can't your scheduling chief help out this model employee? Why are you telling him he can go scratch? If we're all one big happy family, why can't we help him with this child-care issue?' We just kept the phone ringing and the E-mail zinging, and in a week to two weeks he got his transfer."

Asked why he dedicates so much time to furthering his colleagues' interests at the expense of his own—he also has a sixteen-hour-per-week second job, has a college degree in process, holds office in two professional societies, and has a family with young children—O'Neill becomes downright loquacious. "Management sometimes abuses its power and takes advantage of the weak," he says, "and I hate bullies."

He'd like to increase tuition reimbursement for EMS workers. The department offers help toward an undergraduate degree, but nothing for professional education. It organizes some, but not all, of the classes workers need to maintain their state certifications. But those who must attend job-related classes elsewhere pay out of pocket—sometimes hundreds of dollars. Most get no time off and no subsidies to attend skill-building professional conferences, despite the fact that EMS must change as fast as the needs of the population it serves. And the development of drugs and biotechnology is rapid. As hospitals cut costs, sending patients home with more drugs, new types of catheters, and complex life-sustaining equipment, questions arise. Panicked caretakers call 911. EMS workers need to prepare for such situations, experts say. But on salaries hovering between $28,000 and $45,000, most find it difficult to continually underwrite the perpetual education that keeps their skills and certifications current.

O'Neill hopes to forge career paths so EMS workers don't have to jump ship in favor of police, firefighting, nursing, or other alternatives that promise better pay, education benefits, and pensions. He'd like to establish safeguards so management can't force EMS workers to stay on the job and behind the wheel eighteen hours at a clip. But most of all, O'Neill is a competitor who wants to win.

"By nature, I'm a warrior and I can't pass up a good fight." O'Neill grins, referring to his Celtic origins. "I strip naked, paint myself blue, and throw myself headlong into battle." If he took even the twenty-four hours a week he contributes to the union and applied it to his wife and children, his academics, and his martial arts, O'Neill might be happier. And he might break his habit of pitting himself against various IQ tests, which consistently rank him in the top echelon. These quick validation fixes do not last long, for he is overqualified and underchallenged at work. He could polish off his baccalaureate and move on. But his fighting instincts come naturally. "Rabble-rousers run in the family," O'Neill admits. "We sing sad songs about love and happy songs about war. We're a weird twisted people, and I carry that into everything I do."

O'Neill's father was a postal-worker shop steward and an Army medic in peacetime Korea's demilitarized zone. His grandpa Jimmy was active in Ireland's Troubles. And his ancestors raised pugnacity to a whole new level. O'Neill says his family's coat of arms tells the tale of two clans racing toward an island where no one had ever been before. Whoever touched the soil first would get to keep it. Just offshore, the boats were neck and neck. O'Neill says his ancestor cut off his hand and threw it ashore, thereby touching it first. "I can't surrender and I can't retreat," he states with a fiery twinkle in his eyes.

Although his principles are glorious and he does improve his coworkers' lives, O'Neill must know that the battles he wins will be small, and they're sure to come at great cost. His colleagues may rally around his noble goals and cheer him on, but he has a tough sell even inside the union. Their Teamsters local lumps EMS workers with housekeepers, janitors, and truck drivers rather than nurses, physician assistants, or other allied health workers. That's not uncommon; other states commingle EMS workers with supermarket cashiers. Even within the union, the blue-shirts are a minority, 250 versus 3,000. The majority is far more interested in fiberglass broom handles vs. wooden ones, fifty-cent raises, and extra coffee breaks, O'Neill grouses.

Changing unions is another matter entirely. That would require the blue-shirts to open their wallets and fork over cash to pay for attorneys. More important, they would have to identify some other union to take them in. Neither the firefighters nor the police want EMS, even though EMS tends to their burns, their smoke inhalation, their gunshot and stab wounds, and their broken bodies enmeshed in wrecks. Nurses don't want them either, O'Neill says, although

EMS workers here draw blood for routine labs, intubate patients, and start IVs, which the overtaxed nurses would have to do if the EMS workers didn't bother. Finally, the hospital would have to agree with the plan, too, which goes against its self-interest, he explains.

When asked what his role as chief stop steward gets him, the thirty-four-year-old deadpans, "Chest pain." He's not joking.

FATTY FATTY BOOMBALATTI

Heber and O'Neill dash out of their cramped office and head south for an "assist-carry." Rescue is adept at moving very large people, from those who weigh hundreds of pounds to those more than a thousand pounds. In fact, they answer close to 175 similar calls a year, O'Neill estimates. And that is just a glimpse through the window onto obesity, a problem experts say fifty-eight million Americans share, and one the World Health Organization characterizes as "the global chronic health problem in adults."[5]

Soon they're rumbling down the residential street toward the ambulance, its crew, and a small crowd huddled in the frozen twilight. When they park, EMT Ennis Terrell comes over to brief them. At six feet, four inches, with a big gold earring and a rakish smile, Terrell is a natural showman who delights in his very public job. But this evening his voice is unusually diplomatic. "She just moved here, but she can't hold her weight to get upstairs," he explains, tossing his head back at the folks bunched together near a paint-worn tenement whose foundation is cracked and crumbling and whose only lawn is weeds. "She took a cab here, and has been sitting out in this cold all day. She just never considered the steps."

Peering at the group, O'Neill and Heber make out a mountain of a woman in a crocheted cap of fiery yellow, red, and green, swathed in blankets. Terrell tells them she could not even walk through the unfamiliar neighborhood in search of a pay phone. Aghast at her situation, as the hours ticked by, as the cold commenced to sting and bite, she began to cry. A passerby offered to phone a relative. Her sister and nephew responded. But they could not get the woman up the stairs. So she sat. The sun set. And the windchill plunged near zero.

Eventually her sister called the police, who patched her through to EMS, who sent Terrell and Che-heibe Scott, his partner. The patient asked only for help getting upstairs into her apartment, but the two EMTs politely refused. They were incapable of moving her bulk in the first place, and even if they could, they would be derelict leaving her inside, knowing she can't get herself out in case of emergency. Terrell and Scott know obese patients often develop co-morbid conditions that can necessitate urgent hospital visits. High blood pressure, for example, increases the risk of heart attack, stroke, and kidney failure. Diabetes can lead to heart failure, blindness, and amputation. Obesity is also associated with certain cancers, osteoarthritis, coronary artery, and gallbladder disease.[6]

The situation is approaching an impasse. The woman does not want to go to the hospital, and it is against the law to force a competent person to accept care. *She cannot get inside; she cannot care for herself; it's really goddamn cold out; and ethically, we can't leave her on the street,* O'Neill thinks. "We'll Stokes her and we'll ramp her," he suggests. That means substituting their Stokes basket, a yellow and black heavy-duty container rated for 1,200 pounds, for the regular cot, which can only tolerate 325 pounds.

Although ambulance crews sometimes push their luck, a stretcher collapsing under a patient means heartache and possibly a lawsuit, too, Heber explains. Nor does Rescue want anyone on the team getting hurt. Back injuries related to lifting and moving are one of the most prevalent disabilities EMS workers suffer.

O'Neill and Heber plan to build a ramp from the precut lumber they carry. After loading the woman into their Stokes and placing her on the furniture dolly they keep specifically for such cases, they'll roll her up and onto the ambulance floor, lash her down, and beat feet to the hospital.

But Hayducka, their chief, is on the scene, and he kills plan A. He wants something simpler. O'Neill and Heber switch to plan B. "The hardest part of Rescue is not executing plan A; it's having plans B, C, and D at the ready and being able to transition to them as needed," O'Neill says. "What separates the men from the boys is knowing what to do when plan A fails . . . and plan A always fails."

Heber yanks the cot from the bus, shoves it to the side, and radios Dispatch, asking for an ambulance to retrieve it. O'Neill pulls the Stokes out from the truck and lines it with blankets and several sheets. Heber works around him, weaving thick rope through the basket's handles. When the makeshift nest is ready, they join BLS. "Why don't you come with us to the hospital and we can sort things out from there?" O'Neill invites the woman. Terrell and Scott coax her, too. Anxiously she consents.

O'Neill and Heber reach behind the woman's back and grasp each other's forearms, and each holds one of the woman's forearms as well. Terrell and Scott will each brace a side of the woman's upper back. When she rises they can support her and pull her forward. O'Neill counts, "One, two, three!" and they get her up on her feet for the first time in half a day. "Just walk right over this way," O'Neill says, steering her toward the ambulance.

"I'm sorry," the woman whispers morosely. Her eyes droop. Her mouth sags. Her cheeks and jowls dangle. Her light-skinned, chubby, but otherwise pretty face droops like a wilted flower. With each step she staggers, and her weight swims around her as if she were Hula-Hooping a set of Michelin tires.

"Don't worry," O'Neill says gamely. "You're not the only person in the world like this."

The patient's sister, a veritable toothpick by comparison, cries quietly and flits about the tiny procession in neatly creased khakis and a burgundy beret, fretting that they might drop her sibling. The patient's nine-year-old nephew sobs inconsolably. As they approach the ambulance, her blankets begin to slip off. The husky youngster gathers them to his chest and buries his head; his shoulders shake with grief. Although he keeps his fingers near his eyes to wipe away the tears, they come too fast and cascade down his velvety brown cheeks. He's so overcome he gets the hiccups. It's impossible to know if he shares his mother's worry, if he's grieving for his aunt's embarrassment, or if he's suffering some other emotion such an event might provoke in a child. He grieves alone, with nary a hug or a word of comfort.

"These situations are overwhelming to the providers, too," O'Neill explains later. "It becomes an all-hands-on effort, with nobody left to offer emotional support to the family."

As the small parade escorts her to the ambulance, it becomes clear to them that the woman had wet herself sometime during her hours-long ordeal. Her urine has frozen; an icy, irregular banana-colored patch covers the pubic triangle of her green stretch pants.

When they reach the bus, the Stokes is waiting, leaning against the ambulance and resting on the sidewalk. O'Neill and Heber do the slow-motion equivalent of spinning her around so her back faces the bus and she looks toward the crowd. The woman looks wide-eyed and terrified.

"Grab me," Heber says, offering her his arm.

"Y'all gonna drop me," the woman half asks, half predicts.

"No," Heber assures her. "No, we won't."

"Just lean back," O'Neill instructs. The woman shuts her eyes and clutches their upper arms with all her might as they ease her back into the Stokes basket.

Using the corner where the ambulance floor turns down to meet the bumper as a lever, O'Neill and Heber lift the bottom of the Stokes, raise it up, and slide her in. *Give me a lever long enough and I'll raise the entire world,* O'Neill thinks, paraphrasing Archimedes.

Heber takes off in the Rescue truck and drives to the hospital, where he'll lend a hand getting the woman inside. As he drives, he estimates her weight to be between 550 and 600 pounds. *That's just fat,* he ponders. *It's amazing. That's just from people feeding her.*

Scott drives the ambulance. Terrell prepares the chart. Crying from the humiliation, the woman dutifully answers his questions and apologizes. "I'm so sorry," she weeps. "I'm so sorry I embarrassed my family."

"No need to be embarrassed," O'Neill assures her. "We see this situation all the time; this is what we're here for." He chalks it up to the party line, but he takes the extra step of holding her hand all the way to the hospital. If his peers on the B team knew this, they'd bust him mercilessly, because O'Neill is rawhide-tough. But the innate humanity he works so hard to squelch rises to the occasion as he witnesses her distress.

When they arrive at University, Scott backs into a space and hops out to open the bus's back doors. Heber is waiting with a trauma stretcher; it supports more weight than the average gurney. He rounds up a few EMS workers to brace it and climbs into the ambulance to help O'Neill. "We're going to lift the head up and tilt, and you'll slide onto the stretcher," O'Neill tells the woman. It's basically gravity at work, he explains. Rescue prefers to do such transfers outside. They have more room to maneuver, which makes it safer for everyone. One of many unpleasant memories burned into O'Neill's brain is the sight of another EMS squad rolling their enormous patient out of a Stokes, then onto, then over the side of an ER bed. The patient ended facedown on the hospital floor. He won't let that happen.

The woman's natural reaction is to reach out for something to stabilize herself, but O'Neill warns, "Ma'am, you have to keep your arms inside." Their faces turn crimson with effort, but the two raise the top of the Stokes. The patient's family stands by, stiff with anxiety. The sister is so worried that the crew will drop her sibling that she literally shields her eyes, and the boy's tears renew.

The patient slides solidly onto the stretcher in one piece. Her flesh, however, ripples and sways as if she had landed on a waterbed. "Y'all right?" Terrell asks, showing off his movie-star grin and Southern drawl. She nods as he and Scott wheel her toward the ER. "We just got to find one of these rooms," he explains, looking to make eye contact with one of the busy nurses.

As O'Neill and Heber assemble their equipment, they talk about the call. O'Neill thinks the woman's weight problem is genetic, because, if memory serves him, "this woman's brother is a boombalatti, too." (Fatty Fatty Boombalatti is local slang for really fat person.)

"Her brother was living in a multistory wood-frame house that caught fire a few years ago," he recalls. Firefighters figured they could not get the man down the stairway full of smoke without great risk of injury to him or themselves. And he did not have the strength to move his own weight. "So they put him on high-concentration O_2, sheltered him in place with a heat-resistant blanket, and left." In short, they fought the fire around the man while his surroundings broiled.

"They put the fire out, but the building was unsalvageable. It was unlivable—no power, no gas, no water," O'Neill says. "And there's this six-hundred-pound man in the ruins of the building, unable to walk out. Our guys went over, lit the building up, took him out, and brought him to his sister's place. They said the place had cases of Hershey's and bundles of White Castle bags.

"We expend our manpower and equipment on people who don't really need ambulances but just can't take care of themselves. We've been able to put some pressure on our social workers so they can pressure city welfare, because they're paying these people's rent so they should find them acceptable housing. If it's all city-owned, they should be moved to the first floor," he reasons.

In this case, whoever secured the first-floor apartment for this patient did only half of his or her homework. The apartment sits at the top of a ten-step flight, which for this woman might as well be atop Mount Everest.

"I do what I can to make them feel better about what's going on at the moment," O'Neill explains. "But the sad truth is, I personally cannot make a difference in her life circumstances. I am in her life for a little while, and after I do my part, it's up to the doctors, nurses, social workers, and families to follow through.

"I'm not saying she doesn't deserve sympathy, but, emotionally, I don't have anything left to give. I can't make a commitment." He tucks into his chicken Parmesan sandwich, and Heber eats his salami hero in silence, watching the World Wrestling Federation personalities throw their weight around on the TV at quarters.

6

CHECK IT OUT, CHECK IT OUT

RED HERRING

Callahan and Cardona's evening warms up with a feverish, sexually active woman with AIDS and severe stomach cramps, a psychotic middle-aged man who tried to "stick up" the Cozy Corner bar with a "stick," and a middle-aged diabetic man vomiting blood. At 2126 hours Dispatch assigns them a "male, down" on a street lined with towering trees and sprawling Victorian homes. No lights brighten the vintage four-story home's shadowy façade. The chain-link gate creaks in response to Cardona's shove. He jogs up a stone staircase and knocks. No one answers. He thumps harder. Finally, he turns, looks down at his partner, and shrugs.

The house seems familiar, Callahan thinks, scrunching his eyes closed and searching his memory. *Have I been here before?* "Benny, I think the entrance might be round back," he hollers from the truck. "Let's check it out before we do a callback." The two meet on the sidewalk, shoulder their gear, and hike up a dark and quiet driveway.

Toward the rear a yellow porch light glows. It silhouettes a police officer standing with his foot in the door taking notes. Callahan and Cardona's feet crunch on the gravel, and the officer turns at the sound. They nod at each other. The cop stands just outside a well-lit vestibule. Inside, a staircase leads up and a door opens to a ground-floor apartment. A coal black, heavy-busted woman in a floral dress stands in her entryway, arms folded across her chest, jaw clenched, eyes trained on a man contorting himself on the stairs; the EMTs get a first glimpse of their patient.

The officer steps back so the EMTs can evaluate the man.

Their patient hovers faceup over the steep stairs. He suspends his torso between his arms, outstretched backward on a step above him, and his legs, bent and planted several stairs below. Beneath a tomato red baseball cap, his dark round face is slick with sweat, and perspiration makes his black T-shirt cling. But overall he appears robust and tidy. He wears a necklace of beads the color of autumn gourds. "I was strong and healthy," the man bawls. His eyes dart back and forth, searching the officer's and the EMTs' faces for answers. "I don't know what is going on."

"What happened tonight, sir?" Cardona asks.

"I don't know!" the man cries. Nodding at the woman, he says, "Me and her husband were out in the yard cleaning fish, and then I went to bed. I got up to pee and fell down." The man's lips tremble, and he shakes from the strain of his position. "I ain't got the strength to walk, man."

Cardona stares at the woman. *Who is she and what does she have to say about this?* he wonders. She meets his gaze and slowly shakes her head from side to side. Something is amiss already; now the EMTs have to figure out what it is.

"Who are you to him, ma'am?" Cardona asks.

"His cousin."

"I broke my neck in a car accident," the man volunteers.

Those few words carry weight, and the partners glimpse at each other. They might need to immobilize the man's neck and spine with a cervical collar and long board. Cardona probes deeper: "When did you do that?"

"In 1985."

"Shit, that was fifteen years ago," Cardona grumbles under his breath. He tilts his head to the driveway, a signal to the cop that he won't need help, and the officer takes off. "What did you break?" Cardona asks.

"C1 and C2." Cervical vertebrae one and two stand just beneath the brain stem, and a fracture of either can easily be fatal. "They did a bone fusion but it never healed right."

Callahan is ready to return to the bus for additional equipment when Cardona reaches for the jug of apple juice the man has beside him. Cardona wants it out of the way before he squeezes into the tight area to hold the man's head steady. But the patient snatches the jug and clutches it to his broad chest.

"You gotta put the juice down, sir," Cardona insists.

"I want my juice, man," the patient pleads. "It stops me from having the shakes."

"Are you diabetic?" If so, the partners may have to evaluate his behavior differently, and they may need paramedics. When some diabetics suffer from excessively low blood sugar, their brains, deprived of glucose, malfunction. Perfectly sober patients can behave, and even smell, as though they are intoxicated.

"I have sugar."

"Did a doctor tell you that you are diabetic?"

"No, but I need it," the man sobs intently. His shoulders heave.

"Sir, you'd best leave the juice here for now because they won't let you have it at the hospital," Cardona advises. "You are not diabetic. You don't need it as much as you need to have an empty stomach in case you need some medicine at the hospital."

Under the porch lamp's glare Cardona and Callahan exchange loaded glances, a wordless, mutual confirmation that something is definitely odd. The man is alert, responsive, and breathing without difficulty, so he is in no immediate danger. Instead of getting the additional equipment, Callahan sidles by the still-crouching patient and into the apartment, where he talks softly with the woman. She tells him the man suffered a similar episode recently. "He's been drinking and drugging for weeks," she reports. "He comes home, has anxiety attacks, and claims he can't walk." She knows he has been hospitalized in a "mental ward," but she doesn't know where.

In the meantime, the patient continues his battle for the juice bottle. "*I want my juice, man,*" the man repeats, his voice threaded with panic and anger.

"Do you not understand what I just told you?" Cardona asks bluntly. "They might have to give you something at the hospital and you shouldn't have anything in your stomach."

Leaning out of the apartment door, Callahan corroborates their unspoken suspicion: "That's affirmative, Benny." The man probably has a psychiatric problem, possibly substance-induced. But this doesn't negate the fact that the man can't walk, or thinks he can't.

"Look at me, sir," Cardona commands. "Don't close your eyes." He shines a flashlight in the man's face. One pupil is fixed and the other is enlarged despite the bright beam, which is unusual. Although pupils naturally dilate at night to let more light in, they should constrict when hit with concentrated radiance. Cardona suspects one eye is synthetic and something is keeping the other artificially stimulated, most likely cocaine. Cardona nods tellingly at Callahan.

"Let me ask you a question, sir," Callahan says, quietly. "What do you think the problem is?"

"I don't know, man. I can't push myself up. I had to slide down the stairs to get here," he whines, rubbing his thighs strenuously. "My legs, my legs. They're numb. I can't feel nothing."

The partners are confident that the man has ingested some kind of drug. But they're still unsure whether or not he broke his neck, or if the injury is even relevant to tonight's complaint.

"Sir, can you wiggle your foot?" Callahan asks.

The man moves his ankle in a small semicircle. He cries continuously but says nothing about pain.

"Can you lift your leg?"

He complies shakily, lifting one leg very slightly.

"If anything was wrong with your neck or your back, you couldn't move like this," Cardona tells the man.

"What time is it?" the man replies.

Callahan tells him, "Nine-thirty."

"Is it morning or night?"

He may or may not have broken his neck. He's not diabetic. He's under the influence. And he has a psychiatric history. These are just a few of the puzzle pieces through which the partners must sort. Whatever damage the man may have suffered from a previous fracture, his teeming emotions seem to be at the root of his problems tonight, the EMTs conclude. They decide to dispense with the cervical-spine precautions and wheel him to the ambulance in their convertible stretcher-chair. As the partners reach over to help lift the man from the stairs, they urge him to try standing.

"I can't walk. I can't move," the man whimpers. "My leg is numb, man." He rubs his left thigh vigorously then sags and collapses on himself as if boneless. He won't try again; he just sits, a brawny, tearful, 285-pound meat sack. The partners heave him into the chair. Although Cardona says he hasn't been to the gym in about two years, the time he did invest left him with a powerful upper body. A former soldier, Callahan still works out intermittently. Nevertheless, the deadweight is an effort, and in the thick summer heat they both strain like oxen.

They hustle to strap the man in, grasp their treatment bags, and head down the driveway. Then Callahan catches a quick glance of a rubbery scar snaking its way down the patient's ebony neck.

En route to the truck patients are usually too sick to talk or too nervous to be quiet. This man, however, comforts himself by extracting a roller tube of cologne from his pocket, smearing the sweet-smelling yellow oil on his hands, and wiping his palms on his sweating face, soaking shirt, and crisply creased, knee-length denim shorts.

Inside the ambulance, Cardona sits near the patient's head and begins writing the chart. If a patient is stable, he prefers to get his paperwork under way before the bus soars and plunges through the city's rough roads, potholes, and pond-sized puddles and he goes bouncing along with it.

Cardona delves into the chart while he waits for Callahan to report the man's vital signs. He works quickly and meticulously, with three goals in mind. He wants his chart ready for hospital staff signatures when he arrives at the ER and transfers care. He wants to stay ahead of the paperwork so it won't bog him down at the end of his shift. And, he wants high marks on his paperwork. An ambitious perfectionist, he's determined to advance his emergency-services career, in law enforcement or EMS.

As Cardona writes, Callahan parks himself across from the man so he can easily measure his pulse (rate, rhythm, and quality), skin (color, condition, and temperature), lung sounds, and breaths per minute. The size of the man's pupil suggests he's consumed a powerful stimulant. His copious sweating might be a side effect of the drug speeding up his metabolism.

But the EMTs' job is not to speculate or make diagnoses. Instead they examine, interview, and record observations, using the information to alert the hospital and fashion stopgap treatments to stabilize patients before reaching the ER.

"What hospital were you in before?" Callahan asks, wrapping a blood-pressure cuff around the man's bulging biceps.

"I can't remember."

Cardona has not seen the scar, so he doesn't know what to make of the broken-neck story or whether to include it in the chart's narrative. *How much of this story will help the docs help this man*? he asks himself. *When drug fiends are cravin', they'll say anything.* Still suspicious, Cardona asks, "So, where did this accident take place?"

"Fabyan and Lyons," the man replies. The streets mark a heavily traveled intersection notorious for accidents.

"Were you in a halo?" the skeptical Cardona asks. Splinting techniques usually secure vulnerable areas above and below the injury site. A halo brace literally screws into the cranium and rests on the shoulders, rigidly holding the neck in place.

"Yeah."

"For how long?"

"Three months," the man answers. "They did a bone fusion but it didn't heal right."

Cardona doesn't have a stake in the man's past. Personally, he doesn't care if the man lies, intentionally or not. His job is to find out what is really wrong, give the proper care, and maybe save the ER some time. Borrowing from his law-enforcement background, he repeats questions to spot inconsistencies. But this man is sticking with his story, and that raises Cardona's confidence one notch.

At 170/92, the patient's blood pressure is elevated. That can be drug-induced, too, but it's not uncommon for blacks, especially those with poor nutrition, to have hypertension. Stress can boost rates, too. The man's "high blood," slang for the condition, is yet another piece of the puzzle.

The air-conditioning inside the truck cools the metal box to a brisk sixty-eight degrees, but perspiration ripples down the patient's face and coats his neck, arms, and calves. His shirt might as well be a locker-room towel. Whatever the cause, the man's heart is working overtime. Supplementary oxygen will reduce the load. As Callahan sets up the tank and mask, he asks, "What were you hospitalized for, man?"

"Pressure and anxiety."

"And they treated you for how long?"

"Three days."

"Do you recall this happening to you last time?" Cardona asks.

"Last time, I was disoriented and unstable," the man volunteers.

"You take any medications on a regular basis?" Cardona asks.

"Xanax," the man replies. A prescription tranquilizer, Xanax is also known as "sticks." Folks trade it for cocaine in the free-floating drug markets that surface throughout the city, Callahan says.

"Are you allergic to any food or medications?" Cardona continues.

"Anti-inflammatories, penicillin, and aspirin," the patient replies. "I know how to take care of my body. I was a body builder. I won four trophies." And at five-feet, seven inches, the nearly three-hundred-pound man is impressively solid and well cut.

"I was playing video games. Everything was fine," the man weeps. "I went to bed, got up to pee, and I fell on the floor."

Playing video games? Cardona wonders. *He just said he had been cleaning fish.* He might have been doing either, both, or something else entirely. Cardona's not sure if the man is lying or confused. Noting the incongruity, he'll try and figure out what really happened as the assessment proceeds. "Are you blind in your right eye?" he asks.

"Yeah!" the man acknowledges with surprise. "How'd you know?" He doesn't have the presence of mind to recall that Cardona used a penlight to inspect his pupils just seconds ago.

"I checked your eyes," Cardona reminds him.

The patient thrusts his hand deep in his pocket, pulls out a pair of dark, mirrored sunglasses, and shields his face. Next, he extracts a fistful of tightly wrapped bills in various denominations. Lying back on the stretcher, he begins unwinding one after another. Chunky white powder, cocaine, spills from the nest of bills onto his black T-shirt and the ambulance floor.

Callahan's jaw drops but he recovers quickly. "Let's talk real," he says, shaking his head sadly. "You got to get off that cocaine."

"It's not like I'm hooked on it," the man contends, peering sheepishly over the rims of his sunglasses.

"You don't know who you are buying it from or what's in that, man."

"True. But," he continues lamely, "I haven't done any since yesterday."

"With that neck injury, you have a second chance. God blessed you," Callahan says. "Don't do this shit."

Under the ambulance's quartz overhead lights, Cardona spots two seven-inch scars, one on either side of the patient's right calf. *Those mean fractured bones and surgery*, he thinks. Now a surgical history is emerging. *Man, this dude has been through a lot.* "What's that from?" Cardona asks, pointing his pen at the man's leg.

"I was shot in the park last year." Calmly, he recalls, "I been shot four times. In 1990, I got shot in the back. In '91, I was shot in the foot."

"Let's talk about your problem tonight, man," Callahan asks.

And the man begins crying anew. "I have a severe depression. I didn't have no more medication. Last week, I did some heroin." Newark had over 3,800 heroin users admit themselves for treatment in 2000 as well as 1,142 others addicted to alcohol, cocaine, marijuana, and other illicit drugs. Experts estimate seven to ten times as many users need treatment.[1] He turns toward Cardona, the more authoritative of the partners, and begs, "I don't want my family to know."

"We're not the police, man," Cardona assures him. "Your mama probably would be real upset if she knew you were doing this to yourself." He is not surprised at the man's state. To have survived a broken neck and bone fusion as well as four shootings is a lot of trauma for a thirty-one-year-old. *Are the man's drug and emotional problems born of disabilities caused by the accident or is it the other way around?* he wonders.

"Sir, you have a mission in life," Callahan interjects. "God spared you *four* times."

"I know, I know," the man sobs.

"Right now, you're depressed and you're hyped up from the drugs," Cardona explains as he backs out the truck to drive them to University.

"It would be a shame to survive all those injuries and die from the drugs," Callahan counsels.

"I read my Bible every day," the patient offers. "Sometimes I go to church, too."

* * *

He breathes his oxygen and remains quiet for the duration of the trip. After transferring care to a nurse, the EMTs walk away scratching their heads. "My man definitely has a psych problem, and it probably stems from his injuries," Callahan postulates while rubbing his back. Twice he had to lift this patient tonight, which has aggravated old injuries he received lifting and moving just such heavy patients. Callahan has a few surgical scars of his own from on-the-job injuries.

Cardona just doesn't know what to think. "It's a mental challenge to figure out what's wrong in the little time we have with them on the street, as opposed to the ER, which has a lot more time," he says, recalling the six years he worked as an ER trauma technician. When Cardona evaluates patients, he uses all of his observation skills, including those he honed as a store detective who once caught shoplifters. EMS demands "great assessment skills," Cardona says. "But you have to do more than observe. You just can't rely on quick physical assessments. You gotta be able to add it all up. When we first got there, we were about to collar this guy. He'd be crying and they'd be laughing at us in the ER. And you have to know what to project in your narrative. I said that he had broken his C1 and C2, but guess what? He's high as a kite and a psych patient as well.

"You gotta be really sharp because with all the stuff you see . . ." He shakes his head back and forth unbelievingly. Just a week ago, he, Callahan, O'Neill, and Heber extricated patients from a multi-car wreck. One of the drivers was drunk; he was also a paraplegic who suffered his original injuries as a result of another drunken escapade behind the wheel. The frequency of such bizarre episodes is but one of the reasons some of the crews have nicknamed Newark "Pluto," the planet farthest from the sun.

SAY WHAT?

The challenge of assessing patients is sometimes compounded by patients and family members who lack fundamental knowledge of their medical problems. An alphabetical index of phrases the blue-shirts encounter would be incomplete without the following: "Bacardi" for "Procardia," a cardiac medicine; "digestive heart failure" instead of "congestive heart failure"; "high blood" for hypertension and "low blood" for anemia; "mini-Jesus" instead of meningitis; "nipplizer" for "nebulizer," a machine that aerosolizes asthma medications; "peanut butter balls" instead of "Phenobarbital"; "pressure pills" for any type of hypo or hypertension drug; "roaches of the liver" instead of "cirrhosis"; and "sugar" for diabetes.

The malapropisms are funny, but they also reflect a serious disconnection between patients and their caregivers. If the chain of care is working, Fazio argues, patients should be able to master the specifics of their health conditions. After all, patients encounter doctors who prescribe the drugs; nurses charged with educating patients on how to take their medicines; and pharmacists who dispense the drugs. Why, then, are people failing to benefit from all three learning opportunities?

Emergency medical dispatchers have their own collection of gems. People call to report that someone "fell out." The first time EMD Judy Smith heard this, she asked, "Fell out of what?" unaware that the slang meant "passed out" or "fainted." Other callers, unsure how best to describe the urogenital area, report problems "down there." One reported a problem with her "administration," instead of "menstruation." And occasionally callers describe pain in their "vertical veins" rather than "varicose veins."

Malapropisms are *not* limited to the patient population. One dispatcher talks glibly about patients who don't take their "subscriptions" instead of "prescriptions."

Nevertheless, the number of patients who know or claim to know nothing is staggering. More don't know than do, it seems. Many EMS workers have come to see this phenomenon as just another unfortunate fact of life. "Docs don't explain, nurses don't teach, patients don't care," Fazio laments. She, Drivet, Cortacans, and a handful of others make the effort to coach their patients as time permits. But they cannot teach every patient everything he or she needs to know.

The EMS workers speak in a colorful code of their own, too. Many of them love the Pez candy dispensers and the sugary pellets that slip out when the Pez character's head snaps back. Besides deeming Pez an official food group, the EMS workers have made a verb out of the classic candy. Being "Pezzed" means being stabbed in the throat.

The term *shim*, for example, combines *she* and *him*. "A lot of shims get the shit kicked out of them once their trick finds out she's a he," Fazio explains in reference to male patients who pass themselves off as female hookers.

Euphemisms are popular, too. Few patients, for example, volunteer information about their HIV or AIDS conditions, which the blue-shirts call "slim disease." Patients will, however, readily discuss "the virus" or "the package." There are 17,472 people known to be living with AIDS in Newark, and more than 760 new cases a year, which puts the city in the top ten metropolitan areas ravaged by the disease.[2]

Having treated thousands upon thousands of critically ill patients over the years gives EMS workers a sense of who is approaching death. They know when a patient has the "fixing to die" look; their skin looks like "crap," Drivet says. There are other clues, too, such as DIP, their homegrown abbreviation for

"Duty" or "Dump In Pants." "If someone shits themselves, it's pretty unpopular in all cultures," Drivet explains. "So, when it happens, it's a bad sign."

A per diem contributes "Bumsicle," which is a vagrant whose drool has frozen him to the ground.

"KWPs" are knife-wielding psychopaths.

Newark EMS workers have a local rivalry with colleagues from Jersey City, aka "Jerky City." PUHA means pick up and haul ass.

They borrow military terms on occasion, calling visitors who ride along JAFOs—"Just Another Fucking Observer." An NRQ is a person with "No Redeeming Qualities."

Their rich and textured parlance reflects the odd world the B team inhabits at night; they know it's wacky. To John Q. Public, for example, a stabbing seems to be a grave injury. Even if the wound turns out to be superficial, the intent seems horrific. But a stab is a many-splendored thing when viewed through the prism that is Newark. One patient Fazio and Cisternino treated was stabbed eleven times. "My boy here looked like he was bitten by a piranha," Cisternino says.

"But it obviously wasn't meant to be serious," Fazio interjects. "I mean, it was all legs and arms."

People are sensitive to comments about roaches, rats, and other vermin that share their homes. Many abhor the pests and feel embarrassed by them. EMS workers here never warn each other verbally that the walls are crawling with bugs. They might say, instead, "We're among friends," do a discreet Texas two-step to warn the insects away, or decline to put their equipment down on the floor.

They are vicious with each other and themselves, too. Supervisor Keven Cleary, for example, suffered cancer and underwent chemotherapy. A coworker did, too. One way they helped themselves through the ordeal was by calling themselves the Mobile Intensive Cancer Unit.

One of the blue-shirts' survival tools is to render everything fair game. Nothing is sacred. "Irreverence and humor rule!" Fazio cheers: "You have to be able to laugh at whatever they throw at you."

MASQUERADE

By 0105 hours on another hot night, Cardona and Callahan have iced down the goose egg a little girl earned after tripping on stairs at Newark's minor-league baseball park. They've cleansed and bandaged the fatty, lacerated buttock of a pregnant Haitian woman who sat on a broken cinema seat. They've poked their heads into EMD Marion Shabazz's cookout and greeted Asylum and Demona, her pit bulls. She rewarded the crew with plates of mouthwatering fried fish, savory homemade hush puppies, and cans of icy fruit colas. They've examined a chain-smoking cancer patient in the bowels of the Prince Street projects, and listened to his girlfriend's woes; she is recovering from brain surgery.

I feel like I haven't been home in years, Cardona mopes. Having already worked seventy-two hours this week, he is close to being whipped. As if on cue, Dispatch sends them east for a "Female, sick." They drive into some low-rise projects and park on the asphalt courtyard. White-hot lights shine on late-night basketball players. The men trudge several flights up a dun-colored cinder-block stairwell. When they knock on a scarred, metal apartment door, a black woman opens it, pulls a skinny child out of the way, and ushers the men inside. Air-conditioning keeps the apartment comfortably cool. "We don't know what's wrong with her," the woman explains, pointing down the hallway toward a bedroom. The two march past a bubbling, tropical aquarium and a noisy home theater.

Inside the bedroom the EMTs find a whisper-slim woman dressed in white. She lies on a neat double bed with a mirrored headboard. A fan trained on the woman gently blows a breeze over her and ruffles curtains matched to the bedspread. The small room is clean and vaguely redolent of disinfectant. A television chatters in the background.

Meticulously groomed from the mini-braids in her topknot ponytail to her French manicure and pedicure, the patient is a graceful gamine. Emerging from her fashionable Capri pants, her calves, dainty and waxed bare, are a silken toffee. Her eyes open only slightly. Her wrists contort, forcing her palms toward her body.

"Ma'am?" Cardona asks as Callahan takes stock of the woman's vital signs. The patient doesn't answer, nor does she stir when Callahan grasps her wrist to feel for a pulse.

Cardona takes her by the shoulders and shakes her slightly. "Ma'am?"

"Does she have any medical history?" Callahan inquires of the man standing beside her.

Dressed casually in a short-sleeved button-down shirt and a pair of chinos, he has his hands in his pockets and a mystified look on his face. "No."

"Does she take any medications?"

"No."

"What time did this start?" Cardona asks, looking at the man

"I don't know, man," he says, shrugging. "We was at a party earlier tonight. She was drinking Hennessy, Absolute, Bacardi rum mixed into a punch."

"Has she been throwing up?"

"Yes."

Suddenly, the child bolts down the hallway and returns triumphantly. "She was drinking this!" she shouts, handing over a nearly full bottle of Alize liquor. "Mama?" the little girl cries. "What's wrong with you?"

Her mother doesn't blink, much less look her way. Twisting her doll in her hands, the child recounts dutifully, "She was just in the bathroom sitting on the toilet, and I looked in, and she said, 'Just call your father. Just call an ambulance.'"

"She seems to have aspirated something," Cardona notes as the woman gags. He rolls her onto her left side, and extends her arm beneath her head so that she lies in standard recovery position, a pose that helps secretions drain from her mouth and keep her airway clear.

"Why can't she talk?" the man wants to know.

Frankly, the EMTs want to know that also.

"You have to talk to us," Cardona urges, and then commands her, "Sit up!"

The patient, however, lies still—like a doe stunned by a car that has glanced off it.

"I been there before," Callahan says, thinking the woman is plastered.

Checking each vital sign, Cardona finds that the woman's blood pressure is 100/64. Her pulse is 84 and regular. Her skin is warm and damp. Her pupils are midpoint and reactive to his penlight's beam. Her lungs sound clear, and although shallow, her breaths fall within normal range. So far, nothing remarkable except the near catatonia.

"Is she dead?" the child asks, sucking her thumb.

"Mama's going to be OK," Callahan tells the little girl.

"They might have to put a tube down her throat and pump her stomach," Cardona says to the man. "There's such a thing as alcohol poisoning."

"I remember when they stuck Oodles of Noodles in my throat," the child chimes in, remembering her own hospital experience.

Calling the woman by name, Cardona tells her, "We're going to try and walk you." She doesn't look at him. Or move at all. She leans against him like a bag of beans. He pinches the skin on the back of her hand—a quick field test to assess level of consciousness—and she recoils. *She's alert to pain*, he thinks. *So, she's not too far gone.*

Meanwhile, Callahan sets up the stair-chair and the girl's father instructs her to put slippers on her mother's feet. But first she must find them. Doll clutched firmly under her arm, the child rummages through the bottom of a closet for matching shoes, pretty shoes, pink shoes.

"If you can't walk, we'll take you in a chair," Cardona adds, still hopeful his patient will show some independence. The woman cannot or will not sit up by herself, much less stand up and walk.

Cardona lifts her and says, "Try to stay up." But she flops to the side. "We got to carry you out in this thing," he says, resigned. And so they bundle her up, buckle her in, and carry her out, with the child and her father trailing behind. The woman's head lolls. Her eyes flutter. She gags repeatedly. When they reach the bus, Cardona extracts the stretcher and Callahan places the drooling woman on it. They slide her inside the truck.

"Wanna give your mommy a kiss?" Callahan asks the girl. She nods. Lifting the child up, he deposits her in the ambulance. She kisses her mother on the cheek respectfully and clambers out.

Callahan takes the woman's delicate hand in his, calls her name. "If you don't talk to me and tell me what is happening . . ." he says, but his soft tone carries no threat. And he gets no results. He tries another tack: "Let me see you squeeze my hand." She doesn't. "Let me see you lift your foot." She doesn't. "Honey, they gotta know you can follow commands or they'll put tubes in your nose, throat, and hands and you're gonna wish you listened."

He takes another blood pressure—104/68. Her pulse is up to 135.

"Don't spit on the floor!" Cardona shouts with disgust as yellow syrup dribbles out of her mouth. "Here, you can vomit inside of this bag." He puts a plastic emesis bag in her hand, but she doesn't seem to have the strength to clutch it.

"She's no drinker!" Cardona comments sarcastically as he exits the box to drive. *She wanted a little attention, I've see it before.*

Callahan supplements the woman's breathing with a nasal canula: the flexible transparent green tube with two prongs on the end streams four to six liters of 100 percent oxygen per minute into the woman's nostrils. He folds a few blankets and stuffs them under her jeweled ankles, hoping to raise her blood pressure.

The woman finally shows some activity. She tries to pull the canula out.

"Keep that on you," Callahan orders. "It's not hurting you. It's oxygen."

She flails like a bird in a burlap bag.

"If you go into that hospital acting like you're acting," Callahan warns, "they're gonna treat you like you had a stroke. You gotta keep that on. You're not acting like you had too much to drink. You still should be able to talk. You're acting like something is medically or psychologically wrong with you. I hope you do better at the hospital. Can you talk? Let me see you wiggle the toes on your left foot."

She doesn't comply but she does point awkwardly to her stomach.

"You feel sick to your stomach, honey?" he asks. She doesn't answer. "Your stomach hurts?" Again, she has only the empty-eyed look of a dead carp. *She probably doesn't know what it feels like to be drunk,* he muses. *But, she doesn't smell ETOH.* (Even in their thoughts, the partners think in code. ETOH is an abbreviation for ethyl alcohol, the psychoactive element in booze.)

When they wheel the woman into the ER of a hospital at the north end of the city, Cardona reports to the charge nurse, "We think she mighta had a bit too much to drink." And the nurse nods knowingly.

Later, when the partners bring in a demented AIDS patient with ulcerated legs and his bag of Fig Newtons, they check on the woman. She's still lying in the same curtained ER bay, but now she has a tongue depressor stuck in her mouth and soft restraints tied around her wrists.

"Seizures," the nurse tells Cardona. "She's been seizing on and off ever since you left."

Win some, lose some, Cardona thinks. *You can't catch 'em all.*

Callahan takes it a bit harder. *Damn, we was wrong!* he thinks. *It happens. Sometimes in this job you do have a tendency to get complacent.*

Well, stuff like that brings you down to earth. It makes you humble. In retrospect, certain things threw us off. All that talk about drinking. From that point on we just had tunnel vision. We been doing this a long time, but sometimes we're just not right.

Many EMTs consider patient assessment the hardest part of the job. Street medicine allocates precious few minutes to reach patients and analyze and prioritize their problems. Whatever they find can branch out into new investigations and interventions, but always with the aim of controlling life threats and completing timely transport and transfer.

Standardized assessment routines are often compromised by urgent situations that demand on-the-spot, corrective action, at least securing a patient's airway (A), breathing (B), and circulation (C). These are the universal EMS priorities; they supersede all other concerns, with the exception of scene safety. If one or more of these vital functions is compromised, the patient risks permanent damage or death. EMS workers are schooled not to continue their assessment until all three ABCs are in working order.

While the clock ticks, EMS workers evaluate patient consciousness. Is the patient alert and lucid? If not, is this the result of dementia, stroke, overdose, fever, or injury? Is the patient even responsive to commands? To pain?

To come up with a treatment plan, rescuers must discern whether combative or unresponsive patients are oxygen-deprived, diabetic, drunk, in overdose, recovering from seizures, psychotic, or in the throes of another medical calamity.

They must boil down extraneous and inaccurate patient and bystander monologues to the most relevant facts. They have to read between the lines without reading into situations. Take blood on the floor around an unconscious patient, for example. If fresh, it might indicate frank tuberculosis or a burst throat vessel caused by hypertension. Clots can result from interaction with the air or suggest cirrhosis. If the blood resembles dark and crumbly coffee grounds, it points to a possible gastrointestinal bleed. And how much blood is there? The questions go on, but the EMS workers must narrow the possibilities and tighten their focus.

They analyze the physical forces involved in traumas to consider potential bodily harm, how to properly package and treat the patient, and paint a picture for the physician; some hospitals equip EMS workers with digital cameras so doctors can see trauma scenes themselves. At car crashes, for example, EMS workers immediately note whether the patient was restrained or not and consider the spectrum of possible consequences. They scrutinize wrecks for clues. Spiderweb fractures in the windshield or misshapen glass suggest how hard a patient's head smacked against it. The impact passengers absorb is muted or magnified by the vehicle, too—is it a tank or a tin can?

EMS workers also question the potential role of underlying medical problems or substance abuse, even at trauma scenes. Was this person's accident or fall caused by inattention, for example, or did a heart attack, diabetic emergency, stroke, or drug problem precipitate it? Has the accident itself triggered a medical emergency? Car-crash victims have heart attacks, too.

They have to memorize a catalogue of signs and symptoms and be wary of suggestive terms and tunnel vision, distractions that plague overworked systems.

Vital signs (pulse, blood pressure, skin condition and temperature, pupil reactivity, lung sounds, breathing rate, and pain levels) are only a baseline beginning. EMS workers measure them repeatedly to detect and document changes that signify whether the patient needs more help.

Depending on the situation, crews may conduct physicals from the top of the head to the tip of the toes, literally. Squeezing a patient's fingertip and timing how quickly blood returns to the blanched spots reveals circulation health. But taking a pulse by fingering a patient's wrist reveals nothing about how well blood is flowing to a lower-extremity injury—so practitioners must know several different pulse points. EMS workers must also be vigilant for MedicAlert jewelry that tells them if a patient is diabetic, epileptic, allergie, or otherwise medically vulnerable.

An EMS worker's conversational style affects the quality and quantity of information produced. Fazio, for example, studiously avoids jargon. She asks about "health problems," not "medical histories." She never puts words in a patient's mouth. Instead she invites patients to describe how they feel and documents their expressions on her charts. Fazio never questions patients about HIV or AIDS. Harnessing street lingo, she asks instead if they have "the virus," and she knows what they mean if they use other terms, too, such as "the package." She makes sensitive queries only after affording her patients privacy inside the bus.

And she *never* asks for a Medicaid card, which implies poverty. She just inquires if the patient has any insurance information.

Others are considerably more blunt. One expresses a preference for talking to some of his patients "like thugs, so they understand," and thinks nothing of asking, "Yo, motherfucker! What's wrong with you?"

If someone in a crowd complains that the ambulance took too long, instead of soliciting their cooperation or sharing the actual response time—which is usually fifteen minutes or less—he finds it more effective to say, "Shut the fuck up! You aren't the only people in the city. We get here when we get here." He realizes that "some people might say we're not professional," but for him, he says, it works. After all, "everybody's not used to be being treated nice."

EMS workers tailor their inventory-taking and analysis to arrive at a conclusion, then package, treat, and transport the patient to an appropriate hospital, continually reassessing patient status en route.

Crews sum up their findings and alert hospitals by radio as to what is about to arrive on their doorstep. Most follow a basic script. Fast, accurate, and comprehensive, Fazio's crisp, rapid-fire delivery is awesome to behold: patient age, sex, mental status, chief complaint, onset, pulse rate and rhythm, respiration rate and quality, lung sounds, and blood pressure. Until recently, she included race, too, which the chart does as well. Race is significant, she explains, because some conditions are prevalent in certain ethnic groups. Someone complained, though, and management recently changed policy. Race data are still collected and analyzed, but not transmitted by radio. Fazio rolls her eyes at the latest twist in the political-correctness rumba.

After blasting through her primary findings, she segues into her secondary assessment: skin condition and the presence or absence of jugular vein distension, edema, abdominal sensitivity, medical history, medications, and allergies. She tops it off with hospital destination, estimated time of arrival, treatment completed thus far, and what she plans to do. It's a veritable blitzkrieg of information, but it's also concise and well organized.

Some physicians simply concur. Some issue minor modifications. And still others repeat what was said as if the ideas sprang from their head.

Occasionally Fazio modifies her routine to accommodate physician preferences. "Some just tell us to cut to the chase," she explains. "They just want to hear what is wrong with the patients." And that can abbreviate the report to a simple sentence, such as "I have a sixty-year-old in status seizure"—consecutive seizures with no time to recover between occurrences—"and I need an order for Valium." But for the most part it takes years of working with the medics before ER physicians fully trust their field assessment skills.

SING A SONG OF SICKNESS

At 0250 hours, Dispatch receives word about a man shot and sends EMTs Chuck Coles and Pat Vogt and medics Cisternino and Fazio to the scene. Coles and Vogt arrive first at the Central Ward location. They have to peel the five or six bystanders off the patient even to form an initial impression. At the bottom of the horde they find a slim black male lying faceup and terminally still. His eyes wear the glazed look of the dead. His head is awash with blood. Vogt, who has seen the face of death thousands of times in her years serving Newark and Camden, calmly turns back to her bus to retrieve the board, cervical collar, and stretcher.

"Does anybody know where he was shot?" Coles asks, dropping to his knees to feel for a pulse on the side of man's neck. No one answers. The skin on the patient's neck is as smooth and as soft as coffee-colored velvet; he is young, perhaps still in his teens. Coles feels no blood coursing through the man's carotid arteries, vessels that feed the brain, which in turn controls the heart and lungs. He double-checks for signs of life, crooking his neck to look for the telltale chest rise. But the man lies as still as a statue. While Vogt readies the equipment, Coles cuts off the man's jacket and shirt. He exposes the patient's chest so the medics can monitor his heart and maybe even shock it. If he dares ask any more questions, Coles predicts someone will order him to "stop talking and do your job." He's heard it before.

The crowd circles and closes in. Five people become twenty. Animosity hangs thick in the air. "What took you so long?" a disembodied voice demands. "We been waiting a half-hour!"

It may feel like a half-hour because the bystanders don't know how to help the man and every second that they stand there doing nothing intensifies their anxiety. And who knows how effectively police transferred the call? *The Dispatch Center time-stamped the call at 0250 and we were on-scene four minutes later!* Coles thinks. *But there's no point getting into a shouting match.*

Visoskas roll ups in his white Expedition to help control the crowd and package the patient. He's just in time to hear someone toss out a tired and familiar if distressing allegation: "You don't care about him because he's black." Visoskas is as pale as an eggshell. Vogt, defiantly blond, has part Choctaw origins and a golden skin tone. Coles, the color of caramel, is black. Asians, Hispanics, and other minorities are blue-shirts, too, as well as Christians, Muslims, Jews, Buddhists, Wiccans, atheists, and agnostics. The team is nothing if not diverse.

There they go, voicing their opinions, Coles thinks, and sighs quietly. A forty-one-year-old father of three, who grew up in a neighboring town, he considers this "stupidness." One of the few black EMTs at University to complete his training as a paramedic, he'll be taking his final exams days from now. But he can't stop to explain this and take time away from the patient. *People say a lot of crazy things when they are under stress*, he counsels himself, *but it should be clear that EMTs are there to save lives.*

"Do something for him!" a crowd member commands.

With considerable effort, Coles controls his temper. He slips a rigid protective collar around the man's neck, then grasps the bloodied sides of his patient's head to stabilize his spine. Visoskas grabs the man's torso, and Vogt holds on to his legs. Keeping his body straight, they rotate the patient onto his side. Vogt slips the board behind him, and they roll him back onto it.

Get the patient and crews the hell away from this crowd, Visoskas's street sense tells him. *They've been drinking. They're messed up. They're pissed at us when they should be pissed at the guy who shot their friend.* The police are busy doing their "who," "what," and "when." Visoskas feels lucky that they are there at all. It's only recently that the Newark Police Department has begun sending officers on calls, when it has them available. So Visoskas is left to marshal his experience and conflict-resolution training at hostile emergency medical scenes. "Right now, sir, this *is* the hospital," he says softly. The more quietly he speaks, the harder they must work to be quiet and listen. Slowly, he walks toward the group, hands in the air, and implores, "People, people, let them do their job."

Generally, EMS workers here enjoy a slim protective shield from the crowd, but it can dissolve at any moment. Coles worries about Visoskas. *What if the group turns on him?* "Officer?" Coles calls to one of the cops standing on the sidelines. "Can you make some room for us?" The cop does, creating a slim channel for Visoskas, Coles, and Vogt to slide the patient into their bus.

Inside the box, Coles selects an oral airway. He checks that it reaches from the tip of the man's ear to the corner of his mouth, a standard way of measuring the length of someone's throat. He pries open the man's mouth, suctions out a mouthful of blood, and slips the tube in. The curved portion of the hard plastic tube curls around the tongue so it won't fall back and clog the airway. When the medics arrive, they will thread a longer, endotracheal tube into the man's windpipe. Until then, this will keep the area directly behind the mouth open and able to exchange air. Coles fastens a bag-valve mask to his oxygen tubing and squeezes oxygen into the man's lungs, effectively breathing for him.

Vogt brushes aside the thick, yellow-gold chains that hang from the young man's neck. She peels his shirt and jacket back to reveal a lean, narrow torso. His abdominal muscles, small and hard, resemble the smoothest of river rocks. He has an outie belly button. A thick leather belt cinches a grubby pair of waffle-print long underwear and freshly pressed baggy jeans around his tapered waist. A gold watch dangles on a chain from his pocket.

Vogt spots her landmark—the lower third of the sternum just above the heart—interlaces her fingers, straightens her arms, and bears down. By com-pressing his chest, one, two, three, four, five, she pushes blood through the heart's chambers and valves on behalf of his now-impotent cardiac muscle. Coles forces more air into the man's lungs, and Vogt spreads it through his body with more compressions. She drips with exertion. They repeat their two-person CPR technique while Visoskas joins them inside the bus.

He sees streaks of blood coagulating with the viscosity of motor oil as they dribble down the man's face. *It might be a head shot,* he thinks, and he alerts Dis-patch by radio. He also declares the patient an official "trauma code." People who have just died of injury are one of the system's highest priorities, although chances of resuscitation diminish ten percent with each passing minute, and that is if the body has not sustained irreparable injuries. "What's the medics' ETA?" Visoskas asks.

Cisternino and Fazio are just a minute away, Dispatch replies, and seconds later at 0302 they pull up, disembark from the cab, and hustle to the side of their truck, where Fazio grabs the trauma kit and Cisternino grabs the airway bag and heart monitor. She leads, and the two wade through the layers of people who circle the BLS bus, pounding on its metal walls and stretching to peer in the windows. "Is he breathing?" a short, muscular man with dreadlocks pleads repeatedly. But Fazio and Cisternino walk the gauntlet without a word. At a volatile scene you don't want to be the one they fixate on, she explains. After she is safely inside the bus, Cisternino climbs aboard and locks the door behind him, and they collectively shut out the world.

As Fazio begins her assessment, Cisternino stoops to get a bird's-eye view of the man's face. The patient's eyes, a dark bark brown, are wet; his pupils are fixed and dilated. His eyelashes are thick and lush and webbed with blood. His skin is smooth and tender—still boyish. Whatever his injuries, he's dead. If there is any hope of bringing him back, it will depend on a good oxygen flow. Kneeling now, Cisternino sets out to explore for loose teeth, a broken jaw, blood in the throat and nose, or anything else that might jam the man's airway before he intubates.

"Where's the hole?" Fazio asks urgently. "Where's the hole?" Under the blazing quartz lights she scans the man's skin and skims his bloodied surfaces with her gloved fingers, trying to find and assess bullet wounds to his chest and abdomen. "The hole is in his chest! The hole is in his chest!" she shouts, point-ing to a crisp opening in the man's upper right torso.

Cisternino glances up. There isn't any powder burn or stippling on the man's skin, nor can he see carbon-heated particles. *The shot wasn't fired at close range,* he thinks. *Probably eighteen inches to two feet.* From the shape of the hole, about one-half inch, and the way the skin dents inward, he guesses it was a large-caliber weapon, probably a .45 or something similar.

"Did you look at the back?" Fazio asks Vogt. She wants to count the wounds and give the surgeons a heads-up.

"Not yet," Vogt replies; her assessment stopped when she and Coles discovered that the man had no airway, breathing, or circulation—instant priorities.

"We'll do it at the hospital," Cisternino interjects. The chest injury itself is fatal, and anything else they find won't change the course of treatment. Time is running and Cisternino doesn't want to waste a second. "Who's driving?" he snaps. Vogt volunteers. It's 0307 hours when she exits the box. In addition to bagging, Coles takes over compressions, too.

"C'mon, baby," Fazio coaxes the dead man as she sticks a white electrode over the wound. It will do double duty—cover the wound and feed information to her heart monitor. She places a second pad on his lower left chest to complete the circuit, but the monitor shows he is in asystole, no heartbeat at all, also known as "flatline."

"Stop doing compressions so I can intubate," Cisternino, still kneeling, barks. By pumping on the body, Coles makes the epiglottis and vocal cords vibrate, and Cisternino wants everything still as stone. "Shit! It's full of blood!" he bellows, squinting down the man's throat. "I can't see a damn thing. Plus his vocal cords are clamped together." *He must be bleeding into his lungs* Cisternino figures. *His last few gasps of air brought blood up. It looks just like a drowning.* It's hard to wriggle the twelve-inch endotracheal tube through the cords' closed, rubbery gates, but finally he succeeds.

Coles resumes bagging and compressing the man while Cisternino uses his stethoscope to check breath sounds. If he has inserted the tube inside the windpipe, air should be inflating the lungs, and the sounds will be hushed but clear. Instead, the right side of the man's chest is silent, and the left is muffled. That might mean a variety of things, but before he can decipher it, Fazio needs help.

Since the man's heart isn't pumping, no blood is circulating, and that means Fazio can't get her drugs aboard. "No pipes showing," she declares before asking Cisternino, "Can you get something in his neck?"

Normally Cisternino would fish for veins by feeling for the ropy vessels with his fingertips. But the situation is too fragile. His eyes, now mere inches from the man's neck, search the skin carefully. He spots the jugular, about half the width of a pinky finger. It's the main vessel returning blood from the brain. "I got one shot," he replies. "The minute I start poking around I'm going to squeeze the few cc's of blood in there out, because he's bleeding out and I'll lose it and not see it anymore." Cisternino wipes the spot he has picked with an alcohol pad and nails his target with a marksman's unruffled air.

Fazio opens the clamp on a 1,000-ml bag of Ringer's lactate. She readies her vials of epinephrine and atropine, two-heart-stimulating drugs. Cisternino returns to the airway, squeezing the bag-valve mask. Then Fazio sees that something is wrong; the fluids aren't flowing and the drugs are not reaching the man's heart. "What's the matter with this fucking thing?" she mutters, fiddling with the clamp. It flips smoothly but the clear liquid just hangs there.

"Let me know if it's running," Cisternino says, pumping oxygen into his dead patient's lungs all the while.

"It's not."

"You're fucking kidding me!" Glancing up, he studies the bag, lines, and catheter and notes, *It's not clotted. The patient's head is perfectly straight, so the vein isn't kinked. Since the line is good, there probably isn't enough backpressure in the vein.* He tells Cole to lift the bag up to the box's ceiling and squeeze. Finally the fluids begin to flow.

When Cisternino resumes bagging, though, volcanic eruptions spurt from the dead man's body. Watery blood spouts through the tube between the man's lips. The electrode over the hole flutters and blood trickles out. *Whoa, a self-decompressing chest wound!* Cisternino thinks. After looking at the ghoulish fountain quizzically, Cisternino starts singing, "I know what the pathology is, I know what the pathology is.

"The bullet must have hit a major vessel," he tells Fazio. "because there's Kool-Aid coming up through the tube as we're dumping fluid into him." To illustrate, Cisternino squeezes air down the tube and into the lungs. When he releases pressure on the bag, the patient's body should release carbon dioxide through an exhalation. But because the man's lungs are filled with blood and intravenous fluid, what Cisternino gets instead is a clear, pinkish juice. Everything they put in the man just spills out through these holes. Neither the man's brain nor any other part of him is getting the oxygen it needs to live.

Cisternino estimates that at least ten percent of the man's blood has quit his circulatory system and spilled into his chest cavity. It collects there, crowding the injured lung into a smaller and smaller space. Untreated, the volume will displace the windpipe, compress the heart, and eventually compromise the other lung, too.

The bullet pierced the lung, as well. Some of the air the rescuers pump into him during CPR escapes through the hole into the cavity between the chest wall and the lung's membrane. That cavity should be filled with a lubricant that helps keep lung expansions and contractions smooth. But air is caught inside. Normally, the medics would decompress the membrane by inserting a needle catheter and letting the trapped air drain. Ironically, the bullet hole does this for them. *This is a textbook open hemo-pneumo thorax,* Cisternino thinks. It's a rare injury and one he thinks is cool.

Fazio delivers more epinephrine and atropine. *It won't save the man,* she thinks, *but it's the right thing to do.* Cisternino continues bagging the man with one hand, and with a handful of linen in the other he sop ups the Kool-Aid. *We love linen.* One of the most flexible tools EMS workers carry, it's good for bleeding control, as a vomit shield, for cleanup, bandaging, lifting and moving, and, in a pinch, patient restraint. They arrive at the hospital by 0317 hours and, still bagging, wheel the man into the shock trauma room. Nurses and medical students assemble and hook the man up to the various monitors, but he is still flatline. "Anyone who wants to see a textbook case should look at this," Cisternino says, directing students to the man's chest. "It's sad, but it's a neat opportunity to see a self-decompressing, open, sucking chest wound."

"Were there any vital signs in the field?" the doctor asks.

"No," Fazio replies. "He was flatline the whole time."

Patients who suffer penetrating trauma to the torso have the best chance of recovery if the medics reach them while they're still alive. This man died, probably within seconds, certainly before they reached him. Although they plugged his hole and filled his tank, his injuries were overwhelming. "Are you sure there were no vital signs whatsoever?" the doctor repeats, mostly for the benefit of his residents and medical students.

Shaking her head, Fazio says, "Nope." Without signs of life for at least sixteen minutes, the man has been deprived of sufficient oxygen and glucose for too long. Even if the doctor cracked open the man's chest in a last-ditch effort to repair his heart and lungs, it would do no good. The man's cells, the basic building blocks of life, have already begun deteriorating irrevocably.

"Time of death," the doctor says looking up at the clock on the wall, "three-nineteen."

"Gotta bill the dead guy and add insult to injury," Fazio muses as she completes the paperwork over a cigarette. She fills in the standard information and turns to the treatment flowchart. Theoretically, procedures such as defibrillation, medication dispensing, and intubation are documented in real time. To that end, some EMS workers take field notes on their gloves; others jot shorthand on strips of tape they affix to their pants and scribble as they work. But when a job is as urgent as this one was, when all hands are on the patient, it's neither practical nor possible to stop the action and take minute-by-minute notes. *Each* line in the table is a blow-by-blow account of the patient's status and the actions the paramedics take on his behalf. Each line records the time; the patient's breathing rate, pulse rate, and blood pressure; ECG findings; pulse-oximetry readings; treatment selected; dosages/measurement per treatment; how the medics dispensed the treatment; which medic meted it out; and results achieved. In short, a mother lode of data.

Fazio carefully reconstructs events for the treatment table as a cold drizzle falls outside the ER. Cisternino turns his face up to the sky, inviting the spray to soak his skin. He wags his tongue bar at the clouds and dares the lightning to strike him. Vogt and Coles ask for extra time to disinfect their bloodied bus. Shortly thereafter, Dispatch sends the EMTs on another job, but Cisternino and Fazio enjoy a lull. They retreat to their favorite place, a moonlit Branch Brook Park pond that reflects the stunning French Gothic Basilica of the Sacred Heart.

Fazio munches Triscuits, sips the Dunkin' Donuts iced coffee she bought hours ago, and studies a book on pagan Europe, occasionally reading passages aloud to her partner, who shares her interest in the occult. He purloins a sheet from the cabinet, stretches out on the skel bench, and sings softly to himself to the tune of "If You're Happy and You Know It":

> *Got a bullet in my chest. Take it out.*
> *Got a bullet in my chest. Take it out*
> *Got a bullet in my chest; I'm a fucking bloody mess.*
> *Got a bullet in my chest. Take it out.*

Cisternino's boot bottoms are still bloody.

7 *SEE ME, FEEL ME, TOUCH ME, HEAL ME*

When uncertain, when in doubt,
Run in circles, scream and shout.

—A DITTY THAT DISPATCHERS CHANT AT THE EXPENSE OF
THEIR GROUND-POUNDER COLLEAGUES

*O*nce resources have been assigned and rescuers arrive at the patient's side and conduct their assessment, treatment begins. Occasionally, however, situations arise that give pause. One blue-shirt remembers a rail worker who had been checking under the carriages when the train he was working on began to roll. Badly injured and convinced he would die, the man begged the medic to write a farewell message to his wife and three children. *Should I just let him go?* the medic remembers asking himself, moved by the man's desperate condition and plea. *Or should I be aggressive about his care?* Faced with a Hobson's choice, he braced himself to withstand the man's cries and worked him up. The patient survived, albeit with artificial limbs and a probable lifelong dependence on a wheelchair. Choosing when and how to treat makes for a challenging part of the job.

Treatment becomes even more complicated when bystanders, family members, sometimes other emergency-service professionals, and even patients expect EMS workers to zoom off toward the nearest hospital the instant the patient is loaded and the bus doors slam shut—hence a long-standing view of EMS workers as mere "ambulance drivers" who simply scoop and run. Anxious people scream, pound the bus, and even threaten the workers with weapons. They simply do not realize that care is already under way and their hysteria only impedes the EMS workers' ability to perform the job at hand—that is, to abort crisis and prepare the patient for more substantive care.

As EMS has evolved, so has the practitioners' scope of practice. Now they bring a formidable, ever-increasing array of medicines, equipment, and techniques to improve patient well-being. And whatever BLS is trained to find and treat ALS can do to an order of magnitude.

"When you see hoofprints in the sand most people think of horses," Drivet says. "In Newark, the hoofprints may well belong to zebras." Zebras, another *House of God* term, are "obscure diagnoses."[1] According to Drivet, however, zebras really do gallop through Newark, where patients experience everything from hemicorporectomies and pulmonary anthrax to active tuberculosis and rare types of cancer that flourish in bodies ravaged by AIDS. Zebras are one reason why EMS workers flock to Newark, Drivet says. Here, EMS workers get to treat almost everything from the routine to the bizarre.

HAPPY BIRTHDAY

Just after midnight, Buzz radios Callahan and Cardona and sends them to a "possible miscarriage of a patient said to be vomiting blood." In many cities, births are considered sufficiently serious events to merit paramedic attention. Maternity calls in Newark, however, are so prevalent that they would easily overwhelm the small number of medics available to quell the rampage of potential life threats born on Newark's streets every day.

Childbirth, here, is routine for BLS. Callahan, for example, has brought more than seventy-two babies into the world. During his tenure, he has even seen some of the children he delivered give birth to a new generation. Cardona has assisted at more than thirty births, including both of his sons.

"My man is giving us landing patterns," Cardona says, spotting someone in the street waving his arms as if to set down an airplane. He pulls up in front of a white brick tenement where a young woman sits on the concrete stoop, hanging her head between knees. She jiggles her legs and bounces on her toes. The elderly woman standing by her side flaps her hands in distress. Cardona goes immediately to the young woman's side while Callahan gets the stretcher, converts it into the chair, and wheels it to them.

Each partner grabs one of the woman's cigarette-thin arms; she is so slender she practically levitates up to the seat. Her heart-shaped mahogany face is glossy with sweat. Her head rotates around on her neck as if she is possessed, and her eyes roll back, lids fluttering in pain. She rubs her long, shapely fingers, each adorned with delicate golden rings, on her hard round belly over and over. She makes no sound whatsoever.

"How old are you?" Cardona asks as they roll her into the bus.

The teenager doesn't answer, but the older woman does. Technically, the girl is a minor; unless her life is threatened, she needs parental consent to be treated. But because she is pregnant, the law automatically categorizes her as an emancipated minor. Either way, the point is moot, because the elderly woman whispers, "Her mother is dead. I'm her auntie."

"We're going to get a quick pressure before we get going," Callahan tells the patient and her aunt. He wants to make sure she is stable; otherwise he may have to call for ALS.

"Did you vomit blood?" Cardona asks the patient.

She looks everywhere about the box except directly at him. She doesn't answer, but her auntie does: "It was bright red. It was blood."

"She's really warm," Callahan tells his partner as he ticks through the vital signs. Her skin temperature tells him she is in some kind of distress, whether it is a fever indicating infection, exertion from labor, or something else entirely.

"Is this your first one?" Cardona asks.

Again the girl is mysteriously silent. Her face harbors no hostility—no emotion at all, in fact. Only her mute grimaces speak of her pain.

"She has a child already," Auntie reports.

"How many?" Previous births can mean an abbreviated labor. By asking how many children she has had, Cardona can gauge how quickly this next one might arrive.

"One. She had him when she was a young teen, herself."

"How many pregnancies all together, including any miscarriages or abortions?"

"Three," Auntie says.

"Any prenatal care?"

The girl shakes her head.

"I tried," Auntie reports, shrugging her shoulders and turning her palms up. Her shoulders slump as she sighs, "But you can't make them." Of the seventy-four babies born to minors each month in Newark, approximately one-third come into the world without the benefit prenatal care.[2]

"When is the baby due?" Cardona asks.

"I don't know," the girl whispers.

"When was your last period?"

"I don't know," she sighs.

"You *gotta* tell me what's going on!" Cardona cries, exasperated.

Turning her head as far from him as she can, she buries her face in the stretcher, for there are no pillows, no frills in Newark. A note of protest laces her tone, albeit weak, when she insists, "I am."

Callahan gets his blood-pressure reading: it's 130/90, which skirts the border of hypertension. But the number is only a piece of a puzzle. A woman as young and thin as this might have a much lower pressure normally. Her pulse and breathing rate are slightly elevated, too, but she is alert and conscious if oddly quiet. Callahan turns on the oxygen and places a mask over her nose and mouth before stepping out of the back to radio the ER and drive to University.

"Any vaginal bleeding?" Cardona asks.

The patient shakes her head.

"Discharge?"

Again she shakes her head.

"Any problems with the pregnancy?"

Neither answers. When Cardona tries to confirm the address for his chart, the girl offers nothing.

"She lives between her dad and I," Auntie offers.

"Any medical problems?"

"She's got low blood," Auntie says, using slang for anemia, an insufficient amount of iron in the blood.

On the stretcher, the girl writhes noiselessly. Her eyes flash violently. Cardona glances at her crotch and sees a dark stain spreading quickly across the lap of her black jeans. "You might be having the baby, honey," Cardona informs the girl. "Oh yeah, your water's breaking."

Cardona and Auntie help the girl off with her pants, already unzipped to accommodate the belly bulge. Her water, which should be clear, is honey-colored. Sometimes, due to the effort of labor, fetuses will pass their first bowel movement shortly before birth.

Auntie takes hold of the girl's delicate hand. Cardona grabs an obstetrics kit from the cabinet, puts on a pair of sterile gloves, squats over the end of the bench where her feet are, faces her naked bottom, and takes a seat.

The girl begins fumbling with the safety belt that secures her to the stretcher as if she intends to escape.

"Leave that strap alone," Cardona commands. "Oh, that baby's coming now!"

A blank, panicked look spreads across the girl's dainty features, but she utters no sound.

"Sweetie, you *gotta* talk to me." Cardona drapes a sheet over his lap and uses another to cover the girl's belly and upper thighs.

Still looking to the side, the girl spreads her long, brown, spidery legs the full width of the bus. "Baby, don't kick me in my face," Cardona warns the girl, who flails her legs in the air with the energy and range of a Rockette. "Good girl."

As if she wants to split herself open, she reaches for the cabinets with one foot and extends the other to the opposite wall, banging it on the bench where her auntie sits.

"Lift your heinie up," Cardona instructs. When she does, he slides a sterile sheet beneath her. *I don't want the baby coming into the world and landing on something dirty*, he thinks. He gets it in place just in time to catch a slimy yellow discharge the consistency of scrambled eggs spilling out of the woman's moist vagina. It's not uncommon for women to have discharges in their last month of pregnancy, and there are mucal secretions during birth, but Cardona thinks, *That's not normal*. He doesn't know precisely what is wrong, but he does know that sexually transmitted disease is prevalent. More than 120 Newark children contract such illnesses each month; chlamydia, gonorrhea, syphilis, HIV, and AIDs are all on the rise.[3]

The girl lets loose a guttural scream, the first loud, clear sound she has made so far.

"Take slow deep breaths," Cardona coaches. The patient's vulva opens wider. "C'mon, baby," Cardona urges the girl. *"Push!"*

"My legs hurt!" she cries. Rolling her eyes back in her head, the girl moans, "Aggh." Her big doe eyes narrow, then widen with pain as a black, wet, round, grapefruit-sized crown peeps through the vaginal opening. But after a second or two it recedes, and she flops about on the stretcher like a fish out of water.

Cardona smacks her on the thigh. *"Push, girl!"*

Callahan made good time and slides into a spot at University just as the girl begins another contraction.

"If we're gonna move it's gotta be in between contractions," Cardona tells Callahan, and the two fairly yank the stretcher out of the bus before the next one takes hold.

Had the baby been born inside the ambulance, Callahan and Cardona could have cut the cord and placed their names on the birth certificate. It's a sought-after honor and a thrilling note in a job that is witness to so much suffering, but neither EMT is focused on that. The girl seems despondent. Cardona thinks, *She's a potential EDP*. She and the baby belong in Labor and Delivery, but they don't get farther than an ER bay when the girl erupts with a fresh set of screams. A nurse grabs a bottle of Betadine, a topical disinfectant that looks like coffee, and squirts it over the girl's exposed genitalia.

Nurses, residents, and physicians surround the young woman, removing her T-shirt, slipping a gown on her, transferring her to the hospital's oxygen, and hooking her up to various vital-sign monitors. But for the cleanup and paperwork, Cardona and Callahan are done. Still, they can't tear themselves away, and watch eagerly from the sidelines.

"Push, *push!*" says an obstetrician who has been called downstairs.

The baby's head emerges, facedown and covered in blood and mucus. The doctor lifts one of the girl's legs, bends beneath it, and crouches near the baby's face. She inserts a bulb syringe, a palm-sized suction tool with a slim cone on one end, sucks mucus from the baby's mouth and nose, and squirts the brownish discharge on the sheet.

"Come on, girl," the doctor demands, "get that baby out!" A nurse pulls the baby gently by its head. "We need you to push, girl. Sit up and *push!*"

"I can't," the girl cries. Her eyes are wild but her voice is so soft the staff can't hear her.

"What?"

"I can't." And with that she flops back down on the stretcher, giving up.

"Why can't you?" the doctor asks, frustrated by the girl's apathy.

But the girl is spent. Another minute later, at 0028 hours, her baby emerges. He's wailing and wet and covered in vernix, a chalky, white, oily film that protects the fetus's skin inside the amniotic sac. Nurses wrap him in a blanket and take him away to inspect him.

"Get a line in her," the obstetrician barks, as residents hurry to infuse the woman with fluids.

Someone calls from behind a curtain, "He weighs eight pounds, fourteen ounces." (This child is lucky; twelve babies are born with low birth weight each week in the city, and infant mortality is more than twice as high in Newark as it is for the entire state.[4])

A couple of black doctors nearby congratulate each other: *"Mazel tov"*— Yiddish for "good luck."

"What do you want to name him?" one asks the girl.

"I don't care," she answers quietly and turns her face away. "I don't want him." Sitting in a pool of blood, knees up, she retches.

One of the more experienced ER nurses takes a hard look at the mess and grumbles at Cardona, "She didn't need to deliver that here."

He retorts, "I guess *I* have control over that," and squirrels himself away to write the chart while Callahan chats with Auntie.

"All she said was 'I'm sick,' " Auntie tells Callahan. "I been asking her, 'Girl, are you pregnant again?' and she kept saying no. It was clear, but what am I going to do? The girl hasn't been right ever since her mother died." The aunt has had primary custody of the girl since she was a few days old. "I always tried to make sure she had some kind of relationship with her mother, but after the killing, well . . . she just won't talk." (The girl's mother, a prostitute, was murdered many years ago, Auntie whispers, hunching ever so slightly and shielding her mouth with her hand.)

"She's a straight-A student. The school told me to send her to counseling, but the girl just won't talk. She won't say who the father is. She won't even apply for aid for the first baby. I just don't know what I am going to do," Auntie laments. "But that little boy is gorgeous just like his sister."

Having heard the girl say she didn't want the baby breaks Callahan's heart. He believes that much of the trouble in Newark stems from children just not getting the love they need to thrive. And he has a right to be concerned. Here, one out of three children live in poverty, at risk of hunger and chronic illness. Almost seventy percent of Newark-born babies are born to unmarried mothers, and nearly 900 teenagers give birth each year.[5] And there's hardly an easy answer to that. All he can do is love his son to bits and try to be kind and helpful to others. But he just can't stop thinking about this brand-new child's future. Will he languish in the state's care? The hospital is ward to dozens of unwanted babies.

That baby is so beautiful, Callahan thinks. *I just can't see throwing it into the system.* Maybe he *can* do more. Perhaps he and his wife can adopt the boy. They both long for another child but are unwilling to repeat the incredible hurdles associated with fertility treatments. It almost broke them last time.

After work, he peeks at the baby resting in the hospital's nursery. He approaches the hospital's social services department. When he goes home, he brings up the subject with his wife. "At first she thought I was fooling around," Callahan says. By the time he follows up, however, he learns that the girl's family has convinced her to take her new son home.

A few months later, in the middle of the night, Callahan intercedes on behalf of two toddlers about to be dumped into foster care because their mother is being admitted to the ER with no place to leave them. "I just have a thing for kids," he explains. "It took us so long to get our son; I love him so much. He is my world. I just can't conceive of kids having no place to stay."

He phones his mother and summarizes the situation. As predicted, even at 2:00 A.M., Callahan's mother consents. "My mom is a very loving person," he says. "She'll take someone off the street and feed them, let them take a bath. To be frank, my wife has that in her, too." Worried that the two children might be too much for his mother to manage alone, he forfeits his postshift visit to Maryland to stay and help her out until friends of the woman offer to step in.

As for the teenager's infant boy, Callahan says, "We didn't luck out with that one." But he leaves the door open for a different adoption. "We're still thinking about it."

THE HEART OF THE MATTER

> Back in 1969, if you had a cardiac arrest, we just picked you up and took you to the funeral home. Then, we progressed. We'd use two [ECG] leads to determine if you were flat-line. We'd give a little epi, a little atropine. If there was no change we'd go get the telephone book, look up your name, and scratch it out.
>
> —FROM *THE JOY OF DYING*, A PRESENTATION BY PARAMEDIC PAUL EZELLE. HE SUFFERED TWO HEART ATTACKS, ONE OF WHICH KILLED HIM. BUT HE WAS RESUSCITATED.

In September, the summer's intense heat breaks, but the pace of calls is as hectic as ever. Tempers flare and trauma soars. The humidity plays havoc with dialysis patients and people with asthma and congestive heart failure. Shifts are jammed with jobs when Dispatch sends Cardona and Drivet, both matched with temporary partners filling in for their regular teammates, to a seventy-year-old woman with a possible CVA, short for "cerebralvascular accident." CVA is medical speak for the word "stroke," or even the more trendy expression "brain attack."

The BLS truck arrives first. Cardona and his partner, saddled with equipment, clamber up a bleak tenement stoop, shoulder their way through a vestibule, and scale a sixteen-step flight to the second floor. The winding staircase is unlit and cluttered with debris, including an ax. When they reach the top, a single fluorescent bulb quivers dimly. The hallway light is so meager that Cardona yanks out his flashlight just to identify the right apartment. He knocks and is rewarded with the thinnest possible response. He tests the knob and finds the door unlocked.

Inside the threadbare one-room apartment Cardona spies a weak and wasted white woman sprawled on the floor in a white flannel nightgown dotted with tiny blue flowers. Her thin, papery face, pale to the point of near-translucence, is scored with wrinkles. Her hair, the color of faded marigolds, is a nest of tangles. But her eyes, black and bright as a sparrow's, roll toward him immediately. *She's alert*, he sees.

"EMTs, ma'am," he states, crossing the room to kneel at her side. He blinks at the stench—a heady alchemy of urine, gin, and neglect. "Someone's called for help. What's happened here?" he asks, gripping her frail wrist in search of a pulse.

"I'm *so* weak," the woman murmurs, barely audibly.

Through a brief exchange he learns that her name is Hannah, she is in her mid-seventies, and she sank to the floor from feebleness rather than any sudden event. Hannah's speech is whisper-soft but clear. Her muscle tone is weak. When Cardona has her grip his fingers so he can gauge her strength, though unimpressive it's equal in each hand. Both sides of her body respond equally to his other neurological tests, not suggestive of stroke activity.

Cardona lifts Hannah's featherweight frame off the scuffed linoleum floor and lays her gently on her bed, just feet from an ancient white stove. He plumps the lumpy pillow behind her head to make her more comfortable before continuing his exam. Instead of scouting for medications or signs of what might be causing the woman's malaise, setting up the oxygen tank, or preparing her for transport, Cardona's partner stands by with the energy and enterprise of a wax figure.

When Drivet and his per-diem partner arrive, seconds later, Cardona reports, "No history of stroke. But I can't even get a blood pressure of ninety palp." ("Palp," short for "palpation," is a rough calculation of blood pressure, which EMS workers can use in a pinch.) "She says she didn't eat, take her medicine, or drink."

Before he's even crossed the room, Drivet spots his first clue. The woman's arms and legs are mottled; her skin resembles a canvas of bruised figs swimming in cream. Something is preventing her heart from doing its job and delivering oxygen-rich blood throughout her body.

Drivet nods a greeting as he approaches Hannah, takes her wrist between his fingers, and hones in on her pulse. On average, a person's heart beats sixty to one hundred times per minute. Hannah's rate, an impotent thirty-two, is barely throbbing. Instinctively, he calculates her cardiac output, an equation that multiplies the heart's stroke volume by the number of beats per minute. Drivet realizes that her cells are not getting the air and sugar they need to metabolize, nor are they working sufficiently to dump waste products such as carbon dioxide. In short, Hannah is starving and drowning in her own self-made poisons. *She needs to go to the hospital stat*, he thinks.

Cardona's partner holds up the wall and stares at the scene with the dulled eyes of a dead fish. And Drivet's own per-diem partner, new to the system, is still a bit too unsure of himself to jump in. So Drivet, the senior paramedic and a near-legendary caregiver, unhinges the orange vinyl stair-chair and covers it with a sheet. He could delegate the task, lecture the per-diem mopes on idleness, or perhaps even inspire them to take action on the patient's behalf. But Drivet has forged a philosophy throughout his tenure on the street: *Help me to do my job or get out of my way.*

Drivet is rarely confrontational unless pushed, in which case, he says, he quickly reverts to his thirteenth-century Germanic namesake, "Walter the Warrior." But he isn't warm and fuzzy either, and he won't waste a minute of his overcommitted time coaching the mindless, spineless hangers-on. Tired as he is from his two full-time and three part-time jobs, Drivet prefers to take on the extra work and get it done quickly and correctly rather than extend himself for those who lack interest and initiative.

And then there is B-team tradition. Elsewhere, paramedics sometimes lord their training, seniority, and expertise over their basic- and intermediate-level colleagues. On the B team, however, training does not define status. Proving oneself in the field does. When a job needs doing, however menial, it is rare for someone to refuse to pitch in, which accounts in part for the team's tradition of camaraderie.

"We have to take you to the hospital, dear," Drivet advises Hannah. "Can I get you to stand up and move into the chair?" He stands at her side, prepared to help, but first he wants to see what she can do for herself, which will further indicate her strength or weakness. Hannah doesn't get far, so Cardona and Drivet gently lift her under her armpits and into the chair. When they tuck the sheet around her and straighten her nightgown, they see, above her worn knee-high nylons, scraped and bloodied knees. Tenderly, they buckle her in.

Cardona grasps the handles at the top of the chair, and with the two per diems looking on fatuously, the forty-year-old Drivet resigns himself to lifting the bottom of the chair. Their partners scoop up the remaining equipment dutifully, but neither takes the lead to help guide Drivet and Cardona down the stairs. The load isn't especially heavy, but the position is awkward. Drivet's cherubic face sweats with strain as he backs his way down the dark and cluttered stairs with Hannah's bony feet in his face.

As he descends, he has no choice but to inhale the tangy smells wafting toward him, odors of superheated urine and long-unwashed flesh. To hold his breath in this rank, close stairwell while stepping down backward with his hands full of patient is a ticket to fainting. *I hate my life*, he thinks. A college graduate with a degree in business administration, enough postgraduate science credits to attend medical school, sufficient expertise to teach and consult on EMS nationally and internationally, Drivet is still punching his way out of the paper bag that is University Hospital EMS. O'Neill has even dubbed Drivet "Papillon" for his earnest and deserving but as yet unsuccessful attempts to escape.

Drivet is enmeshed in a classic love-hate relationship. He's passionate about the variety of challenges that the urban setting affords. In the past twelve months, for example, a traveler's tantrum left an airport gate agent with a broken neck; a gunman sprayed a crowd with bullets; a plane spiraled out of control and plunged into a crowded residential street; and a college dormitory went up in flames. Drivet had trained and then applied his disaster-management expertise at the 1993 World Trade Center bombing, and he has coordinated EMS backup for several dignitaries. For fun, he also runs a ninety-member ski-patrol force at a northern New Jersey resort.

While he'd rather be chief of thoracic surgery at the Maryland Institute for Emergency Medical Services Systems, perhaps the nation's preeminent trauma center, his role as physician-surrogate in dangerous and dynamic circumstances has been rewarding. But after nineteen years he wants a more substantive challenge. And it wouldn't hurt if he could whittle his five jobs down to one, maybe two. With any luck he'll earn one of the hospital's coveted flight-medic spots that have just opened up. Nothing would please him more, however, than a full-time spot on one of the EMS teams that back up federal law-enforcement agencies. Toward that goal, he has taken on leadership of another urban county's tactical EMS unit and joined the military's Counter Narcotics Tactical Operations Medical Support Group as faculty. But until the next phase of his life crystallizes, he is caught in Newark's seductive purgatory.

He backs down the stairs gingerly. There . . . is . . . no . . . escape from the strain or the stench—at least until he gets a breath of what passes for fresh air in Newark, outside the apartment building, where garbage cans fester in the tired summer heat.

He and Cardona transfer Hannah to a stretcher, slide it into the bus, and secure it in place. At this point, Drivet could give the order to get the vehicle in motion, but EMS is no longer the scoop-and-run profession it was thirty years ago. Emergency-medicine practitioners, from first responders to physicians, have learned that seconds count. The days of just rushing to the hospital are long gone.

When EMS workers identify distress or extremis, they should be equipped and trained to start treatment and stabilize their patients. Without even leaving the scene of a crisis, paramedics can regulate breathing, control bleeding, correct blood-sugar imbalances, begin to address heart-muscle damage, and initiate other critical-care measures that might be delayed if they just rushed to plunk down patients at the nearest hospital. As the number of people in the U.S. without primary-care physicians or insurance nears fifty million, many ERs are dangerously overcrowded.

Moreover, when EMS workers arrive with stable patients whose airways are secure, whose bloods are drawn, whose tubes are inserted, etc., physicians and nurses can proceed even more quickly to definitive care.

Drivet connects Hannah to his LIFEPAK 10 immediately; the heart monitor integrates an electrocardiograph, a defibrillator, and an external cardiac pacer, among other cardiac-care tools. He reaches into the neckline of her gown to stick the electrodes beneath her right and left clavicles; her skin is tissue-thin, deeply wrinkled, and flaccid. As he pulls the gown back to place the third electrode near her left waist, he sniffs and sees a watery diarrhea as well as mottling on her belly. "Ooh, she's got some feces here, too!" he shares cheerfully with the crew, as if he had found her pockets stuffed with gold doubloons. Pausing, he gloves up.

"Hannah, we're gonna start an IV on you and take you to the hospital," he tells his patient.

Like an artist choosing a paintbrush, Drivet selects a fourteen-gauge needle—one of the biggest, bluntest sharps he carries. The larger the needle, the more it hurts. But the brief pain is an unfortunate by-product. The larger the needle, the bigger the hole, and the faster it can infuse saline into her system and prevent vascular collapse. "We're going to fill your tank up," Drivet promises. Hannah merely nods.

While Drivet ties a sliver-thin rubber tourniquet around Hannah's emaciated left arm, neon green waves are already oscillating across the LIFEPAK's screen, reflecting her heart activity. Cardiac tissue has a property called "automaticity," which means its cells are uniquely capable of generating coordinated electrical impulses to flood the heart's upper chambers with blood and squeeze it into circulation from lower chambers. The per-diem paramedic glances at the undulating lines and concludes, "Second-degree, type two."

At this diagnosis, Drivet cocks a discerning eye at the screen and recognizes third-degree atrial ventricular heart block. Having managed thousands of calls per year, he has the depth of clinical experience to interpret the electrocardiogram more accurately. "Hmmm," he says thoughtfully, as if he never heard the per diem go wrong. "Complete heart block."

The heart has three primary sites of electrical activity, and Hannah's first two sites aren't working well if at all. Some nodes are firing, but not in relation to the bottom chambers. Her heart can only manage twenty to forty beats per minute, explaining her low blood pressure, blotchy skin, and lethargy.

Drivet knows his heart rhythms. In fact, it is not unheard-of for ER doctors to consult him on occasion. What he doesn't know, with his limited equipment, is whether the woman suffered a heart attack in the area where the heart generates its electrical impulses. Scar tissue may be blocking the normal electrical pathways, or she may have another problem entirely.

Regardless of the cause, which is not his job to decipher, Hannah's existing heart rhythm can kill her within minutes. *She just may brady out*, he thinks, worried about the fine line between "bradycardia," an excessively slow heart rate, and no heartbeat at all. Then, even his most valiant resuscitation efforts might fail. Turning to Cardona, who is strapping an oxygen mask over Hannah's face, Drivet says, "This is an evolving situation. I'm going to keep you guys with me."

Cardona nods. He sets the oxygen tank's flow meter to fifteen liters of 100 percent oxygen per minute and leaves to take the wheel.

Drivet's partner clips a pulse-oximetry monitor on Hannah's finger. It grips the fingertip like a clothespin but feels like a neoprene thimble. The monitor's sensors detect how well the blood is saturated with oxygen.

"I'll start the IV," Drivet tells his partner. "You look at this for a minute." He nods casually at the LIFEPAK. Perhaps a second look will give the new guy a chance to reconsider his conclusion.

Despite the taut grip of the rubber tourniquet wound tightly around Hannah's reedy arm, which should cause enough pressure to plump up some veins, he finds nothing to stick. He can't even palpate a vessel. His best bet is to try the other arm, but that means turning it over to his partner or negotiating his way to the other side of the bus. The working space is barely five by eight feet, and even that is packed with supply cabinets, benches, canvas bags stuffed with portable equipment, med trays, hanging bags of intravenous fluids, lengths of oxygen tubing, his supine patient, and his partner, too.

A five-foot-ten-inch, 240-pound man, Drivet is nevertheless a miracle in stealth. He practically beams himself from one side to another, tourniquets her right arm, and watches a ropy blue vein appear. He wipes Hannah's flesh with an alcohol swab and waits just long enough for the sterilizing agent to evaporate and lessen the impending sting. "Here comes the needle," Drivet warns. "Don't move. It hurts like hell."

Hannah flinches anyway, and although Drivet gets the plastic catheter sheath in place on his first effort, some wine-dark blood dribbles out. "I need a four-by-four," Drivet announces, sending his new partner on a cabinet-by-cabinet search for absorbent gauze bandages. In the meantime, Drivet attaches a yellow-tinted vacutainer, which speeds extraction of enough blood to fill five tubes for lab tests. He also smears a pinky-sized reagent strip in the small spillage on her arm. The specially prepared paper reacts to blood glucose to indicate her sugar level.

His partner tears open the gauze packet and hands it to Drivet, who swabs Hannah's arm dry, pulls a sheer, biooclusive dressing from his IV tray, and secures the catheter in place. "Do you know what your blood pressure normally is?" Drivet asks Hannah as he unclamps the shutoff valve on the saline bag and frees the solution to slip into her vein. His question is deft; it elicits information and prompts the new medic to strap a blood-pressure cuff onto the patient and inflate it.

"130/70," Hannah reports.

"I got 112/50," the rookie interrupts. It's not surprising that a thin, elderly person's BP is lower than average, but this is hypotensive. "Her rate is *so* s-l-o-w," he says, pressing the inside of her wrist. Looking quickly at the LIFEPAK, he tells Drivet, "It's thirty-two (beats per minute). You don't want to pace her, do you?" Pacing, one of the most aggressive field treatments ALS offers, uses the heart monitor to course electricity through the chest wall and prompt the heart's electrical cells to increase contraction speed and intensity.

"No, she seems stable," Drivet says, stalling. He wants another few seconds to assess Hannah's status before undertaking what he knows to be a painful intervention. Pacing also causes musculoskeletal twitching, which can be agonizing. "Hannah, you have *no* chest pain?" he asks, probing further. "I know we've all asked you thirty-eight times."

"No," she assures him.

"No shortness of breath?"

"No."

"Does your belly hurt?"

"Yeah," she confirms, wincing for emphasis. "I got to pee."

"OK, but wait just a minute," Drivet implores her, while thinking, *This woman is very sick.* For him, that is saying a lot. In his overscheduled, nineteen-year career as an urban, SWAT, and wilderness medic, Drivet has easily seen tens of thousands of patients. Turning to Cardona, he says, "Just get us a med channel"—on the radio—"and let's get out of here." Drivet is even-tempered by nature; his voice is calm but his tone connotes urgency.

As Cardona speeds them toward the hospital and hooks them up with a doctor through Dispatch, Drivet continues interviewing his patient. "Hannah, do you have problems with your blood sugar?"

"No."

"It's a little high," he notes as he examines the reagent strip. Its colormetric scale shows 240, about twice the upper limit of normal. *She doesn't take very good care of herself*, he thinks. *I wonder if she is also an undiagnosed borderline diabetic?* But before he can go further with the thought, his partner hands him the black telephone receiver so he can give report.

"Hi, Doctor, it's Walter. We're en route with a seventy-five-year-old female. Apparently she called 911 complaining of generalized weakness. We found her on the floor of her apartment. She's awake and alert. Blood pressure is 112/50. Her heart rate, which concerns us, is thirty-two.

"It looks like she takes very bad care of herself. We got an IV and routine labs. We have her on high-flow O_2 and she is satting good"—meaning the concentrated gas and mask are helping the oxygen molecules reach throughout her body. "She has some mottling in her lower leg and left arm. Because of her heart rate and mottling, would you like us to pace her?"

"Sounds good, Walter," the doctor confirms. "Go ahead."

"OK, we'll start with a heart rate of sixty and we'll do milliamps up to capture," he suggests. "Can we give her some medication for pain if she can't tolerate it?" The doctor allows him to use his discretion and dispense morphine or Valium.

"Hannah," Drivet says, catching her attention by tapping her forearm gently. "Your heartbeat is really slow. We're going to bump you up a little bit. If this is uncomfortable, you let us know. We'll give you some medicine to make it feel better. You just relax.

"I'm just going to cut off your nice clothes," he says soothingly, almost buoyantly, a hallmark reflecting his command of the situation. Besides, he sees no benefit in upsetting patients, bystanders, or colleagues with displays of temper or anxiety.

Peeling back her flowered nightgown, almost stiff with soil, he sees her sunken breastbone. Hannah's skin has yellowed and her bosoms are two flaps of pancake-thin flesh. "I just have to lift up your breast and put this on your chest," Drivet explains as he rearranges an ECG electrode to accommodate one of the three-by-six-inch white pacing pads. He sticks one just below her left armpit, on her bony rib cage, and places the second over her right upper chest. Both pads connect to LIFEPAK with white, three-foot wires.

With his drug box at his side in case she needs a painkiller, Drivet takes a breath. "Here we go," he alerts her as he dials sixty beats per minute on the LIFEPAK. Gradually, he increases the amplitude until the sixty milliamps of raw current provoke Hannah's heart to synchronize with the machine at a healthful pace.

Drivet compares what Hannah is feeling to using wet fingers to touch both terminals of a car battery for a fraction of a second, which is about how long each jolt occurs. Hannah spasms. And shudders. And spasms. But she doesn't complain.

"I know it's really uncomfortable," Drivet empathizes, surprised that she is tolerating the intrusion so well. "But it really is necessary."

Drivet flicks his eyes between Hannah and the LIFEPAK screen, looking for capture, the point when her ECG overlays the pacing spike on the machine and he feels a pulse beat with each of the spikes. Just as they approach the hospital, Hannah's heart's waves conform to the normal rate and rhythm on the screen.

Cardona parks the bus and opens the back doors to help them unload. But Drivet puts the brakes on: "Just stay still here for a moment." He wants to confirm capture and get another set of vital signs before transferring Hannah to a new environment and another set of caregivers. The added information will tell him how effective the treatment has been so far, and add meat to his chart. "Let's get another pressure before we go in," he reminds his per diem. "You got pulses or not?"

"I don't feel them," the young medic confesses.

"I'm going in for a femoral pulse," Drivet cracks. Since his partner can't find a pulse at the wrist or neck, Drivet needs to palpate a major artery near the groin. Probing there will not only give him information about her circulatory system's status but may even point to other vascular problems, such as an aneurysm. "Pop in and close the door," he tells Cardona, so passersby can't gape inside the bus.

The three men hover over their infirm, vibrating patient. Drivet is preparing to dig his fingers into the old woman's urine-soaked and feces-encrusted groin when his partner cries, "I got it!" The carotid artery in Hannah's neck is throbbing.

"Got a pulse?"

"Yeah, I got a sixty," the medic exclaims.

"You're doing 157 percent better!" Drivet tells Hannah.

Next, his partner reports that Hannah's blood pressure has beefed up to 138/72.

"Really good!" Drivet says. "Excellent." Checking the IV bag, Drivet announces, "I need another one of these cocktails." And Cardona's partner finally sparks to life, yanking a fluid pouch from a shelf and handing it to Drivet. After he restocks the IV, Drivet fashions a makeshift carrying case for his blood tubes by stuffing one into each finger of his used glove, which now resembles an empty udder.

Still a pale, almost almond color, Hannah is less ghostly white. "Hannah, you feel better?" Drivet asks.

Despite clear improvement in her circulation, Hannah shakes her head. It doesn't surprise Drivet that she still feels poorly. Years of ill health, poor nutrition and hygiene, and a possible drinking problem have rendered her vulnerable. Her rack-thin frame still convulses with each jolt from the LIFEPAK as they wheel her into the hospital.

Drivet hands the blood tubes off to one nurse and gives report. Watching another struggle with the hospital's pacing machine, he discreetly assists, which gives him pause to wonder about Hannah's prognosis.

A student at another medical center twenty years ago, Drivet spent as much time in the stacks and the hospital as he did in the back of the bus. His mentor pummeled him with complex questions and demanded details, diagnoses, and keen medical insights that began with the patient's symptoms in the field and carried through admission and discharge.

"Do I really need to know all that?" Drivet asked once or twice.

"Of course you need to know that. You are practicing medicine!" his mentor bellowed. "To the library with you!"

Drivet still loves medicine enough to buy and read, for pure enlightenment, the densest medical textbooks he can find. Give him a free minute on the job and he's likely to hightail it to University's medical-school bookstore or plunge nose-deep into a volume dedicated to some facet of emergency services.

After he brings a patient into the ER, it is still his custom to stay a few minutes, help the staff, study ECGs, or ask for help evaluating X-rays. He queries physicians about diagnoses and treatment plans. Many times, he follows up on patients, too. He chooses interesting cases, researches them independently, and discusses them with hospital-based colleagues. But tonight—and too many nights, given the exhausting volume of calls—transferring Hannah is as far as it goes.

Drivet, whose ex-wife dubbed him "the King of Detached Concern," contents himself with knowing that he did everything possible for his patient while she was in his care. It's how he copes when the nightly influx of ill and injured gets to be too much. It's how, he says, he avoids putting a bullet in his head.

Cardona completes his chart, thinking, *Hannah just bought herself a pacemaker.* The two per diems put fresh linens on the stretcher. Drivet, who endeavors to keep an even keel, feeling neither joy nor sorrow, has already moved on to the next target.

PRIME TIME

Cisternino is on a low-carbohydrate diet; he has already lost eighteen pounds in two weeks. He's tired and cranky but ekes out fun wherever he can. Last night, he tells Fazio, he played an aggressive game of beer pong with fellow students at Ramapo College. "It was OK," he justifies, because he played with Budweiser, which he describes as "water with a drop of beer flavor." Two cans of Bud only counted for six grams of carbohydrate, practically his whole day's allotment but well worth the expense.

And Fazio delights him in return, describing her future stepson's ingenuity at mastering Oodles of Noodles, his recent most favorite food. Family is on her mind. Her wedding is fast approaching. Cisternino's long-term relationship, however, feels fractured beyond repair. The stress of the job and perhaps even the personalities attracted to this type of work make family and romance exceptionally hard to sustain.

At 2020 hours, Dispatch sends them to a possible DOA.

"If the patient is under age twenty-five, it's probably an overdose," Fazio predicts, invoking "EMS algebra"—the street medics' law of averages and a game of chance they play to forecast bogus calls. "Chances of it being an overdose or death by violent crime are pretty high."

They reach the designated street but spend a minute scanning several building fronts, few of which are numbered. They settle on a squat, tired-looking edifice of yellow brick and taupe cement. Children ride bicycles on the sidewalk outside where adults gather and smoke.

Airway bag, defibrillator, and drug tray in hand, the medics march up the stoop, twist and squeeze themselves through a double-door vestibule, and wind their way through a narrow hallway. They go directly to the apartment whose door is ajar. Cisternino walks in first and finds himself inside a kitchen. A maroon-tinged film of filth sullies once-white walls. The kitchen and the sitting room are combined, and before the medics can get through it to the bedroom where the patient is, they must pass by a trio of elderly men seated on lawn chairs around a television. The silver-haired men, dressed in plaid flannel jackets, are positively riveted to *Judge Judy*.

Inside the bedroom, a few feet from the door, a young woman, a neighbor who lives next door, lies dead. EMTs Ennis Terrell and Che-heibe Scott are already there, and so are two cops. When the EMTs see the medics, they just shake their heads. The woman has been dead for hours.

She lies on the floor, the color of weak tea. Her hair is short and bushy. Her eyes are closed. Her mouth, open, makes a small "o." She wears a wrinkled white T-shirt and a peony pink windbreaker. Tiny, child-size hands protrude from her sleeves. Her lips are purple. She wears black jeans that are wet at the crotch, white anklets, and black sneakers.

"RMA?" Cisternino jokes, using the abbreviation for patients who Refuse Medical Attention.

The woman appears to be deep in sleep, but the signs are clear to these experienced professionals. She is dead, and she can't be resuscitated. "I would have no qualms about laying my cup of coffee on her belly while I write my chart," Cisternino jokes to make the point.

"It's gone beyond anything we can do," Terrell says, confident that the medics will issue an official pronouncement of death.

Still, protocol requires them to confirm the death with a reading from the heart monitor. Cisternino unwraps three ECG leads. When he lifts her shirt to attach them to her chest, he sees stretch marks from childbirth striating her belly. He sticks the white electrode beneath her right collarbone, the black one under her left, and the red one to her lower left chest. Once the heart monitor confirms asystole, and other signs are noted, he radios an ER doc at University to arrange an official pronouncement.

Never at a loss, Fazio makes the death a lesson. Turning to the EMTs, she goads them into reporting the findings concisely and professionally. "Criteria for pronouncement?"

Scott and Terrell look at each other.

"Give me the signs," Fazio says, tapping her foot. Certain signs of death automatically render rescue attempts futile: decapitation, hemicorporectomy, and decomposition, for example. The EMTs should be able to rattle them off, if only to justify why they haven't initiated CPR.

"Well, she's stiff," Terrell states. And it's true. The woman's jaw is fixed in position. When Fazio tries to close the woman's mouth, it's not especially pliable. Rigor mortis usually sets in between five and eight hours after death, as proteins collect in the joints, but room or temperature or environmental conditions can affect that. Twelve to fifteen hours later, the proteins begin to disintegrate and rigor gradually disappears.

"Lividity," Scott contributes. And that's true, too. The skin on the woman's forearms and back is claret-colored and mottled. She has lain on the floor long enough for blood to begin leaking from her capillary beds as gravity draws it down. Left undisturbed for more than six hours, all her blood would settle in the tissues closest to the ground, so the upper half of the body would blanch pale and the bottom half would deepen to a solid port-wine.

The deceased woman's skin is dry. And although the apartment is not air-conditioned, and it's hot and humid outside, her body is cool to touch. "Dead bodies cool approximately one degree per hour," Fazio explains, but that also depends on clothes.

"This didn't just happen," the rookie officer, a black female, half asks, half postulates. She cocks her head toward the TV-watching oldsters and continues dryly: "They *say* they thought she was sleeping. They noticed she hadn't moved in a while."

"They don't give a shit about her," Terrell snarls. "They're still looking at the TV, laughing!"

The rookie shakes her head, dumbfounded. A woman wearing a bandanna and soiled denim jacket pokes her head into the room and moans.

"Here comes the concerned family," Cisternino mutters.

"Get her out of here," the cop tells her partner. Then she goes back to her notes: "She's twenty-five. History of drug abuse."

"It happens every day," Terrell sighs dispiritedly.

"How long does it take for the smell?" the rookie asks.

"It depends on the temperature of the room," Scott answers.

"As long as there are no maggots, I'm all right," Terrell volunteers. He's learned not to stare at the dead or their faces will haunt him when he tries to sleep.

"Oh, but the smell of burning flesh," Fazio says with a brief shiver, "that's really the one I don't like."

"Yeah, and it stays in the truck for a long time," Cisternino agrees.

Every EMS worker has a weakness, Fazio asserts—"some injury, sight, or smell that we can't stand. Decomposition is pretty gross; gases bubble up under the skin. But on the bright side, if there is a bright side, they are hardly recognizable as human, so it's easy to detach."

"For me it's the eye," Cisternino confesses, recounting multiple encounters with dangling eyeballs. "If the optic nerve is intact, can they still see? And what is their brain thinking?" he wonders aloud. "I've been told as long as the nerve is intact, the eye should be able to function, but because it's no longer in position to receive signals the way the brain is accustomed, I don't know. No one's been able to give me a really good answer. Not even an ophthalmologist."

Once the crew officially pronounces a victim dead in the field, they leave the body in the custody of the reigning law-enforcement officer. He or she makes arrangements with the medical examiner and any additional investigation. Thankful that they don't have to charge the dead woman for her pronouncement, they begin packing up their equipment. (The department has not traditionally billed for such services, but limiting revenue recovery to the patients it transports is not sufficient to meet the cost of preparedness. Within months, regulations will allow it to charge for pronouncements to help recover costs associated with the EMS workers' time, travel, and expertise.)

A homicide detective sticks his head in and asks, "Natural? Any signs of trauma?" Police investigate all deaths, except for those of natural causes, that a nurse or doctor has attended. Noting the woman's history of drug abuse, the crew dismisses the young woman's death as "voluntary."

"Most drug users know someone who has overdosed," Cisternino explains. "So they know death is a possibility." He throws the heart monitor over his shoulder, stashes his clipboard under his arm, points at the dead woman, and addresses her: "You, stay cool."

As they file out, the old men remain seated around their color TV, enjoying a snack. Curious neighbors crane their necks inside the apartment, asking what happened. Tossing his silvered head toward the bedroom where the corpse lies stiffening, one of the senior citizens replies nonchalantly, "Oh, Leila died."

It doesn't faze Fazio that the woman has been dead on the floor for hours while her friends and neighbors relaxed casually mere feet away. "The worst thing I've seen on this job," she says, and she has seen heinous murder scenes and vicious cruelty, "is the total disregard for human life."

Scott and Terrell go on to their next call. Fazio and Cisternino go out for barbecued chicken.

8   STEP ON IT

It's not all lights and sirens. It's not all glory, high-profile jobs. Your day-to-day bread and butter is the sick baby, the cold and flu, the 'I just don't feel right.' It's not always an all-balls-out adrenaline rush.

—GEORGE BURR, SEVENTEEN-YEAR B-TEAM VETERAN, 2000

*E*mergency medical dispatcher Jimmy Smith, who joined the department in 1970 as an "ambulance driver," remembers: "We were considered the lowest of the low. All we had to have was a standard and advanced first-aid card. When there was a patient to pick up, we'd drive over to the hospital and wait for an attendant to come down. They sat in the back with the patients even though they were less qualified than the drivers were. I remember one attendant banging on the door between the compartment and the cab, shouting that the woman was in labor. I had to pull over to deliver the baby."

AMBULANCE DRIVER

Even when driving is the crews' main focus, because mildly ill patients do not need much intervention, the jobs can be taxing.

Early one brittle-cold morning, a woman dials 911 and requests an ambulance because her three-year-old son is having "difficulty breathing." Dispatch escalates the call and sends Drivet and Tommy Opperman to a shadowy grouping of garden apartments in the Central Ward. The woman, fashionably dressed, elaborately coiffured, and spectacularly manicured, invites the crew into her threadbare living room, where a small boy stands staring at a blaring giant-screen TV. Drivet kneels to befriend the boy and examine him.

The boy is sick with a common head cold. With painstaking grace, Drivet explains this to Mom and lets her know he's not in danger. He offers to bring the boy to the hospital if that is her preference but also offers her the confidence to monitor her son at home with a thermometer and children's cold medications. Mom has no thermometer in the house. She has no children's medications, or Tylenol, either. Mom wants to go to the hospital, so she starts to scoot the child into the subfreezing night in his thin cotton T-shirt and jeans. Politely, Drivet prompts her to find a jacket for her son. The zipper is stuck halfway down, but Drivet makes a game out of dressing the boy, closes the coat, and carries him to the bus. He is past the temptation to question the mother's priorities and beyond the impulse to intervene more aggressively on the boy's behalf. That level of negligence isn't even worth mentioning to the Division of Youth and Family Services (DYFS), EMS workers say; DYFS is already overwhelmed with much worse. Authorities substantiated almost 1,200 cases of child abuse in Newark in 1999.[1]

It seems inevitable to the crew that one day the boy will call to casually summon the ambulance, having learned to do so at his mother's knee, which is probably where she learned it, too, they imagine. "We don't have enough money, manpower, or legal authority to enforce a change of lifestyle," Drivet says. And thus, the sick status quo limps on generation after generation.

About 0100 hours on a humid summer night, Dispatch sends Callahan and Cardona to treat "a man, bleeding." They arrive to find that their patient has disappeared but not before dumping his children on the street corner. Standing under a street lamp waiting for her father, a twelve-year-old girl wears a turban on her head, a scowl on her face, and a baby boy on her hip. She is rack-thin and yet voluptuous where men are most likely to look. Her top and skirt, a striking tie-dyed blue, cling to her developing body like a second skin.

Callahan and Cardona quickly conclude that neither the girl nor her infant stepbrother are sick. But they cannot leave them unprotected at this drug-dealing crossroads. They confer with a cop, who raises his palms, backs away, and declines to become involved. Chief Visoskas authorizes them to take the children to a nearby hospital; at least there they'll be safe. Along the way, Cardona coaxes some information from the sullen girl. She gives up her father's cell-phone number and a predetermined code word she uses so he will know she needs him. After three tries, Cardona gives up. He elicits her grandmother's number. He reaches the girl's grandmother, apologizes for the late hour, and tells her where he is bringing the children.

At the hospital, Cardona gives report, suggests that the nurse call DYFS, and leaves to write his chart. The nurse ignores the twelve-year-old girl; she may not even realize the girl is a minor, but she doesn't bother to check. Instead, she plays with the baby. Under the bright hospital lights she finds, to her surprise, slivers of glass in his silky hair. The nurse glances up at the girl for an explanation.

"Someone took a baseball bat and hit my dad's windshield," the girl explains. "Me and my brother were sitting there."

When the nurse removes the boy's soaking-wet diaper, the glass inside sparkles like a cache of diamonds, but his behind is uninjured. Another nurse gets the baby a bottle. No one asks the girl if she's hungry, and she doesn't ask for food. But she is. She hasn't eaten in at least one full day.

According to a 1999 survey published by Zero Population Growth, a national nonprofit environmental group, Newark's seventy thousand children are growing up in what is probably the country's least kid-friendly city. The EMS workers are not permitted to criticize the parents. They can, and do, rescue dogs, cats, and other neglected pets, but they can't take the children home with them. And they can't improve the children's living conditions. Instead they bite their tongues and harden their hearts, just a little, with each case.

Over time many blue-shirts begin to view their work with a certain doomed quality, a feeling that their yeomen's efforts are as successful as Sisyphus pushing his boulder. Unable to effect long-term change, frustrated by stacks of paperwork, short of sufficient feedback, and constantly rushed, they limit themselves to helping patients during the thirty minutes it takes to reach, stabilize, transport, and transfer. Nothing more, even for those who most need advocates.

THE MIXING BOWL

The shortest distance between two points is a straight line, and Dispatch has GPS and AVL to help abbreviate transport times. The tools help, but the city and its environs are fraught with obstacles in the form of one-way streets, unsigned streets, unlit or dangerously dim streets, and seven crowded highways whose interlacing boggles the mind. The New Jersey Turnpike, for example, is one of the busiest roads in the nation. Called to jobs on the 117-mile turnpike, EMS workers must wind their way through inner and outer lanes, for cars and trucks, respectively; eastern and western spurs; ramps; access roads; and interchanges galore. One interchange even has its own nickname: "the mixing bowl."

Abbreviations in the department manual help keep things straight—or do they? NSI, SNI, NSO, SNO, NSW, SNW, NSE, SNE, and more! There are toll-booths with inside or outside entries and exits. Even the ramps are complicated: NWT, for example, runs from the northbound western spur to the tolls. But there are TNW, TS, TSI, and TSO, too. Each exit has its own alphabetic jumble to negotiate anew. U-turns are coded Z/1000. Crossovers are UU/1000. And this is just one of the roadways. Sometimes finding a job feels like a swim in alphabet soup.

With fifteen hospitals in or around its twenty-four-square mile territory, University EMS workers often complete each job in less than an hour. Outsiders sometimes misconstrue their speed, and dismiss University as a scoop-and-run operation. There may be a kernel of truth in that image, albeit a dusty, thirty-year-old kernel that harks back to pioneering first efforts in the early 1970s when Newark's first EMTs nicknamed the city the "Wild West" and dubbed themselves "cowboys." Now the buses are well equipped; crews have ten, even twenty years of experience; the scope of practice is broader than ever; and the relentless pace has honed them to sleek efficiency.

In other parts of the country, however, ambulance trips can take much longer. In Sweet Grass, Montana, for example, a volunteer corps of twenty EMTs serves residents of the 2,400-acre county, where temperatures can plummet to minus sixty-four degrees Fahrenheit and diesel fuel can freeze. Snowfall of more than two feet can slow the four-wheel-drive ambulance response times to an hour or more. Paramedics in Nevada say it can take two and a half hours just to reach a ranch office, where they must then pick up a map and drive another twenty miles before first laying eyes on their patient. The "very rough, hasty, single-trap roads" and "198-mile trips" make them "laugh at the golden hour" and sympathize with patients suffering back problems. "We just got a helicopter in the last two months," one medic told colleagues from around the country at an NAEMT dinner. "But in any kind of weather, we lose radio contact, so it can't fly." EMS workers serving the 1.4-million-acre Yakima Valley closed area (Native American land) can only go so far in their vehicles before strapping on snowshoes to hike a ten-foot-high snow base deep into the forest for some patients.

Ambulance drivers drive ambulances. But the title is as archaic as it is unfair. We might as well label pilots "plane drivers." Emergency medical services and the transportation involved is more than rolling patients from doorsteps to hospital entrances.

It's getting to the scene, sometimes lights ablaze and sirens screaming, in a city besieged by car theft and reckless drivers, some as young as age ten and some willing to speed faster than 120 mph. It's ensuring safe passage through centuries-old buildings or poorly planned ones. It's the physical strain of laboring under thirty to eighty pounds of equipment, and patient weight also, with too few hands to distribute the load. It's rushing to addresses that do not exist and navigating murky obstacle courses such as homeless people pushing overloaded shopping carts down the center of major byways, streets studded with unwanted furniture, drunks and downed tree limbs. It's zeroing in on distressing problems, marshaling resources to quell crises in real time, and doing it all while operating heavy machinery, not infrequently during weather extremes. It's living twelve hours a day, plus commuting time, in a vehicle—and caring for their trucks with the attentiveness and affection that GIs have for their rifles.

OH, THE PLACES THEY GO

Cisternino and his per-diem partner race to a highway job at 70 mph trailing their comrades on the rescue truck. It's 0100 hours and it's spring, at least officially. But the winter's frost, reluctant to retreat, still chills the April night air. Suddenly, Dispatch changes the assignment and directs them to a municipality north of Newark for an "EDP, possible jumper." The medics who cover that town, employed by a different hospital, are busy handling other crises, so B-team medics will fill in. (Authorities should have plans to cover crises when customary resources are occupied. The most efficient, most reliable way to do this is hotly debated, often without much public contribution. The time it takes to raise and import a substitute crew multiplied by the distance from the incident equals added delays in patient care.) On command, Cisternino turns his truck around and heads to the suburb, hoping that the town's BLS service, which its fire department provides, will arrive first and cancel the request.

A history buff, Cisternino can't help but appreciate the stunning contributions architects have made to Newark's cityscape. Preservationists have protected quaint eighteenth-century farmhouses and older structures, too. Developers protected the character but converted Tiffany and Company's first sterling factory into a condominium. North Newark's mansion-lined streets always enrapture him, even though he is driving through them for the umpteenth time, as he is tonight. Master builders crafted these small castles from fieldstone, brick, or stucco, and adorned them with turrets and balconies and dozens of rooms. Leaded-glass windows sparkle in the moonlight. Velvety lawns and lush landscaping showcase each home in a frame of newborn green.

When he shows up at the designated location, there's plenty of confusion but no patient. An animated, half-hysterical woman spouts drunken gibberish, and police try to translate. One of the officers whispers to Cisternino that she is a "mister-if-you-have-a-bottle-I'll-be-your-friend" type. That doesn't discount her report, but it does raise questions. "You *might* have an EDP on your hands," the officer says, unsure if the woman is the patient or if it is the friend she is babbling about.

She was drinking with two friends, she explains, when one climbed onto the rock outcropping near the side of a train trestle "to take a leak." He lost his balance and tumbled into the dark void. That was twenty minutes ago.

Looking over the edge of the bridge, which allows cars and foot traffic to cross over some railroad tracks, Cisternino senses only a dark abyss. As he scrutinizes the scene with his naked eye, he sees only a limitless black hole. He feels a hollow breeze blow over his head. He smells the first of the season's weeds and the rank dampness of still water. He hears nothing from the silent chasm below.

When the cops walk toward the middle of the trestle and shine their flashlights over the brink, everyone peers down. There, half-submerged in a ditch of coal black water dotted with flotsam and jetsam, is something that looks awfully similar to a person in a fetal position. *It's the perfect mission for Rescue,* Cisternino thinks. *O'Neill can rappel his way down, stabilize and package the patient, and rig his ropes to haul the two of them up to the ambulance.* But Dispatch assigned Rescue to the turnpike job, so Cisternino and company must fend for themselves.

"A guy hung himself here about eight or nine years ago," the cop recalls, nonchalantly. "Damnedest thing, him hanging between two districts." The trestle straddles two towns. As if that does not sufficiently complicate this call, now that they have found a patient more or less on the train tracks, a third jurisdiction—a public-transportation agency—comes into play.

"Hopefully," someone says, carefully eyeing the third rail, "the Transit Authority has shut off the electricity and closed down the tracks, or we'll all be hamburger."

The officer figures that the nearest entrance to the train tracks is a mile or two into the neighboring town, which he must now contact. After getting directions, Cisternino drives his bus there; the cops follow and call for a volunteer emergency squad and the fire department to meet them there, too.

Once Cisternino arrives, he hops out of the bus and straps the airway bag over his shoulder. "Just be glad it isn't July," he yells to his per-diem partner as he starts trekking across the railway bed's four-inch stones. "It would be mosquito hell, not to mention West Nile virus."

The size-thirteen, high-top, zip and buckle, black leather combat boots he wears offer some protection against a turned ankle. (They come in handy with the rats, too, because they give the bold rodents something to gnaw on before they get to his flesh, he says.) But the going is treacherous, and the farther he hikes the darker it gets. Cisternino whistles while he walks. His shaved head and multiple earrings gleam in the moonlight. He sets an ambitious pace for the ragtag group that follows. His partner scrambles after him with the trauma kit;

firefighters from one town are next—lugging a long board, collar, and head blocks. The vollies (volunteers), from yet another town, trail behind, chatting with police and cutting pale yellow swaths through the night with their flashlights. The makeshift group now numbers fourteen, six of whom are cops from various districts. They slog over the stones for three-quarters of a mile. The surefooted Cisternino doesn't miss a step. The worn sneaker, old tire, dented cans of beer and soda pop, rusty license plate, and other debris do not disrupt his focused march, or that of his partner, who has paraded plenty as a soldier. Everyone else gets distracted or temporarily derailed.

When they reach the pit under the trestle and the patient obscured within its shadows, the vollies circle his pale white, waterlogged body, fix their lights on him, and begin giving what B-teamers sarcastically call "the stare of life."

A slight man dressed in a plaid shirt and jeans, the patient lies curled on his right side in a watery depression. Cisternino steps down into the pool. Six inches of cold, stale water cover his boots. Bending over the man, Cisternino wraps a collar around his patient's neck and then holds the man's head still.

He talks briefly with the patient, just long enough to discover that he is conscious, his airway is intact, the eyeball that's visible is both blue and bloodshot, and he stinks of body odor and booze. His condition, after a fall of thirty to forty feet, makes Cisternino think, *This is just the luckiest guy I've seen in a long time.* "OK, let's get him out of here," he says, and the firefighters join him in the ditch.

Cisternino continues holding the man's head steady and directs the firefighters to logroll their soggy charge onto the board. In a clumsily choreographed moment, the three step up and out of the ditch, fighting not to lose their patient as the chunky gravel dances beneath their feet. Once on level ground, the rescuers put a foam block on either side of the man's head so he won't aggravate any cervical-spine injuries. Under the flashlights' dim glow, they tie him to the board with cravats, partly so he won't fall off and partly to keep him still. The alcohol and probable head injury make for a potentially combative patient, experience tells them.

"I don' need thish!" the patient slurs on cue. His beard resembles shredded wheat.

He's got hundred-proof breath, Cisternino thinks. *I need a couple of olives to go with that!* Cisternino and a firefighter hump the patient out. The trek back feels longer with the additional 150 sodden pounds, and a Monty Python scene flashes in his head. He pictures a serf trudging through streets with his cart full of bubonic-plague victims. "Bring out yer dead," Cisternino chants in a perfectly pitched medieval monotone. "Bring out yer dead."

Police glance through the man's wallet as they round out the procession back to the bus. They find the patient's name (Bob), birth date (he's in his fifties), and Social Security number. One remembers arresting Bob recently for burglary and concludes, "He's just another troll hanging out under the bridge."

Once they reach the ambulance and crowd inside, the EMS workers strip Bob of his wet, silt-drenched clothes. They want him naked for two reasons. First, they want visual clues to any potentially serious fractures. Second, they want to help him fight hypothermia. But the man does not go gently into patient care. "Fug yer mudder!" he growls, employing his wiry biceps to swing gnarled fists. His words betray a mouthful of rotten stumps, and gaps where teeth are missing altogether.

Thankfully, Cisternino probably won't have to intubate the man. Poor or no dental care, as is often the case in his patient population, means teeth have a tendency to crumble at the cold touch of the laryngoscope blade.

Bob continues to protest, and patients have the right to refuse care. But he must be competent to do so. Because Bob is drunk and the probable victim of a head injury, he forfeits these rights via the doctrine of implied consent. EMS operates under the assumption that people want lifesaving care, and if their thinking is disturbed by substance abuse, low blood sugar, a brain tumor, or head injury, their right to on-the-spot self-care decisions is compromised. Caregivers must act in the patient's best interest.

Someone cranks up the heat while another covers his ghostly pale strip of a body with a sheet and several blankets. It's hard not to notice Bob's half-inch penis nesting in a patch of beer-colored hair shot with gray. It becomes a target for one crew member who begins to resent Bob's vile behavior. "That's what happens when you're cold and wet," the rescuer mumbles. "You shrivel up to nothing."

Soon it is so hot inside the bus that the crew members swelter. Dripping with sweat, they seem to be melting. They note injuries on Bob's upper shoulders, head, and knees. Cisternino orders an ECG; it reads normal. His partner struggles to insert an IV, but Bob is so combative that he dislodges it even though he has been tied down. When that happens, the solution disperses and puddles under his skin, causing his arm to swell. Depending on the patient and the fluid, this can mean anything from a harmless inconvenience to tissue necrosis. In Bob's case, the medic must simply try again.

Bob crosses his legs and clenches to avoid having his ankles tied down. He strains to pull up his head; he fights the oxygen mask, collar, and head blocks. It doesn't matter that the crew tries coaching him through each aspect of care with calm voices, simple information, and appeals for his cooperation.

When they arrive at the hospital and enter the trauma center, a doc greets them: "Hi, sir. What happened?"

With his partner giving report, Cisternino turns to walk out to his bus. "God protects children and stupid people," he mumbles. In the background, he hears Bob skirmishing with the nurses. "Time for Bob to go on a respirator," the doc says, unwilling to fight this patient, either. "Let's paralyze and intubate him. Send him to CAT scan and X-ray."

An ER nurse strolls by, looks casually at the man flailing about in his pallid, emaciated, and hirsute nakedness, and continues walking, licking her ice-cream sandwich.

SLINGING LIZARDS

The B-teamers put a hard twenty thousand miles a year on their buses. They keep their fleet glossy on the outside and at least broom-clean on the inside, which some say isn't good enough—but they don't want to add bumper-to-bumper disinfection to their responsibilities, too. Some buses are in better condition than others, but wear and tear manifests in failed brakes, broken air-conditioning, cabinet doors that swing wildly during cross-city journeys and won't snap shut, and the sharps boxes that tumble from the wall, spilling their infectious contents across the floor. These buses are only fit for "slinging lizards"—*lizards* is slang for old people—between nursing homes and hospitals, one says.

MCHALE'S NAVY

Drivet has pet names for his ambulance. On days he dreams about becoming a NorthSTAR flight medic, he dubs his bus "Groundstar." Most days, he christens it the *S.S. University* and cloaks himself and others in a tongue-in-cheek fantasy that borrows liberally from his passion for all things military, Tom Clancy novels, and a touch of *McHale's Navy*. He's not far off course. As Drivet steers the *S.S. University* into the darkened streets, the dashboard instrumentation is aglow. The blue-uniformed professionals, ensconced in slate-colored corduroy captains' chairs, wrangle radios, read tangerine-and-lime-colored digital displays, scan pale liquid-crystal screens, and punch codes into the GPS. The cab resembles the bridge of a patrol boat floating through the city's troubled waters.

OPPOSITES ATTRACT

Externally, anyway, Opperman and Drivet are polar opposites. Opperman arrives early to work. Drivet always manages to defeat some crisis just barely in time to beat the clock. Opperman is tall and lean. Drivet has more trouble keeping the goodies off his waistline.

Neither appreciates having to add janitorial duty to their taxing shifts. A good sport, though, before he clocks out Drivet lumbers from bus to bus inviting his pals to give him their garbage and thinking, *Eighteen years as a paramedic, and I can empty garbage cans myself*. Opperman, on the other hand, perpetually tidies up. He begins and ends each shift with a six-inch dust broom and pan in hand, collecting catheter tips, safety pins, needle caps, used electrodes, and miscellaneous screws off the floor, then using the Leatherman tool he bought himself to tighten loose screws in the door. In a word, he's neat.

Opperman is a natural mechanic who keeps his aging, burgundy Camaro in mint condition. Drivet pushes his red-hot-red Saab as hard as he drives himself; and he neglects it much the same way he shirks his personal needs. Stuck in traffic en route to a call, Drivet is more likely to address a slowpoke with "Sailor, what is your malfunction?" or "C'mon, Governor, get out of the way." Opperman is prone to invoking spicier language.

"The first ones to say what took you so long to get here," he theorizes, "are the ones who don't move their cars when we're sitting behind them with our lights and sirens."

"The magic finger is more effective," Drivet cracks.

"We need a bigger dashboard," Opperman states bluntly one night. His side is empty and pristine.

"I live off the dashboard!" Drivet replies, as if he were just slapped on the cheek with a glove. As if a line bisected the truck, Drivet's side has all the comforts of home, all of which he shares generously—a *Men's Health* magazine, his wool cap and gloves, a coffee cake, a chocolate cake, a Tastykake, half a chicken-parmigiana sandwich, a book—and at his feet are a few napkins, a bottle of water, a bottle of Sprite, a bottle of Snapple, and a box of oatmeal cookies. "If we get in an accident I'll more than likely have one of these items impale me, but at least while we're getting extricated we'll have something to eat."

CREATURE COMFORTS

Chief Piumelli and Bill Heber have worked for University Hospital EMS for twenty years apiece, too. "In 1981, there were only four ambulances, and one of them was a green Dodge Duster," Heber recalls. Now the fleet has more than thirty vehicles.

"Yeah, the Duster had one strobe, a big cone siren. It was a two-door, like Al Bundy's car, with a yellow streak of lightning down the side," Piumelli laughs, thinking of the TV sitcom *Married . . . with Children*. "I remember

'Supervisor' was written on it like 'S-u-p-e-r-v-i-s-o-u-r.' " By this time, the six-foot-four-inch, nearly 300-pound man is cracking up at the misspelling and nearly doubles over.

"I remember one night, when I was riding around with a supervisor as extra personnel, we got a call for a pedestrian struck," Heber says. "We found him on the hood of a car, unconscious. We put him on a backboard, rested it on the Duster's front hood, and rode him over. Back then, we used to pick up multiple jobs, end up with three to five patients in an ambulance. Ah, the things you could do before the Department of Health." He chuckles. "We had no heat or air-conditioning, no portable radios. If you opened the bench you could see the ground 'cause the floor had rotted out. Driving down the road one night I heard this *bang bang bang*! I said, 'Mario, you hear something? What the hell was that?' " Heber pauses to re-create the perplexed look he wore on his face.

"I stopped, took a look," Piumelli jumps in. "That grinding noise? It's your big oxygen bottle that fell through the floor. We were dragging it down First Street!" He lets loose a ferocious belly laugh, although he recognizes that by smacking the compressed, combustible gas against the asphalt, catastrophe was in the waiting. It's pure luck that he and Heber are more than memories today.

The crews sometimes take for granted that even twenty years ago their ambulances did not boast the creature comforts and tools they enjoy today. Now they have climate control, AM and FM radios, cushy seats, cup holders, double-width doors for loading and unloading, voluminous scene lighting, GPS systems, sophisticated telemetry, and cabinets to store over four hundred pieces of equipment and supplies. Many countries have no ambulances, and still transport patients by donkey, camel, bicycle, etc.

Legitimate complaints about the buses loom large. "With one being the worst and ten being the best, mechanically, I'd say they're a seven . . . but I've seen them as bad as a three," one of the more knowledgeable blue-shirts says. "The guys now think they're atrocious, but they're a lot better now than they used to be. As to cleanliness, though, that's a failure. That would be a four."

The fleet has six ALS ambulances, fourteen BLS buses, two Rescue trucks, a neonate pediatric intensive-care truck, a mass-casualty response unit, a command-post vehicle, and several support vehicles and supervisor trucks, too. Activating more trucks would reduce response times and lighten what is inarguably a heavy workload. For example, between midnight and 0700 hours, except for units stationed in a bordering town and on city outskirts at the airport, only four medics and six EMTs are on hand to care for Newark's 273,500 residents.

Although the service has added units over the years, an administrator concedes, "We have trouble putting ambulances on the road." It takes money to activate more trucks. (A heart monitor alone can cost $20,000.) And that money is hard to come by. For example, University has provided twenty-four-hour EMS coverage to Newark International Airport and its thirty-four million passengers a year in exchange for a "donation," which has not increased since 1985.

MY HOUSE

It's hot and steamy, still light outside, when Dispatch sends Callahan and Cardona to help a "sick" man near headquarters. A carful of people pulled up to a senior citizens' building, opened the door, and shoved the man out, a bystander reports. Cardona kneels at the head of the pallid, skeletal man, who lies slumped on the asphalt driveway.

"How are you doing, sir?" Cardona asks.

The man blinks his eyes and looks at him but offers no response.

"Where do you live, big guy?"

The man continues lying quietly, as if content to bake in the evening sun. The bitter stink of alcohol wafts up from his skin.

"Why don't we help you up?" Cardona asks. He and Callahan reach under the man's sweat-soaked armpits and raise him to his feet. The man's hair, once black, now threaded with silver, is short but stiff with grease. The back of his scalp is crusty with matted blood.

"Are you staying anywhere, man?" Cardona tries again as he walks the man a few feet to the bus.

Callahan has opened the ambulance door and is ready to give the man a hand. "Bring that foot up," he coaches the man to step inside the bus.

"I haven't done anything," the man slurs.

Cardona sits the man on the bus's bench and patiently explains, "Sir, we're here to help. It's a little bit hot to be laying on the ground." Beginning his examination, he asks, "Where'd you hit your head?"

But Callahan's movements nearby distract the patient. "Please don't do that," the man begs, huddling inside his black T-shirt and gray sweatpants.

"It's just a blood-pressure cuff, buddy," Callahan says. "I just want to check . . ."

"Does your head hurt?" Cardona cuts in.

The man nods. Tears well in his soft brown eyes. He fingers a white band around his wrist.

"When were you in the hospital?" Cardona asks.

For a moment the patient just hangs his head and sags against the wall. He closes his eyes and thinks. "Last week," he says, finally.

"What for?"

"I hurt my head."

"Relax for me," Cardona says, looking at the wound. The thick row of stitches beneath dried blood is neither fresh nor clean. Bruises cover the back of his neck. "C-spine hematoma," Cardona tells Callahan. "We're gonna get that looked at for you, sir. How old are you?"

"Forty-four."

Callahan finishes measuring the man's blood pressure and quips, "120/70— hey, that's better than mine!" With that, he excuses himself to take the wheel and drives them to University.

"Do you live anywhere or are you staying out on the street?" Cardona asks. He is persistent because, if the man is homeless, he can recommend that the hospital connect the man with Social Services.

A scowl creeps across the man's face. "Leave it alone, man."

"Do you have any medical problems?

"Seizures."

"You take medication? Those pills, the pinkish ones? Dilantin?"

"Fuck you!"

"Listen, you're in my house. Show a little respect, huh?"

"Yes, sir," the man acquiesces. His bony shoulders sag.

"I have a few more questions while we're on the way to the hospital," Cardona says. "Besides seizures, do you have any other medical problems?"

"Yes."

"Do you or are you supposed to take medicine?"

The man just hangs his head and refuses to answer.

"We're not the police, man," Cardona assures the man. "We're from the hospital and we're here to help you."

"I got lung cancer. And I'm a vet."

"How many tours you do in Vietnam?"

"It's none of your business! Don't ask. You don't have the right to ask," the man glowers. "FUCK YOU. *Fuck you.* Fuck you. Don't never ask me!" He leans toward Cardona with menace and wags his finger. Then he slumps over like a rag.

"Sir, if I offended you in any way I apologize," Cardona says. "There is just some information we need to help the hospital take care of you. Do you have pain anywhere besides your head?"

"My whole body," the man sobs. Then he springs to his feet and thrashes out with both arms.

"Hey!" Cardona barks. "Why you busting up my house?"

"It's not your house."

"Yeah? Well, I have to work here twelve hours a day, so to me, it's a second house."

As they pull up to the hospital, Callahan leaves to get a wheelchair.

Then the man lunges. Cardona is shorter but infinitely more muscular and able to hold him off. His voice sharpens as he cautions the patient, "Don't grab me, don't you . . ."

Callahan comes back and reports there are no wheelchairs to be found but he'll snatch the first one available.

"I'm going to get you inside. Give me just a minute," Cardona tells the man. "Things don't happen overnight. Take it easy. Let us help you." He looks at the man hopefully, black eyebrows arched.

The man sticks his hand out in friendship and the two shake. But seconds later the patient is restless, up on his feet, and moving toward Cardona.

"You don't have to put your hands . . ." Cardona's voice, previously soft and paternal, escalates into a roar: *"I'm telling you, man, for the last time. Don't put your hands on me!"* Many EMS workers would restrain a patient who presents a threat. And Cardona is the first to admit he enjoys a good fight. "Part of growing up in the city is fighting," he says. "People will test you." But Cardona saves his fists for self-defense, especially around Callahan, who takes pride in his ability to talk violent patients into cooperating. Sometimes, however, heartfelt dialogue just doesn't work.

Alone in the box with a drunk, mentally unstable man, Cardona finally gets tough. He thrusts his head forward, squares his shoulders, and speaks firmly: "I've been nothing but nice to you, but don't confuse it with fucking weakness." Then he puts his hand on the man's shoulder and forces him to sit down again on the bench.

"Get off of me," the man cries, although Cardona is already back in his seat. "Please, please, please."

"I told you to wait," Cardona snaps back. "Keep your mouth shut now."

Callahan returns with a chair. He opens the door and, sensing the tension, calls the patient's attention to himself. "Yo, I respect the fact, man. You earned this care." He coaches the man out of the truck. "One step down. You want to put your hand on my shoulder?"

The man leans heavily on Callahan's tall frame.

"Here's your hat, man," Callahan says, offering the man the crushed baseball cap he had been lying on. Sympathetically, he adds, "My brother is a vet."

"Fuck you!" the man responds, four times over. He whirls violently and narrows his eyes to threat-filled slits. "Don't fuck with me, man."

"No, man, we're gonna do the right thing for you," Callahan assures him. Even the rich bass tones of his voice are comforting.

"Shit, man."

"Please watch the language," Cardona interjects.

"You want to fuck with me?"

"There's a bunch of ladies and children here, and you got the best people to take care of you," Cardona says.

"You helped us in the sixties, now we're gonna help you," Callahan says.

"I did the best I could do."

"You did a fantastic job," Callahan says while offering the man a seat in the chair.

"He goes in and out of this violence," Cardona whispers to his partner. "Two seconds ago he was shaking my hand."

The patient launches a fresh volley of curses and balls up his fists. "That's it!" Cardona says. "I can't deal with it. He's getting restraints." *I don't think he is stable.* For the hospital staff's safety, Cardona plans to tell the nurse that the patient cannot be trusted.

"We all have problems," Callahan continues soothingly. "You did your time over there. You earned it."

Cardona gives his partner an exasperated why-are-you-encouraging-this-guy look. *This guy came back from the war with who knows what problems,* Cardona thinks. *Now he's probably getting disability checks and "friends" of his, like those guys today, pick him up, pal around with him until he spends every dime of his benefits on booze and drugs. Once they've juiced him completely, they dump him.*

"Damn it. I fuckin' earned it," the man cries. "Fuck yourselves and have a good life."

I feel sorry for these guys who did their time in the war, Cardona thinks. *But one day, someone is going to kill him with that mouth.*

HIGH-SPEED, LOW-DRAG

Cisternino and Fazio compare their bus to a sports car. "We trim the fat," Cisternino says. When a nurse sneaking a cigarette outside his hospital's ER asks to peek inside their shiny white bus, he's readily admitted. Once he's inside, his jaw drops. "This is set up better than our ER!" he croaks. The medics have streamlined and positioned their equipment and supplies so as to reach most anything without much strain. For example, asthma meds and airway supplies are stationed near the cab, where patients lay their heads.

Efficiency might well be one of the B team's guiding principles; it carries over into everything. EMS workers here prefer to do quick assessments on-scene, take any necessary lifesaving action, and then quickly get back on board the ambulance. "We don't set up there, so we don't clean up there," Drivet says, as opposed to volunteers, who sometimes wrangle everything, including their cumbersome stretchers, inside patients' homes.

"If I have to do an IV and if I don't get it the first time, now I'm committed to try and try again. Then I have to transfer them to the gurney, and there's the potential for it to rip out while moving," Drivet explains. "But if I don't get the IV in the ambulance, my partner puts the vehicle in drive, and starts to go. If things go very badly we're already en route to hospital."

Some EMS pros look askance at this practice. But the Newark blue-shirts don't feel they have much choice, given their extraordinary number of assignments. The only way to survive the constant stream of patients is to be what Drivet calls high-speed, low-drag.

FEATHERWEIGHTS WALK

Studies have shown that paramedics are not especially accurate at estimating patient weights, which is important for calculating drug dosages. It's not uncommon for patients to be too embarrassed to be honest and underreport. It's an EMS worker's luck that featherweights often walk to the bus. Obese patients often can't. Generally, transport devices such as the Reeves, the stretcher, and the stair-chair are only guaranteed to some three hundred pounds. Unintentionally, patients continually test carrying-tool integrity as well as the EMS worker's spines and joints. In Newark, two-member teams often go on calls alone. The notion of two adults carrying a three-hundred-pound person down narrow, winding stairs is implausible, and even more so when burdened by up to eighty pounds of routine equipment (twenty-six-pound heart monitor, a twenty-two-pound airway kit, a thirteen-pound medication bag, transport tools such as Reeves, long boards, or stair-chairs, etc.).

And much of the existing infrastructure is in gross disrepair. An embarrassing number of once-elegant buildings sag, abandoned and condemned. They are dangerous but commonplace refuges for homeless people, drug addicts, crack whores, people down on their luck, and others who need emergency aid. Crews also respond to calls from residents making their homes in decrepit row houses well over 150 years old. As they wind their way up the narrow and fragile staircases, loud creaks, sharp cracks, and eerie moans announce their arrival. Half-dressed strangers inhabiting individual rooms in homes that used to belong to whole families stick their necks out and gawk as the blue-shirts analyze how to distribute the burden of body weight, equipment, and patient. It is more than some structures can bear.

One night, EMT Ennis Terrell and his partner were carrying a patient when worn floorboards suddenly gave way; he hung by his armpits between stories until O'Neill and Heber pulled him out. The preferred strategy now for the tougher cases is to summon Rescue and let O'Neill and Heber pull out their dolly, build ramps, or deploy ropes and pulleys to get everyone in and out without mishap. But the crews are so independent-minded that they tend to do the work themselves; thus some of the back injuries.

In an ideal world, EMS workers would haul every piece of equipment they might need to every call. In fact, their job requires it. But with equipment weights easily exceeding sixty pounds, it simply doesn't happen—especially in busy urban centers where too few workers are assigned to too many jobs. Management's answer is to quote standard operating procedure and shift the onus to the EMS worker.

Responding to upwards of a dozen trips per shift, many of which require hiking up flight after flight, is too much to handle with such onerous loads, especially when they are also expected to carry down patients as well. "Any time you have to go up in a building, it's best to bring everything. It sucks to get up there and get caught with your pants down," one B-teamer says. "It's got to happen from time to time to remind you not to get lazy." Eliminating one or two things is a gamble some take on occasion if they believe it will save their backs and lessen the chance of lifting and moving injuries.

"It's a bit of an art," Fazio says, describing the effort involved in entrance and egress. "Girls here carry heavy shit." She makes a point of highlighting obstacles before her coworkers, especially newcomers, literally trip up. Stairs seem perpetually underlit, overcrowded, steep, narrow, and abundant. There are doorjambs and doormats to traverse; ill-tacked carpeting, rugs, and plastic carpet protectors; and icy, dim, cluttered, and otherwise unsafe streets, too.

Wishful thinkers honk as they approach an address—praying patients will get themselves dressed, ready to go, and out to the street. Fazio says she's warned her dad, whom she says weighs more than three hundred pounds, "The first thing you do if you ever have chest pain, before you even call 911, is get downstairs." She loves him but she lets him know that he is a paramedic's "logistical nightmare."

Even if there were more hands to help, the spaces EMS workers operate in are often constrained or precarious. For example, elevators in senior-citizen high-rises are sometimes too small to accommodate a flat stretcher. Lying flat is exactly what's needed if a patient requires CPR.

HAVE IT YOUR WAY

At 1415 hours one silver-gray winter day, Drivet and his per-diem partner JoAnn Rusk are plotting how to fill their bellies, waiting on line at a Wendy's drive-through, when Dispatch sends them to an eighty-year-old female with chest pain in the Ironbound section of Newark. "Jingle fucking bells!" Drivet grumbles. "That's about as far away as possible." As he maneuvers out of line, he smacks his head with his palm, fearing he'll soon discover it's one of those times where he won't get to eat throughout his noon-to-midnight shift, much less the late-night trip home.

The radio meteorologist reports that a storm center is brewing. With -15-degree windchill and 30-mph winds, Newark digs in for the big chill.

"2108," the dispatcher broadcasts, calling Drivet's bus.

"2108," Rusk replies.

"I got 1107 coming to you." At least Drivet and his partner won't be alone on this job; extra hands are always handy when treating patients with breathing and circulation problems.

Drivet forces his way through traffic as thick as "lung butter," slang for the yellow mucus patients cough up.

"2108, your status?" the dispatcher asks at 1420 hours.

"We're heading south on Route 21 by Route 280," Drivet replies into the dashboard's handheld radio.

"Your AVL isn't working at this time, so do me a favor and just report your status."

"Received," Rusk replies.

Most of the blue-shirts are suspicious of the AVL. Administrators added it, supposedly to increase efficiency. Dispatchers use it to identify and assign the closest appropriate, available ambulance even as emergencies occur. Combined with the buses' mobile data terminals, the AVL has reduced radio traffic. Ironically, the technology has also become a pawn in the ongoing conflict between Management and the EMS workers. Management has employed it to detect wrongdoings, and EMS workers have countered by using it to argue their innocence. Either way, the technology often seems broken. Although Management says the buses have backup units, Dispatch instructs the blue-shirts to report when they receive a job, when they head toward the job, when they reach the job, when they arrive at the destination hospital, and when they are available for a new assignment.

"Pretty hard to get around down here, isn't it?" Rusk says, dismayed by the bumper-to-bumper traffic.

"Yeah," Drivet replies, expertly snaking his way through congested streets, both sides of which are lined with parked and sometimes double-parked cars.

EMTs Scott Williams and Evelyn Gamble, Unit 1107, catch up to them. Between the loud staccato blasts their siren issues and the ear-piercing wailing and yelping of Drivet's bus, the unrelenting cacophony coerces enough drivers to clear a path, and soon they arrive at their patient's street. The ambient noise is deafening, but the EMS workers pay it no mind; they carry on conversations and listen with one ear to Dispatch and another to commercial radio.

Finding no building to match the assignment, Drivet and Williams leave their heated buses, where the temperature is a balmy seventy-two degrees, where they cook inside their turtlenecks, sweatshirts, and winter-weight coats. Momentarily, they contemplate being flash-frozen; they pull on woolen caps, rub their hands together, exhale and watch their breath condense, and divide up. Walking briskly up and down the street, they search for a number that corresponds to their directions. No luck. Drivet radios Dispatch and asks them to confirm the address. Minutes later, Dispatch issues a correction, and the four EMS workers grab their gear and enter a nearby building.

They burn off their chill by climbing a narrow stairway dressed in ratty red carpet and loose area rugs. When they reach the fourth floor, a puffy-eyed, sallow-skinned woman of middle age is waiting for them by her apartment door. She introduces herself as the patient's daughter.

Drivet is first inside the small but spotless residence. The decor of the tidy apartment is primarily portraits and sculptures of Jesus and furniture clothed in plastic upholstery covers. A small, chubby woman with a head of thick white hair lies in a hospital bed off in a side room. Dressed in a pastel-flowered nightgown, she has pulled the covers up above her nose. Only her glittering black eyes and pink, porcelain-smooth forehead are visible.

Between Drivet's rudimentary Spanish and the bilingual daughter, the crew learns that the woman has renal cancer (although she doesn't know it). Drivet examines her gently and assesses her vital signs. She is stable but for poorer than average oxygen saturation and a slightly elevated pulse, both consistent with her complaint. Rusk charts the woman's medications, including steroids that help account for her bloated appearance. As Drivet assesses the woman, he's thinking about how to get her down the stairs. "Ma'am, last time you took her to the hospital, did she sit in the chair?" he asks the daughter, pointing to the portable stair-chair.

"No, because her leg was broken in eleven pieces."

Her comment ignites a more detailed physical exam, during which Drivet determines that the leg has probably healed by now. Still, it will be easier for the patient, and therefore everyone else, if they use the Reeves. Williams scoops up the chair, runs downstairs, yanks the Reeves from his bus, stuffs the chair in its compartment, and climbs the four flights once again—this time huffing and puffing. Inside the apartment, he stretches the Reeves out on the floor beside the hospital bed as much as space permits. He lays two blankets down, followed by three sheets. "She's gonna have to be hot for a while, because it's cold out there," he mumbles to himself.

Each EMS worker grasps a section of the patient's bedsheet and lifts her off of her bed. They can't help but grimace with effort. The woman's appearance is deceptive; delicate strawberry-and-cream complexion aside, she weighs three hundred pounds easily. She moans as they move her, "Ai! Ai! Ai . . ."

"Ma'am, what hospital do you prefer?" Drivet asks.

"Elizabeth General," the daughter answers.

Great, Drivet thinks. The hospital she wants *is* minutes from Newark, but it's also one they can no longer travel to since the new policy went into effect earlier this year.

Patients have the right to a medical screening exam, management says, but not necessarily at the hospital of their choice. Medicare regulations drive the policy. The federally funded insurer pays only to treat patients with a medical necessity who are so infirm as to be unable to get the hospital by private or public transportation. And it only pays for transport to the closest appropriate hospital. Besides, the department's primary obligation is to have enough ambulances in Newark to care for Newark's residents, an administrator explains. And, that can best be accomplished by keeping the buses inside city limits. Management explained this to area hospitals and community groups recently, it says, but left it to the EMS workers to inform patients and their families.

"They are saying we can't go to there today," Williams tells the patient's daughter. Predictably this upsets her. "You can't take her there because . . ."

"Well, she can't go anywhere else!" the daughter interjects with arms crossed in defiance. "That's where her doctor is. That's where her records are. I told them when I called 911, 'I need an ambulance to go to Elizabeth General.' "

Drivet sees conflict fermenting and wants to avoid an argument. *"Ask REMCS to send a field supervisor,"* he commands with a whisper. Turning his attention to the patient's daughter, Drivet soothes her: "Let's not get upset about it yet. We'll take her downstairs and by then we should have a supervisor here."

"They did this to me before," the daughter complains. "They took her to St. James, and I had to transfer her out of there."

In an effort to turn ambulances around faster, we now have another disgruntled customer, Drivet thinks. *The system is already overworked. All this for a few minutes that won't make that much of a difference.* Powerless to change things, he carries on with resignation.

The crew has the woman wrapped within layers, with the Reeves rolled around her, fastened with Velcro strips. The staircase is too narrow to permit all four caregivers to share the load. Although females here are expected to pull their weight, chivalry is not entirely dead. Williams and Drivet each grab an end, while Rusk and Gamble gather the equipment.

"Your speed, Walter," Williams says. His good intentions are a nevertheless clumsy way to highlight the fact he's not only in better shape than Drivet, but a good fifteen years younger.

"Just drag her for now," Drivet replies. They slide their heavy package over the carpet and doorsills toward the top of the landing. After a brief respite, Drivet grips the Reeves handle tightly and backs carefully down the stairs. Williams lifts at the other end. The flights are steep, the carpet is hazardous, and the landings are narrow and cluttered. After two flights, Drivet asks, "You wanna change hands?"

"Yeah," Williams gasps.

Drivet twists himself around and tries reorienting himself to lessen the strain. It's useless. The space is too tight. "Wait," Drivet says, "I'm not gonna be able to do this. Hold on." And he repositions himself once more.

"Ai, Dios mío!" the patient cries, Spanish for "Oh, my God!"

"How you guys doing?" Rusk asks.

"Just great," Drivet answers sarcastically, as he steps carefully over two loose area rugs, *except for the fact that my c-spines are fusing.* By this point even Williams's face is scarlet with effort. Drivet pauses to rub his aching lower back. People whose careers involve heavy lifting suffer debilitating osteoarthritis later in life, studies show. In fact, nurses suffer greatly . . . and they work *in* the hospital, with colleagues and orderlies to assist.

Finally everyone makes it through the vestibule, down the steps, and over to the BLS truck. As all four put their hands on to hoist her onto the stretcher, the woman pleads, "Ai, ai, ai!"

Inside the bus, Williams pulls the Reeves out from under the patient, like the old tablecloth trick. He tucks it away and sets up the oxygen mask. Gamble helps the woman sit up, and connects her to the heart monitor. Drivet studies the strip and concludes that it shows nothing significant. Whatever hospital she ultimately goes to will be by way of the BLS truck. Gamble rebundles the woman, tucking the sheets and blankets over her turquoise and white lace robe. As she buckles her in, Williams spots an administrator driving up in his white Suburban, his dashboard crowded with toys.

"I'll talk to him," Drivet says, stepping out of the bus.

"You better watch it, Walter; he's on the warpath," Williams warns. "No one is preparing for the storm, so he's been ordering everyone to make sure their units are fully stocked and telling managers to get off their computers and do some real work."

The administrator unrolls his window, leans an elbow on the door, and cocks his head toward Drivet.

"Hi," Drivet begins, leaning down toward the vehicle. "We've got a cancer patient who wants to go Elizabeth General. Her doctor and all her records are there. She refuses to go anywhere else. She's BLS. Her daughter said, when she called up, she told Dispatch she wanted to go to Elizabeth General. She says if she had been told 'no way,' she would have called a private ambulance service."

"OK, Walter," the administrator replies. "Hey!" he shouts to Williams. *"Don't get lost!"*

"I won't," Williams promises.

"*No shit*," the administrator adds. "We got ten jobs lined up." With that, he guns the gas and drives deep into Ironbound.

Williams asks Drivet for directions as Dispatch assigns double shootings, strokes, and other emergencies over the radio. By 1458 hours, Drivet and Rusk are back in their bus, available for the next call, and daring again to think about food. "What will it be?" Drivet asks. "The lovely McDonald's or the delectable Kentucky Fried Chicken?"

Suddenly, the administrator's voice booms over the radio. "I want a quick turnaround time," he commands. "No hanging out in the ER."

Rusk gives Drivet a pregnant glance before saying, "Duh."

THE DOPPLER EFFECT

One evening, Dispatch sends Cisternino and Fazio to treat a stabbing in the West Ward. It's rush hour and the sun is setting after a searing afternoon. Cisternino literally zips in and out of traffic, jumping the vehicle to the left, to the right, blitzing past children who jump rope on the sidewalks. Explaining how it is possible to go so fast in such a large, encumbering vehicle, and to clear narrow passages, he shrugs and says, "The Doppler effect—the faster you go, the thinner you are."

Research is under way regarding the safety of ambulance travel and how to improve it; the current body of knowledge is inadequate. One 1993 study concluded that people in ambulances risk injury five times more than those riding in civilian vehicles. And the collision risk for ambulances is thirteen times greater. Human error on the part of drivers (both ambulance and civilians); ignorance of the rules pertaining to emergency vehicles, which differ from place to place; inadequate maintenance; and the chilling effects of adrenaline all share the blame.[2]

"Every time we rush across this city to answer a call, we take our life in our hands," a B-team veteran says, and he's not kidding. O'Neill's former partner, George Burr, broke his neck in one such incident.

Drivers, sometimes entranced by strobe lights, plow into emergency vehicles. EMS workers can be distracted, almost hypnotized by the defeaning, repetitive sound of the siren, too. In his *EMS Magazine* article "Wheels of Fortune," John Erich explains, "Under stress, drivers tunnel. They focus too much on what's directly in front of them, and stop scanning from side to side and utilizing their peripheral vision. Potential hazards, however (dogs and joggers, for example), don't stop coming from all directions just because you're preoccupied with one."

Experts argue that lights and sirens exacerbate the problem, especially when used for noncritical calls; they cite studies showing that at least two-thirds of ambulance crashes happen when lights and sirens are in use—about twelve thousand emergency vehicle crashes a year. It takes considerable skill to subdue one's sympathetic nervous system and learn to choose cool and calm over fight-or-flight.

SHAKESPEARE IN THE NUDE

Transport is not complete without transferring care, and ERs are notoriously busy. Occasionally, the ER is quiet but for the sounds of rustling paper, beeping monitors, hissing oxygen, and chatting nurses. Now would seem the perfect time for Cisternino to turn over care of his patient, a thirty-two-year-old woman with asthma and HIV. He and Fazio picked her up from a street corner in a neighborhood he calls "a truly shitty section with high, high crime." When the woman first stepped into the ambulance, her eyes bulged with the effort to breathe. Tears streamed down her high, rounded cheekbones. She clutched her concave chest with a bony hand, unconsciously signaling respiratory distress.

She's doing much better now, because of the efforts Cisternino and Fazio made and the risks they took going to fetch her. Cisternino wheels her into the medical side of the ER and sets her up in an asthma chair. (University treats so many patients with asthma, that they have dedicated chairs with regulators and tubing hooked to super-sized oxygen tanks buried in the wall.)

Once she is comfortable, he approaches a nurse and asks to transfer the patient. She ignores him, so he repeats his request. He could strip down to his tattooed birthday suit and do a rain dance while reciting Shakespeare in Japanese and still not get her attention, it seems. After waiting several minutes, he tries again, asking another nurse, "Can you take report on this asthma?" She neither looks at him nor otherwise acknowledges his presence. It's as if he is not there. He waits and waits. He walks twenty feet to the other side of the nursing station, where a doctor and several nurses and residents sit casually talking, exchanging jokes, and discussing their vacation plans. "I have a patient here to turn over," he offers up. It's hard to ignore Vincent Francis Cisternino, a towering, muscle-bound, bald man in uniform with surgical jewelry piercing his tongue and his ears. But they do. *I tried twice. That's my limit*, Cisternino tells himself. He is calm on the outside but roiling internally. *Now I'll have to sit here until she decides to notice*. He takes a seat and waits.

Cisternino's experience is not uncommon among EMS workers. Some nurses, especially former EMS workers, are attentive and helpful. But many snarl some variation of "Why did you bring him here?" or just refuse to make eye contact.

SUNSHINE AIR

> We don't take all the credit up here. It's big; it's loud; it's noisy.
> But the people who get there before us do a lot of the work.
>
> —CAROL BACON, R.N., FLIGHT NURSE

Debra Conte, a five-year veteran of the Summit Police Department, demonstrates CPR on a pink plastic dummy while the crisp khaki-uniformed recruits who jam the auditorium think, *Why do I have to learn this? I came here to be a cop—I don't wanna be a first-aider.*

Conte, who earned her EMT certification while training at the police academy, knows what they're thinking and aborts their complaints by appealing to their loyalty. "You *better* pay attention," she warns, "because it may not be Mrs. Smith who needs your help. It *may* be your partner." The recruits collectively hush.

The petite, athletic woman pauses the lesson when her boss, Sergeant Rich Weigele, who also works as a paramedic, introduces Terry Hoben, air medical coordinator for University Hospital. Hoben has come to teach the recruits about NorthSTAR, the state's Northern Shock Trauma Air Rescue service: how and when to summon the flying ambulance, how to set up landing zones, and how to safely send it on its way.

Hoben, whose twenty-one-year EMS career began as a volunteer in suburban New Jersey, has stretched his skills around the globe. On harrowing Middle East and African rescue missions, he has treated embattled refugees. On U.S. soil, he's equally active. When the town of Bound Brook, New Jersey, succumbed to ravaging floods, and Hoben was cut off from work, he skippered a boat and whisked townspeople to safety.

Hoben zips through his presentation. The recruits are awash in facts, statistics, and history. The bulk of NorthSTAR's patients are victims of car and motorcycle crashes, fires, and explosions. Others need interfacility transports—for example, patients with cardiac problems who urgently need the higher-level care bigger hospitals can provide.

NorthSTAR's whole raison d'être is getting patients to trauma centers as quickly as possible, because, according to studies done at the Maryland Institute of Emergency Medical Services Systems, those who undergo surgery within sixty minutes of sustaining a critical injury have a significantly higher survival rate. Everyone in EMS, from the first responder to physicians board-certified in emergency medicine, focuses on that time period known as the "golden hour." Trauma centers have board-certified traumatologists, attending surgeons, fourth-year medical students, physician assistants, specially trained nurses, respiratory therapists and anesthetists, X-ray technicians, and ER technicians. At University, Dispatch alerts the trauma team by pager; it stands ready, willing, and able to care for the severely injured twenty-four hours a day.

As recently as the 1970s, few people considered air medical treatment and transport economically viable, Hoben says. But impassioned believers, with lessons culled from the Korean and Vietnam wars, persisted. Test programs began springing up all over the country, and New Jersey, often at the tail end of EMS initiatives, quietly crept onto the bandwagon in the late 1980s.

More than half of air medical crews throughout the U.S. pair nurses with paramedics, Hoben says of the personnel configuration that NorthSTAR also uses. "The two disciplines are distinctly different. But once they work together they influence each other's styles," he says. "Nurses lean on medics in the field where they're confronted with hair-raising scenarios that they've not been exposed to."

That's something Carol Bacon, a flight nurse, concedes. Although she earned her B.Sc. in nursing and toughed out five years of hospital-based trauma nursing before joining NorthSTAR five years ago, Bacon admits, like many of her colleagues, "I had no idea what paramedics did. The scenes are uncontrolled, chaotic. You have to deal with the police, family members, small children, drunks, the fire department, and a tremendous amount of noise. You have to block out all this sensory input and stimulation to focus. You cannot imagine what it's like to have all this going on and make split-second decisions. Out there everybody's looking at you. Medics are sort of on their own. Of course, they can call the docs, but they have to have an idea of what is going on and what to articulate."

Conversely, medics lean on nurses during interfacility transports, Hoben says. Patient care can be complex, especially when NorthSTAR transports people with nine medication drips, arterial lines, and intricate catheters.

A third discipline fleshes out NorthSTAR's patient-care triad—pilots. Hoben weaves into his lecture a plea for some of the recruits to consider careers as air medical pilots. Risks historically associated with air medical flights may deter some. So many EMS-related helicopters crashed throughout the 1980s, and so many fatalities occurred, that EMS managers across the nation almost phased out air medical transport altogether. From the outset, air medical programs followed basic aviation safety guidelines, says Dawn Mancuso, executive director of the Association of Air Medical Services. "But we still had things to learn. When calls would come in, patient information was shared with the pilots, and that could inadvertently influence their decision to fly even in dicey weather. It's hard to say no to a very sick baby. We discovered a lot in those early years and were able to make changes that greatly improved our operations."

The pilots and air medical crews who work NorthSTAR feel secure. State troopers first, they qualify to fly NorthSTAR, and its southern New Jersey component, SouthSTAR, at a Sikorsky training school in Florida. Two pilots fly each mission, to enhance safety. Their mechanics are civilian employees of the state police who inspect and conduct routine maintenance on the birds five days a week. And the mechanics stay on call throughout the weekend.

By watching the air medical niche almost implode, NorthSTAR learned that no one benefits when pilots or air medical crews are pushed to their limits. NorthSTAR is so cautious that colleagues on the ground jokingly refer to it as "Sunshine Air." Weather minimums include eight-hundred-foot ceilings and two-mile visibility during the day, and thousand-foot ceilings and three-mile visibility at night. Pilots can decline to fly in sustained winds over forty knots or precipitation that affects visibility.

Sensitivity to weather is a bit of an issue between EMS workers who serve on the ground and those in the air. Ground crews drive to patients' sides regardless of rain, sleet, snow, ice, hurricanes, extremes of hot and cold, and other weather anomalies. Because weather can exacerbate certain illnesses—for example, asthma and congestive heart failure—ground-pounders have many more patients than the air medical crews have. Five patients in twelve hours means "getting killed" for the air medical crew, compared with twelve to twenty-five patients on the street. Nevertheless, the air medical crews say that one patient on the helicopter is equivalent to five on the ground, because the urgency and complications are so intense, not to mention the stress of vibration, noise, and other flight-related conditions.

Still, fewer patients mean more downtime, a priceless perk—especially for those in EMS who often work multiple jobs. Downtime, however, does not necessarily mean lounging about on a couch in the crew's rooftop quarters. Hoben delegates plenty of work. Flight medic Bill O'Brien spends hours lining up public-safety lectures, such as the one Hoben is giving today. And Nurse Bacon keeps track of supplies.

Hoben outlines some of the preconditions recruits should consider before summoning NorthSTAR. (EMTs, paramedics, firefighters, docs, nurses, and public-safety officials can also request the bird.) He teaches the recruits that crises are not always obvious. For example, a patient may not exhibit signs of internal bleeding after a substantial ejection or rollover, but if the vehicle has tumbled and ended up crushed in a ditch, the mechanism of injury may be reason enough to call.

Sometimes the decision to summon NorthSTAR is a judgment call, Hoben explains. Traffic, in the most densely populated state in the country, can turn a few miles into an eternity. And extrication times, road conditions, and other factors may mean that NorthSTAR is the most expeditious route to care. As an example, Hoben tells recruits that air medical crews have flown two-minute flights to and from Newark's neighbor, Jersey City. It has even flown *within* Newark's borders to airlift patients from impassable, snarled traffic jams on the city's many highways and byways.

His prepackaged slide show comes to life when the presentation moves outdoors. Suddenly the skies roar with the sound of dual gas turbine engines capable of generating a 155-knot speed. Willowy swamp grasses fringing the parking lot bend flat from the downward pressure of the bird's rotor blades. Gusts sweep grit from the ground and propel it through the air, stinging the faces of those who did not heed Hoben's warnings to step back and turn away. The pilot drops his shiny white Sikorsky S-76B neatly onto the police academy's parking lot.

When the blades stop spinning, the pilot, Bill O'Brien, and Carol Bacon disembark. The blue-eyed, blond-haired air medical crew, outfitted in royal blue, fire-retardant jumpsuits with shiny silver zippers, makes a stunning impression, despite what the ground-pounders have nicknamed them: "the pajama-clad heroes of the sky." The police recruits break formation to join a wide-eyed crowd of visiting fifth-graders; everyone swarms the bird and peppers the crew with questions.

Officer Conte leans toward Sergeant Weigele and whispers, "My limo is here."

Few are aware of the phenomenon taking place in their presence. Sergeant Weigele and Hoben chat briefly and discover that O'Brien and Bacon were the crew who treated Officer Conte one glacially cold January morning just over a year ago. Without Weigele and Hoben's chat, Conte would not recognize O'Brien or Bacon. She has no memory of that day, the day she nearly lost her life—the day a Mitsubishi Montero driving at least 35 mph struck and carried her before screeching to a stop and launching her onto the pavement.

Now, some fifteen months after the accident, Conte walks with a slight limp, her words get jumbled on occasion, and her speech is slightly slushy. Constant numbness and tingling irritate her left hand and foot. Her left side jerks a bit and lacks the muscle tone it once had. She lets doctors inject her calf and toes with Botox, a botulin derivative, to stop the spasms. And she still devotes much of each week to physical therapy and recovering her strength and balance.

While the crowd mills about, Weigele and Hoben organize a makeshift reunion. O'Brien, Bacon, and Conte drift toward one another with mutual awkwardness. Once introduced to the air medical crew, however, Conte is tongue-tied—a shell of her wisecracking self—momentarily, at least. "If it wasn't for NorthSTAR," she gushes, stepping up to shake hands, "I wouldn't be here." Her long-lashed, deep brown eyes are awestruck; she seems much a Little Leaguer meeting a baseball champion.

"Good to see you on your feet," O'Brien replies, taking her hand in his. *It sounds so cliché*, he thinks, *but I feel like saying, "I was just doing my job, ma'am."* Like his ground-pounder colleagues, O'Brien finds that expressions of gratitude are infrequent, especially from the critically injured. That thanks "are nice" is as far as he is willing to go. Generally, he says, gratitude makes him uncomfortable. A tall muscular man, with pale pink skin and tired blue eyes, O'Brien has the "aw, shucks" feeling most EMS workers do when the notion of "hero" lights up a patient's eyes. Their hard-core bravado is not intended for public consumption. O'Brien casts his eyes to the ground bashfully, and he and Bacon shift the subject and quickly throw credit to the EMS team who assisted Conte on the ground.

"Open yer mouth," O'Brien commands.

A grinning Conte complies.

"Oh yeah, that looks familiar!" he jokes; NorthSTAR flies some six hundred patients a year. But Conte's status as a cop and the emotion surrounding her accident were distinctive. "We were going to have to sedate your fellow officers," O'Brien jokes.

"Yeah, well, I had this party for everyone and I realized, everybody in this friggin' room saw me naked," Conte confides, having realized that what was once her private collection of tattoos is no longer secret. "*Everybody* saw my ass. If I woulda been awake I woulda said 'No way!'"

"Oh," O'Brien assures her, "that's another guy who saw you on your back. Last time I saw you I was staring down your throat." It's a truthful enough statement, but even if he had seen Conte's colorfully illustrated birthday suit, it wouldn't have made much of a dent. "After years on the job, you see but you don't see," O'Brien explains.

Conte shows them her latest tattoo—one that commemorates her accident. The illustration has three elements. An angel floats on top of her shoulder, representing her deceased mother. "My mother must have taken her eyes off me that day, just for a moment," Conte says. "She was probably playing golf up there in heaven." The angel watches over Saint Michael, who Conte says "is the patron saint of cops." And Saint Michael, in turn, watches over a boy. He represents the youngster on the street corner whom Conte guarded the day she got creamed.

"Nice," O'Brien remarks. "So, how are you doing?"

"I'm still in therapy," Conte confesses with a hangdog air.

"That's OK," O'Brien reassures her. "We were surprised you made it."

"I'm coming along," Conte says. "I've got so much metal in me, my husband can melt me down." With a titanium rod in her femur, a plate in her ankle, a blood-clot filter in her aortic artery, and a shunt in her brain, she's only half-joking.

"Or, he can sell you for scrap!" O'Brien cracks back, and the laughter they share is hearty. Conte's shyness starts to fade and goes to hell altogether as they joke about the size of the tube O'Brien thrust down her throat.

Just then, a reporter nosing for news cajoles the small group into posing for a photo. After the journalist jots down some details and leaves, Conte musters up the nerve to ask O'Brien and Bacon, "Do you guys have any T-shirts or pens?"

With a promise to send her a shirt, the EMS workers and the patient shake hands again and part.

Picturesque and rich, the suburb of Summit, New Jersey, is also a busy transportation hub. Pedestrians, motorists, and bus and train commuters hustle, and the police department places officers around town to help. At 0700 hours on the ice-cold morning of January 28, 2000, Conte contemplates the subzero temperatures as she prepares herself in the station-house locker room. Her traffic post begins at 0730 hours and will last forty-five bone-chilling minutes. Her first battle today will be with the weather.

Conte dons her long underwear, bulletproof vest, winter uniform, jacket, and hat. She hates looking like "a pumpkin" but pulls on the Day-Glo orange vest and gloves, too. A bike officer, Conte normally works uptown. But it's too cold for cycling today, so she drives Car No. 6 to the intersection of Broad and Elm, where it's up to her to tame the beast otherwise known as rushed and snarling traffic.

After absorbing as much heat as she can, practically leaning against the blower in her car, she plunges into the flow. A short time later, however, she feels the cold's nasty sting. *I want my morning coffee bad*, she thinks. Soon she'll be downing a steaming cup with Tony Crowe, her friend and fellow officer. He's counting down to a coffee break, too, while helping a stranded commuter a few streets away.

Kari Phair, Conte's friend from the local emergency squad, is two miles away, defrosting her driver-side door before leaving for work. *It's butt-ass cold*, the pixyish blonde with dark eyes, spiky hair, and pink cheeks thinks. If she can get into her van at all, Phair plans to drive past Conte and wave hello before heading to the office.

About 0740 hours a teenage boy pauses at the crosswalk, and waits for Conte's signal. She holds her neon-sheathed hands up to work the traffic and accommodates him. The next thing she knows, she's headed to a long-term rehabilitation center in central New Jersey. Months have passed, time lost to her forever.

She never sees the wine-colored SUV barrel down on her. She misses the impact; it's forceful enough to knock the gloves off her hands. She's oblivious of riding the hood of the car, flying through the air, and crashing on the street one hundred feet from the collision. She doesn't hear the long bone in her thigh crack, her rib shatter, her ankle smash. She misses the blunt smacking of her brain against her skull—first when the SUV strikes her, then as her head hits its hood, a third time as she soars like a projectile, and yet again when she hits the pavement. Conte, a woman who relishes action, misses it all because she is unconscious.

The boy waiting to cross stands drop-jawed, riveted with horror.

A rubbernecker who sees the accident drives past the white-haired, pink-cheeked Crowe and his stranded commuter, unrolls his window, and shouts, "You've got an officer down at Broad and Elm!"

Crowe knows it's Conte. He excuses himself from the commuter, heads to the intersection, and radios headquarters. The police dispatcher calls "Car 6!" over the radio repeatedly—but Conte doesn't respond.

And Phair, addicted to the police scanner she keeps to stay informed as an emergency responder, hears the dispatcher, too. She sticks her flashing blue bubble light on top of her van and zooms toward Broad and Elm. *Deb will be sitting there with a broken arm or two, screaming obscenities,* Phair tells herself.

Crowe arrives first to find Conte facedown, utterly still, unresponsive. Her legs are twisted oddly. *She looks like a broken doll,* he thinks as his fair skin crystallizes in the cold. He tries feeling a pulse but can hardly find a patch of skin beneath all the clothes. *Mother of God, she's dead!* he thinks. On closer inspection, he sees Conte, barely breathing, blowing bubbles in her blood even as it freezes on the asphalt. Terrified that she won't survive, Crowe confirms the accident with police dispatch, and asks them to summon Summit's volunteer emergency squad and the local paramedics. Concerned with rush-hour traffic delays, Crowe asks for NorthSTAR, too.

CENCOM, the EMS dispatch service for this part of New Jersey, gets the word out to the volunteer ambulance service by 0749 hours and passes on the request for NorthSTAR nine minutes later. The air medical crew's pagers go off immediately: "Pedestrian struck, Summit, Union County." The pilot is first down the hallway of the air medical crew's quarters on University Hospital's rooftop. He pushes through the double doors that lead to the STARport and hops aboard the Sikorsky to warm up his equipment.

Meanwhile, Crowe covers Conte with blankets from the trunk of his squad car. He fights the urge to pick his friend up in his arms and cradle her. In his helplessness, the Dublin-born officer turns to God. *Hail Mary, full of grace, the Lord is with you,* Crowe prays. *Blessed are you among women and blessed be the fruit of your womb. Holy Mary, mother of God, pray for us sinners now and at the hour of our death.*

Cops arrive en masse. Some block the intersection; others initiate crowd control; others gather witnesses. Conte's lieutenant jogs over to Crowe for an update. And Phair, jammed in traffic, struggles through the next few blocks until police see her blue light and make room for her to pass. Phair stops at the scene and grabs her EMS responder kit, but she can't get out of her car; the door has frozen shut. She pounds on the horn until a cop helps free her. Stumbling from her vehicle, Phair sprints to her friend's side.

Phair tries adhering to prehospital care standards. She knows she should glove up to prevent contamination from possible blood-borne pathogens, but she is so shaken that she abandons the safety precaution and thinks, *Screw it!* Crying, she yells into her friend's ear. "Oh my God, Deb! It's Kari. I'm here."

"Don't touch her!" Crowe roars. Color floods his frozen cheeks. Thus far Conte has been immobile, and he worries that a rough gesture, however well intentioned, will shake the life out of her.

Phair leans down to check Conte's breathing but hears only gurgling sounds and hard-won breaths maybe four times a minute.

A volunteer EMT from a nearby town stops to help. While they wait for the ambulance, the volunteer holds Conte's head still between his hands to prevent further injury to her cervical spine, and Phair takes a set of vitals.

It's almost the height of rush hour. The local EMS crews have not yet arrived. The volunteer squad is already out on a call, and raising a team of stand-ins takes time. *Her only chance is to get to a trauma center,* Phair thinks. Using her EMS radio, Phair calls CENCOM: *"I need NorthSTAR, and I need it now!"*

She stoops to palpate her friend's head and identifies a deep gash on her forehead, a cut near her right eye, and an ugly wound on her scalp. Conte's hairstyle, which she and Phair jokingly call the "bitch bun," is loose, knotted, and wet with blood. Phair gives in to her worst fears and pulls up the blankets to check if Conte's legs are still there. She spots Conte's gloves a good twenty feet away. Her friend's hat is nowhere in sight. "How hard did he hit her?" Phair asks, incredulously. Before she even gets a reply, she blurts out, "Who hit her?"

"We've got him," Crowe assures her, nodding toward an SUV with a broken headlight, crushed grille, and badly dented hood. Phair is nauseated. Clearly, Conte took a massive hit.

"Is he all right?" Phair asks weakly. An EMS worker's job is to care for the ill and the injured, regardless of their legal status. Crowe tells her the driver is stunned but otherwise unhurt.

Phair pulls shears from her kit to cut through Conte's Day-Glo vest, jacket, and belt to help prepare her for transport. The paramedics will need to inspect her "trauma-naked" body for other signs of injury. (To make patients trauma-naked is to remove their clothes so that EMS workers can rapidly spot bleeding, punctures, deformities, or other life threats. Sometimes the EMS workers will leave a patient's underwear on, but not always.) To everyone's surprise, Conte, who has yet to respond to any stimulation, reaches back to protect her gun. Phair tries again, to no avail. "Tony, she's gonna fight me on this," she tells Crowe.

Crowe bends within inches of Conte's ear and yells, "Deb, it's me, Tony. I've got your gun!" The urgency in his voice underscores the soft Irish brogue that threads his normal speech. Conte's hand relaxes just enough for Crowe to grab the weapon.

The fire department arrives, lugging a long board, a collar, and head blocks. Phair removes Conte's gold necklaces, a crucifix and a Chinese character that means "all life." The rescuers wrap a cervical collar around Conte's neck and logroll her onto the long board.

"Let's get her on some oxygen," Phair suggests to the police. Fortunately, Summit police carry automatic defibrillators, oxygen canisters, and related supplies. But no one has an oral airway to keep the tongue from occluding the back of the throat, blocking the flow of oxygen. And no one has a portable suction unit. Without them, the rescuers have no tools to clean and protect Conte's airway. Besides, Conte has her mouth closed rock solid—a classic sign of head injury.

The volunteer ambulance arrives at 0755 hours.

By 0804 hours, O'Brien and Bacon, dressed in leather bomber jackets, sunglasses, and shiny white helmets, are on board NorthSTAR. When Newark International Airport's tower clears the area's busy airspace and grants them permission, the pilot lifts off. Dispatch coordinates landing-zone logistics between the pilot and the Summit Fire Department. To set down, NorthSTAR needs a square, about 110 feet wide by 110 feet long, free of trees, high-tension wires, cars, people, and their cigarettes. The police choose Tatlock field, a schoolyard playground about one mile west of the accident.

Medics arrive on-scene about the same time, too. One almost falls to his knees in shock when he realizes his friend Conte is the victim.

"What do you think?" Phair asks, hopefully.

"I don't know," the medic answers. "It doesn't look good."

Phair sees he has tears in his eyes. The shock starts to overcome her, too. "I can't do this!" she cries. "You *have to* handle this, because I can't." Usually Phair doesn't show emotion, she says, "but people saw it that day. I couldn't get two words out without crying." Phair may wear her despair more boldly, but most everyone has to force themselves to stay on track with rescue procedures that are otherwise a straightforward matter of routine. Conte's husband, also a police officer, arrives. It seems that all of Summit's PD, FD, and EMS are there rooting for Conte, desperately wanting to be useful.

After loading her in the BLS ambulance, the medics finish stripping their patient for closer examination. Someone cranks up the heat to help Conte, in shock from blood loss and lying on the frozen pavement, fight hypothermia.

Most important is finding some way to secure Conte's airway. Deprived of oxygen for even a few minutes, brain and heart tissue can deteriorate irreparably and die. But all the plastic airways in the world won't make a difference now, much less an endotracheal tube. The medics can't get anything past Conte's clenched teeth. They can't even get a suction tube in her mouth to cleanse it of blood, broken teeth, or vomit.

If they try and pry open her jaw and she fights them, the EMS workers may well lose a finger. It happens. Some medics, like Drivet, are skilled at nasal intubation, which offers an airway when the mouth is compromised. Not all medics are confident enough to risk performing it on a head-injured patient, however. It's a difficult skill to master, and then there is the common misperception that medics might miss the precise pathways to the lungs and accidentally damage the brain. Research simply does not bear this out, but the notion, however misguided, intimidates some.

One medic does his best to oxygenate her with a bag-valve mask connected to an oxygen tank. He squeezes the flexible, football-shaped plastic tube every five seconds.

Another searches for broken bones. A broken femur can kill if it severs blood vessels; one-third of the body's blood can leak into the leg instead of circulating and nourishing the vital organs. Conte's left thigh is already twice the size of her right. Other fractures appear probable, but there's no time to splint even the obvious injuries. The long board will serve as a body splint. It's more important to start an IV and replace some of Conte's body fluids before she bleeds out entirely.

At 0814 hours, forty minutes after the accident, the ambulance and North-STAR meet on Tatlock field. O'Brien and Bacon duck out of the aircraft, carrying their airway and drug kits. They climb inside the bus, where two medics, two EMTs, and what first seems like a thousand others are waiting to brief them.

O'Brien's first impression is that the emergency workers are experiencing "controlled hysteria." *They're on the ball on the outside but they're probably screaming on the inside.*

O'Brien and Bacon assess Conte according to scales that classify level of consciousness. Her scores are stunningly low. Conte is unresponsive and combative, another sign of head injury. The downed officer stiffens her limbs and thrashes about, which poses additional risk to her spinal cord.

They focus on Conte's airway, breathing, and circulation. By now, her respiration pattern has changed. It's rapid, shallow, and more akin to grunting than true inhalations and exhalations. Head-injured patients tend to breathe too fast or too slow, and either extreme interferes with the lungs' ability to blow off carbon dioxide (CO_2). When excess CO_2 accumulates, it can trigger brain swelling. Patients with excess CO_2 or unstable airways blocked by injury, blood, loosened teeth, etc., can vomit and choke, especially if their teeth are clenched. They can also inhale their emesis into their lungs and develop pneumonia.

People who puke in the helicopter have "a tendency to projectile-vomit, which is *bad* for the flight crew," O'Brien explains. They are transported flat on their backs, and when they throw up, they do so literally. "There's really no place for the vomit to go. It hits the ceiling forcefully and rains down on the crew. We have no place to hide."

He tells the ground crew he wants to intubate Conte. They know that flight medics have access to drugs that paralyze the body, relax the muscles, and enable aggressive airway management. Anxious for their friend to get help, Phair and others clear out to give O'Brien and Bacon room to work.

Because the drugs stop the body's movement, patients literally stop breathing on their own—for about five minutes. That gives the crew sufficient time to insert the endotracheal tube. Then, using a bag-valve mask, they breathe for the patient, infusing oxygen into the lungs and securing a pathway for carbon dioxide to escape. Medics call this procedure "rapid-sequence induction."

Before O'Brien can thread the tube down Conte's throat, he and Bacon have to deal with her tightly clamped jaw. Bacon prepares injections of lidocaine and succinylcholine, and pushes them into Conte's catheter. Seconds later, her muscles go limp. Her teeth unclench. Her jaw becomes pliable.

Don't screw this up! O'Brien thinks. *All eyes are on you.* A paramedic of twelve years, with a five-year track record on NorthSTAR, O'Brien nevertheless feels some pressure. When police, firefighters, or fellow EMS workers fall victim, he gives them the same care as other patients, but, he says, the calls are always a bit more emotional. O'Brien wants to get the tube in without complication and preferably here in the ambulance, which offers extra room and lighting.

The drugs take effect as planned, and because Conte is still unconscious, she has no gag reflex. At O'Brien's direction, Bacon exerts pressure on the ring-shaped cartilage just below the Adam's apple. He has no trouble opening Conte's mouth, slipping his steel laryngoscope over her tongue, using its tiny light to spot her vocal chords, and sliding the slim, flexible stylette and sheath into her trachea.

He removes the stylette and uses a syringe to inject air and inflate the tube's cuff, which anchors the tube in her windpipe and seals off her esophagus. He adds an entidal CO_2 detector to measure carbon-dioxide output and ties the tube into place so it won't dislodge. Using her stethoscope to listen to lung sounds, Bacon verifies that the tube is channeling air into Conte's lungs and nods at O'Brien.

Bacon is concerned, too, but less so than O'Brien. She has witnessed patients sicker than Conte survive. Bacon believes she will make it.

The air medical crew assesses, medicates, intubates, and moves Conte to the helicopter within twelve minutes. It's cramped inside the four-by-six-foot space, but would be even worse if they had another patient; sometimes they carry two.

Once on board, they shift over to liquid oxygen and hook Conte up to their ProPac, which monitors her ECG and records vital signs. They drape her in a papery aluminum wrap to conserve heat, then add a wool blanket and a heavy canvas cover, too. The helicopter has heat but it's always cold, the diminutive Bacon says. She wears long underwear even in warm weather.

At 0826 hours, NorthSTAR lifts off. The noise is thunderous and all-encompassing, but the crew is accustomed to it. During the seven-minute flight, Conte needs no further intervention. Bacon monitors the pump, and alerts a trauma center in Morristown, New Jersey, via radio. O'Brien has access to a portable ventilator for long trips, but he chooses to squeeze the bag-valve mask and breathe for Conte the entire flight. Periodically they reassess her condition, but for the most part Conte is on what O'Brien calls "cruise control."

They land at 0832 hours. O'Brien notes Conte's vital signs on the chart. Her heart rate has increased from 97 to 113. It's working hard to sustain her pressure, which has fallen from 148/76 to 128/79.

The hospital's trauma team is waiting on the helipad to meet them. O'Brien and Bacon transfer Conte to a stretcher. The doctor listens to Conte's lungs to confirm that the endotracheal tube has been placed correctly; it can shift with movement. O'Brien and Bacon, along with the hospital staff, roll Conte into a dedicated elevator, down a cream-colored hallway, and into a resuscitation room. After some paperwork, the flight crew's role is over.

From the University's 911 dispatch to landing at the trauma center *at least* forty-three minutes have passed, but it's almost an hour since she was first struck. Conte suffers a brain bleed and significant swelling. She slips into a two-week coma, then spends weeks on a mechanical ventilator. She suffers pneumonia and then a blood clot, which requires surgery. The right side of her brain is injured and the left side displays strokelike symptoms. The neurological damage she sustains will leave her memory spotty. The tissues around her kidneys swell. Both legs are broken as well as a rib and her wrist.

Conte spends months in a wheelchair and months more in residential rehab centers with therapists of every kind helping her win back her life and control over the left side of her body, too. But without EMS she wouldn't have had a fighting chance. The normally acerbic officer bubbles over with gratitude.

She still has months of healing ahead before working her way back to being a cop. In the meantime, she teaches basic lifesaving skills to recruits, and volunteers to coach other trauma victims. And every day the self-described "stubborn Guinea" counts her blessings. "It's a very thin line between what I coulda been and what I am," Conte says. "I coulda been a vegetable."

Many consider air medical positions to reflect exceptional achievement. To qualify for NorthSTAR, paramedics must have a stellar record of performance on the ground for at least three years. Preferred candidates have college and advanced degrees, too.

They then undergo an intensive eight-week training program with classroom and clinical components. They ride University's Rescue truck to study kinetics as well as the care and extrication of patients who are entrapped in vehicles or otherwise hard to reach. Candidates spend long days in burn units (including tanking and debridement sessions, where burned flesh is scrubbed off). It's gruesome but necessary because they transport a significant number of burn patients. "Sometimes they're conscious," O'Brien explains. "They want to know what to expect, and we try to prepare them."

O'Brien and his fellow flight medics take on the additional training, responsibility, and risks associated with flying because they want new challenges. They get no extra pay. Like their colleagues on the ground, many hold second jobs, if not more.

Drivet, Cisternino, and a number of other medics want to step up to the challenges NorthSTAR offers when Personnel posts job openings. The two friends are among twenty competing for three available spots. As the weeks, then months tick by, each undergoes interviews. Advancing through the application process keeps their hopes alive. Discreetly, they seek out one another's status. The best of colleagues, and good friends to boot, neither wants to succeed at the other's expense. Drivet and Cisternino root as hard for each other as they do for themselves, but as the process drags out, the competition and wait begin to feel interminable.

9 PAPER STORM

B-teamers often say they chose their profession because it lets them work outdoors and make substantive decisions in real time away from a boss's prying eyes. Squeezing out some four hours a night to shuffle paper, too, leaves many feeling more like secretaries or supply clerks than physician extenders or surrogates.

Almost every aspect of the job has a form. After swiping in at the start of each shift, blue-shirts sign a communication log, which holds them responsible for the department's handheld radios, batteries, and pagers.

Every night paramedics must inventory their portable pharmacies and sign a narcotics log. One of the dark sides of the health-care business is the proximity to drugs and the temptation to use them to combat fatigue, stress, and depression.

Twice a month the blue-shirts must verify that their ambulances are in order. Two-person BLS units are responsible for checking at least 427 items, from engine fluids and hydrogen peroxide to working windshield wipers and eight-by-ten-inch bandages. Paramedic crews inspect 440 items, from several types of laryngoscope blades, handles, and spare batteries to various endotracheal tubes, nasogastric tubes, even binoculars. If they spent a minute finding and checking each item, the task would take more than seven hours.

At the close of each shift, paramedics must also submit a tally sheet, which restates who did what, when, and what outcome was achieved, even though the charts capture these data and dispatch records do, too.

If the radio or pager fails, crews must submit Radio Failure Reporting forms.

Fast Track forms are on hand for unusual incidents or complaints by or about EMS. One afternoon, Opperman and Drivet log in with Dispatch, get a bite to eat, stop into an automotive parts shop, and pay a visit to the medical-school bookstore. Eventually they realize that things are uncharacteristically quiet. They drive to quarters and ask Chief Piumelli to investigate. He discovers that Dispatch had forgotten to enter them in its computer. Whenever a unit is out of service, the crew needs to report the length of time and explain why. It's not good enough to prepare one report that both partners sign. They *each* have to write up a form. Dispatch has to explain itself, too.

There are Social Service Referral forms to help patients unable to care for themselves get more substantive assistance from social workers and city officials than EMS can provide.

"Some people's houses are full of garbage—food all over, dishes over the top. I kid you not," Henry Cortacans says, bobbing his head for emphasis. "It's stacked against the walls. Just piles of things. It's pretty disgusting—rats, roaches, unhealthy. It's unsanitary to live like that. And a fire hazard. We have quite a few of them here."

"Garbage houses" are not unique to Newark, but its population density means that EMS workers encounter obsessive-compulsive hoarders every so often. Fazio has seen several in her tenure. One she remembers well was discovered when a neighbor could no longer tolerate the stomach-turning odors wafting from a nearby house. "You couldn't see through the windows, it was piled so high," she recalls. "What these people do is tunnel through." EMS workers entered the home and burrowed through shoulder-height refuse until they reached the source of the sickly sweet stench—the basement. Several dogs there had died from starvation. The homeowner had been admitted to a veterans' hospital a month previously, they later discovered.

"And there are elderly who can't take care of themselves," Cortacans adds. "We had this one guy who *called every day for five years!* But there was nothing wrong with him. He'd say he had difficulty breathing and then ask us to take the laundry out, turn out the lights, or move his couch."

Terry Hoben, air medical coordinator, designed the Social Service Referral form a few years back when he was a training supervisor. He had a reputation for stopping his colleagues in the hall and updating them on their various referrals. But Hoben earned a promotion, and the blue-shirts lost the man willing to champion the cause of those who float through the EMS portal perhaps under false pretenses but clearly in need of care. "Now," one blue-shirt admits, "we don't even know if the forms ever leave the building."

Shift Exchange Requests require EMS workers to find a replacement, and justify why they want to swap shifts.

Vacation Requests follow suit.

Employees also receive a *Policies and Procedures Manual* of several hundred pages, which managers supplement with a crushing cascade of memos. One administrator is so prolific that the blue-shirts have dubbed him "the Paperwork King."

CLOSE, BUT NO CIGAR

When Piumelli began working BLS for University in 1981, patient-care reports were just an idea. "When we first evolved to charts, nurses hesitated to sign them," he recalls. Quality Assurance, Continuous Quality Improvement, and other such esoteric terms were not standards, just newfangled business ideas. "Used to be, we went years without looking at a run sheet," Piumelli remembers. "Maybe we'd pull one every five years."

In the mid-eighties, the state's Department of Health and Senior Services directed EMS administrators throughout the state to select criteria for improvement, regularly audit at least ten percent of their charts, and demonstrate progress, a former state official says.

Administrators state that the department has had a quality-improvement program since it took over EMS responsibility from the city, but the blue-shirts say they can't recall participating in any consistent program until recently, when one of the street medics was promoted to an administrative position. With his colleagues' assistance, the new administrator drew up a list of criteria to automatically trigger some charts for review. The list includes "meat and potato" practices, Cortacans says, such as acute traumas not brought to University; serious burns not brought to the regional burn center; Do Not Resuscitate cases; intraosseous infusions or attempts (a technique usually used to infuse infants in cardiac arrest through their still-porous bones rather than their delicate veins, which can be challenging to find under the best of circumstances); needle thoracotomies (chest decompressions) or attempts; external cardiac pacing; respiratory and cardiac arrests; certain irregular cardiac rhythms; patients who spontaneously recover breathing and circulation after cardiac arrest; use of IV infusion pumps; bystander use of automatic defibrillators before ALS arrives; intubations; the use of midazolam, a sedative that diminishes memory of unpleasant procedures; unexplained on-scene times exceeding thirty minutes; clinically questionable paramedic decisions to release patients to BLS crews or patients who refuse medical attention; and ALS treatment that occurs without contacting the supervising physician.

Some items on the manager's list are mandated by the state; others are there to ensure that medics meet the hospital's performance standards. The federal government has an interest in records and practices, too, in part for research purposes but also because some EMS workers have been very bad apples, putting the rest of the barrel under close scrutiny. For example, those who have been at University for a while say there have been EMS workers who actively discouraged patients from going to the hospital, hoping to save themselves the work of transporting and charting.

If all those charts do not add up to at least ten percent of the total charts per day, the manager directs his staff to also select every tenth chart at random.

EMS systems around the country have myriad ways of handling case review. Some rotate crews through QA positions so their employees can learn from each other's strengths and weaknesses. University's administrator recruited a few blue-shirts who excel at chart writing, such as paramedic Henry Corta-cans.[1] Each week, Cortacans spends a few hours reviewing his peers' charts for legibility and completeness, and makes a few extra bucks.

After noting anything incomplete or illegible, he forwards the charts to his boss, who then decides on a score. The highest mark is zero, which means "Report exceeds standards, treatment acceptable." The lowest grades, three and four, trigger corrective measures. The administrator then kicks the charts back to the blue-shirts and requires them to acknowledge his comments by signing the QA form or making a timely appointment to rebut his determination.

Thus far, the quality of charts is increasing, but so is the level of discord. Fazio becomes apoplectic one day when she gets low marks for her chart documenting a tough but successful resuscitation. It was 0655, the end of her shift one night not long ago when Dispatch sent her and a partner into a high-rise to care for an unconscious male. She arrived at 0659 and found her patient, an obese man, dead. His family had not seen him alive for hours. Even if she could resuscitate him, she worried, the lack of oxygen he suffered would probably render him "a six-hundred-pound cucumber." She suggested pronouncing him, but, via radio, the doc insisted she treat the man. Fazio and her partner spent more than forty-five minutes working on their patient. They managed to get his heart beating. With the Rescue crew's help, whom Fazio says "pulled like sled dogs," they brought him to the hospital by 0757, well after shift change. After transferring care and completing her chart, she went home. Although Dr. Gluckman drew a smiley face on the chart and wrote "Very nice job," the administrator blackballed her paperwork because she did not include the patient's final disposition. "We're supposed to call the hospital before we go home," she explains. "We knew he was alive. I was just so friggin' tired I forgot to put it in there!" she recalls, furious that she could work so hard and get castigated for this one error.

BEATING THE CLOCK

"Patient has chest pain if she lies on her left side for over a year."

"Healthy appearing, decrepit 69-year-old male."

"She has no rigors or chills, but her husband states she was very hot in bed last night."

"The skin was moist and dry."

"Occasional, constant, infrequent headaches."

"The patient refused autopsy."

"Discharge status: alive but without my permission."

"The pelvic exam will be done later on the floor."

—EXCERPTS FROM "ACTUAL WRITINGS ON HOSPITAL CHARTS," AN E-MAIL POSTED ANONYMOUSLY ON AN EMS BULLETIN BOARD AT QUARTERS, OCTOBER 2000. AUTHOR'S NAME DELETED.

Quality-assurance experts recommend that EMS workers take their time and organize their thoughts before committing pen to paper. (If they don't, the type of mistakes shown above may well occur. When Drivet treated a feeble, ill man in a nursing home last week, he found notes on the facility's chart that said the patient was "alert but lethargic.") The advice presumes there is time to synthesize information, but with such high call volumes, other paperwork, equipment checking, supplies restocking, gas replenishing, and other routine activities, there isn't much of a buffer between jobs.

Patient charts and billing forms, which come with a five-page instruction book, can be challenging. The type is small enough to give Superman a headache. The billing sheet evokes a nightmarish return to math class. There are permutations of care dispensed to select, notations regarding which crew dispensed what, distances to calculate between patient pickup and dropoff, and other items to choose from column A and column B, as if the bill were a Chinese menu. Failure to fill in the blanks means performance demerits, but seeking the information during treatment, transport, or transfer can bring the wrath of the federal government.

In the ten-minute cushion between calls, crews must find a nurse or doctor willing to sign the chart and assume care of the patient. Then they remake their stretchers, clean up the medical detritus inside their trucks, wash their hands, and, occasionally, pop a smoke. Most try to make progress on their charts, too, but often they cannot complete them before Dispatch assigns them to another job. Almost inevitably, paperwork builds up.

Fazio attacks unfinished work when the city quiets down between 0500 and 0700 hours. Sitting in the cab (because headquarters provides no desks, no quiet, well-lit offices—just an ersatz wood table for meals in the kitchen), she tucks into her stack of paperwork, sustaining herself with sips of what's left of her third or fourth extra-large cup of Dunkin' Donuts coffee. She searches the cinnamon sunrise that splits the horizon's seam for inspiration and writes.

Plenty of her colleagues do last-minute paperwork during the "witching hour," too. Some have been too busy to catch a break. Others are inveterate gamblers rushing to beat the clock. And some are just downright superstitious. By engaging in Something That Must Be Done, they hope to shield themselves from that last emergency—the one Dispatch assigns when the ground-pounders' eyelids are heavy, when their backs ache from heavy loads, when their behinds have gone numb from hours on end conforming to ambulance seats, when even the cheerily disposed become downright surly.

Not only can Dispatch assign them a job five minutes before they swipe out, but the department can, sometimes at the very last minute, force blue-shirts to stay behind the wheel up to six hours longer for a punishing total of eighteen hours on the job. Although they are duty-bound to care for their patients, most can't afford to wait around for hours to discover what disposition the ER will assign. The majority have second jobs whose bosses expect them to show up on time, spouses counting on them to assist with child care, class to attend, or lectures to give. Some have been working back-to-back shifts at assorted hospitals or have been hustling without pause to meet life's demands. Desperate for hot showers and cool sheets, they confront more patients, more charts, more billing mazes. With each passing hour, fatigue increases, and so do mistakes.

NINETY-FIVE WAYS TO FAIL

The EMS workers here are largely cynical about QA, a contentious process which they view as little more than an exercise in dotting i's and crossing t's, something done to mollify bureaucrats and reduce litigation as opposed to substantively improving patient care. That's insightful, according to a former state official, who says, "When the state began implementing QA, it had nothing to do with patient care and everything to do with hammering people on documentation."

Recently, Fazio and Cisternino treated a woman they nicknamed "Biohazard Lady." An AIDS victim with dementia, this combative patient spit, drooled, cried, bled, urinated, defecated, and generally made treatment a Herculean task. She even pulled out the intravenous catheter in her jugular vein. "It looked like a Stephen King novel," Fazio recalls. "Blood was everywhere!" Though she was a challenge to sedate and intubate, the medics accomplished this *and* drew blood for labs—to help their ER colleagues expedite patient care. Fazio expected to earn a high rating for this case. Instead, the administration rebuked her for not having used a carbon-dioxide detector, a color-changing device that reflects whether the patient is exhaling appropriately.

"It was hard enough to tube her!" Fazio says defensively. "Have you ever tried intubating someone who is thrashing and spitting and emitting infection from every orifice? I'd like to see him get a CO_2 detector on her, too."

Cortacans would rather eat glass than find fault with Fazio and Cisternino, whom he considers "superior caregivers" as well as friends and mentors. "The B team is my heart," he says. "They are truly a family who watch out for each other, help each other out, back each other up; they're excellent prehospital-care providers." They watched him work as an EMT; they encouraged and helped him to become a medic. And when he graduated, he says, "They fine-tuned me." He knows how skillfully Fazio and Cisternino intubate. He knows the two often operate in cramped, dynamic conditions without much if any help—circumstances far different from those of their hospital-based colleagues. In spite of his respect for them, apart from his friendship with them, Fazio's defense is beside the point, Cortacans explains.

The hospital requires that *all* intubated patients get $ETCO_2$ detectors, because endotracheal tubes can shift, and if they move enough, air may not flow into the lungs but into the stomach. Apart from causing the patient to vomit and possibly choke or aspirate, there is a risk of oxygen deprivation and its attendant consequences. Mandatory use of $ETCO_2$ detectors is intended to make the technique more successful for *all* caregivers who intubate—especially those with less skill. And Fazio and Cisternino, adept as they are, are not exempt. When procedures are impossible to execute, that needs to be explained for the record, Cortacans says.

The way employees manage the deluge of paperwork can hobble if not cripple an EMS service entirely. Each patient-care report is a potential lawsuit; each chart and its authors are subject to subpoena in criminal and civil investigations. (About five percent of University EMS jobs result in complaints, and seven to ten EMS workers here get served every month.) Industry-wide, the stakes are so high that some enterprising instructors send their EMS students to court to observe trials. Others create scenarios and have students write corresponding charts. Employers are even hiring attorneys to audit their charts and grill their EMS workers in mock trials. Lawyers say and EMS workers know that if a procedure is not written down on the chart, it wasn't done. Should this AIDS patient or her family sue, the department could not produce a chart that justifies why they did not use a CO_2 detector.

Although it's clear that the chart might better withstand legal scrutiny had the medics written that the patient made use of the $ETCO_2$ detector impossible, this case also speaks to weaknesses in the department's QA system. Rarely do managers or objective experts accompany blue-shirts on jobs and coach them in real time. Rarely do blue-shirts sit as a group, much less with their Dispatch and hospital-based colleagues, to review tapes and charts and analyze a patient's experience from their initial 911 call through to discharge. The department has no on-site resources to help blue-shirts deconstruct and examine tough cases when events are fresh. And measures of quality—for example, patient outcomes, customer-service ratings, and benchmark comparison—are underdeveloped compared with the percentage of documentation errors. Bucking a national trend in EMS, the department does not do customer-service surveys, although the hospital's other patient-care departments do. "They're too expensive," an administrator explains. "But we do investigate complaints."

"QA here is nothing more than Monday-morning quarterbacking," a blue-shirt complains. "And hindsight is 20/20."

In addition to revamping criteria for evaluation, the administrator initiated staff meetings to improve communication and let paramedics know what he expects from them. But he only holds staff meetings during the day, hours that the B team does not work. Although such scheduling disrupts their child-care arrangements, other responsibilities, and time off, and although he offers no compensatory pay, he expects blue-shirts to attend, and he factors attendance into their performance reviews. On principle, most of the medics refuse. In lieu of compensation, they are lobbying to have at least half the meetings held when they are on campus.

Under the title "Chart Report Shortcomings," the department's QA form lists ninety-five ways that an ALS chart can be deficient and zero ways that it can be exceptional or otherwise impressive, which strikes some as a witch-hunt. There is no place on the chart, except for the Paramedic Rating System, or grade, in fine print at the bottom of the page, that sets aside even a possible opportunity for commendation. "Why don't they give us some praise on occasion?" a B-teamer protests as others grumble in agreement. Management points to a few blank lines on the bottom of the form for comments, and some charts do get the occasional "Good job" written on them. But overall, the blue-shirts say, praise is so thin as to be starving.

An administrator posts a chart that compares and contrasts A-, B-, C-, and D-team documentation scores—generating a little competition in the hope that underperforming crews will kick up their efforts a notch. B-teamers say this smacks of treating them like children. It incenses them that they can be among the most hard-core EMS workers and yet be publicly ranked beneath their peers.

Managers point to charting improvements as evidence that their techniques are effective. But several blue-shirts feel alienated. Many say they no longer strive to write insightful charts they are proud of but find uneasy peace in mediocrity. Even Drivet, the de facto team leader, the paramedic people respectfully call "the Commander," the practitioner even managers call "the Yoda of EMS," has become discouraged and disenchanted. "Now I don't even write adequate charts," he says woodenly. "I just check the boxes and give them the minimum data set."

GOOD FOR THE GOOSE

Ironically, there are papers that the blue-shirts want management to track, too—for example, records of their awards. Administrators say that when a job is well done, "we make sure our employees know about it. We post things on bulletin boards and file them in their charts." The bulletin boards do boast a congratulatory note every so often, but these are exceptions to the rule, the blue-shirts say. As for any catalogue of accomplishments, the blue-shirts believe none exist. Fazio once had her car stolen. She had made the mistake of keeping several awards in her glove compartment. When she requested photocopies of the originals, she says, management told her it had no records.

Another EMS worker dares anyone to walk up to management, which some call the anti-morale office, request his file, and look for the section entitled Awards and Accomplishments. "You won't find one. I am one of the most decorated people in memory. There is not one mention of it in my file."

Still another blue-shirt says he reviewed his personnel file recently. Management had taken disciplinary action against him. With help from the union, he fought the charges, and management agreed to rescind the penalty. When he examined his file, the disciplinary notice was still there, but there was no copy of the retraction. Moreover, "all the warnings and bad notices were in there, but there was no record at all of any of the awards I had received, nor any 'Adda boy!' letters that I had received in the past from patients," he states. "Thank God *I* keep copies."

10   *REALITY BITES*

When EMS workers say EMS is a young man's job, what they mean is
that it takes a youthful strength and naïveté to do the work. After twenty years
of building an experience base and honing their knowledge, skills, and intuition, they are primed to give care, but it gets harder to stomach the bullshit and
the physical punishment, too.

At twenty-seven, paramedic Henry Cortacans is still a young man. After six
years as an EMT and two years as a paramedic, he continues to be enthused by
his job. Yet Cortacans has already been injured, by a car thief who slammed into
his ambulance at 70 mph, pinning him so tightly that he had to be extricated by
O'Neill and Heber. Worse, his peers disrobed, examined, and treated him. To
show their affection, his teammates later teased him shamelessly about his
impressive physical assets. He was hospitalized and out of commission for a
considerable period of rehabilitation.

He has also sustained bruised ribs and a black eye from riding a 250-pound,
muscle-bound seizure patient like a mechanical bull. The patient panicked when
Cortacans's partner pumped up the blood-pressure cuff, and pummeled him without mercy. Cortacans called a Code 5 and sprang to his partner's aid and was

thus "Scrappy" for taking on the challenge in spite of the odds. He has also been treated for smoke inhalation, after rescuing a family from an intense house fire.

With all that behind him, Cortacans is still a "pup" by the veterans' standards. Although he has yet to cook in the field for a while, he exhibits the valor, dedication, and intelligence to take care of business and to take care of himself—well enough so that he can fight the good fight again and again. Fortunately for Cortacans, he comes from a close family. His parents, immigrants from Uruguay, emphasized brotherhood and other humanistic values. He goes to church regularly; he prays daily; and most of the time he comes to work eager and able to help the human race.

Whether he will stay on the streets or move on is unknown. Odds are, his B-team buddies would venture, he'll leave. The best and the brightest always do, they say, reciting a list of friends and mentors who have left EMS, or Newark, for bigger, better things.

WHEN YOU WORK THE BOX, YOU EAT OUT OF A BAG

Headquarters provides the EMS workers with a soft-drink dispenser, a caffeine machine, a refrigerator, an icemaker, and a microwave. Traditionally it has had a stove, but that was hauled away last year, and the blue-shirts await a replacement. Years ago, they took pride in their communal cooking, not unlike firefighters. Fazio isn't the only one with a lingering taste for the holiday spreads and Heber's wife's homemade pierogies. Some, such as Opperman, bring meals from home. If and when he catches a break, he pops his Tupperware into the microwave and may get halfway through lunch or dinner before Dispatch sends him back out.

Many do not make the time or have the energy to brown-bag. When they get a chance, the graveyard shift swings by any number of typical fast-food eateries and some lesser-known establishments such as Amin's Fongyip Chinese Halal Cuisine. Burt's is popular, too; it serves what Cisternino calls "heart-attacks-on-a-bun" (eggs, potatoes, cheese, and hot roast beef with onions piled high on a thick Portuguese roll). "It's really good and greasy, but you have to schedule an angioplasty afterward," he quips.

The constant pace builds an appetite, which gore doesn't diminish. A construction crane knocks a twenty-eight-year-old father of four off scaffolding forty feet high. He plummets to the asphalt and lands with a force so extreme it probably pops his lungs like two paper bags. The crew can't hear any breath sounds. They figure the blow tore holes in the man's lungs through which air escapes into the surrounding membranes. They grow fatter until they squeeze the lungs and heart so severely that the vital organs can no longer expand and contract to circulate air and blood. His chest cavity might be filled with blood, too, but that can only be treated in the hospital with a chest tube.

For now, it will help to deflate the swollen membranes so they can supplement his minimal breaths and give the organs room to work. A new paramedic struggles to shove ten-gauge needles into the man's meaty chest to decompress what is probably nothing less than a bilateral tension pneumothorax. He quietly codes. Minutes later, the EMS workers are eating shrimp with garlic sauce and yellow rice in the Portuguese part of town. "It's a basic human need," one says. "Gotta feed yourself."

Nothing makes them feel more disenfranchised than people who call 911 to complain "Don't they have something better to do?" after spotting an "ambulance driver" eating a sandwich in his bus or crews meeting up to enjoy coffee during rare periods of peace. The blue-shirts wish management would educate such callers that the food they wolf down may be the only energy source to fuel hours and hours of lifting, carrying, problem solving, and rushing. They get no meal breaks.

For the most part, food has to be tasty, fast, and able to energize them. Convenience foods and comfort-eating meet some of their needs but also influence weight gain, an industry-wide problem. Studies associate obesity, high triglycerides, and cardiovascular disease with shift work.[1] One has found that shift workers with unhealthy waist-to-hip ratios have numerous hormonal abnormalities characteristic of stress reaction, for example, cortisol, insulin, testosterone, and growth hormone.[2]

Some of their emergency services' colleagues take perverse pleasure in labelling many EMS workers as "fat." From there come allegations of uncontrolled eating, laziness, and a general discounting of professional contributions. Surely not being allowed a meal break during a twelve-hour shift, intense schedules, impractical hours that limit access to healthy foods, little control over work circumstances, and constant immersion in human tragedy offer more substantive and realistic explanations for the phenomenon than accusations of gluttony and sloth do. The EMS lifestyle is harsh. Without practical alternatives, super-sized colas and sugary snacks offer quick bursts of energy to stoke the workers' near relentless activity. And what could be more soothing than fried chicken with mashed potatoes and gravy?

When it comes to food, most veterans have an emergency plan. If Drivet has time at the top of his shift, he stocks his portable provisions locker with Ring Dings, Starburst fruit chews, JuJyfruits, and cheese puffs—no healthy alternatives, which he dismisses as "bird food." When hunger bugs Heber he drives to an all-night Exxon station for Pepsi and Funny Bones. Opperman counts on Yodels and chocolate milk from Krauszer's. Fazio and Cisternino (when he's not losing weight) are partial to Goldfish crackers, Pepperidge Farm chocolate Milano cookies, huge bottles of Fiji-brand water, and extra-large coffees from Dunkin' Donuts.

Cisternino's years as a weight lifter left him with an appetite for vigorous exercise. He likes to work out and can still press 335 pounds. But work, school, romance, and the occasional bit of steam he blows off leave little time. Fazio says Cisternino is the only person she knows whose weight can fluctuate sixty to seventy pounds every year. He puts it on bit by bit; he takes it off all in one shot. This year, he's experimenting with a high-protein diet of his own design. When rested and cheerful, he cooks 101 varieties of chicken, and brings it to work. He spouts all kinds of great diet news. "I'm excited," he says with a childlike grin. "Mustard has no carbohydrates!" But when he's dragging between jobs, short on sleep, and hungry, food is not funny.

At 0100 hours one morning, Cisternino realizes he hasn't eaten since he can last remember; now he's ravenous. Piumelli stands by their truck cursing and wiping some patient's vomit from his trousers. Cisternino is too hungry to laugh. But others do, and Piumelli threatens to tear off their limbs and beat the EMS workers with them while they're still wet. Hankering for a fresh chef's salad, Cisternino and Fazio plan to zoom over to Top's, a twenty-four-hour diner in East Newark (a distinct town of its own). Then Dispatch assigns them a job in the opposite direction. Fazio drives while her partner copes by pouring designer protein powder into his water bottle through a flier he has folded into a makeshift funnel. Most of it ends up in a fine mist all over his pants. His face shrinks into a tight angry mask. After another attempt, he abandons the idea of a protein shake, and pours the powder down his throat. He washes it down with swigs of tepid water.

"I can't imagine that tastes very good," Fazio commiserates.

"No, it sucks actually, but I've got a raging headache right now." After another throat full of powder and swallow of water, he lights up his eyes and says, devilishly, "Mmmm. Tastes just like candy." Then he coughs and he hacks and he chokes. "This fuckin' guy better be fuckin' dead," he says of the patient they're en route to pick up.

Some nights the crews get tantalizingly close to something to eat, but food eludes them like a mirage. As hunger pangs strike, they indulge in paranoid fantasies. Drivet swears Dispatch has every decent eatery programmed into their computer-aided display; whenever the crews get within fifty feet of a good restaurant, an imaginary citywide "FoodCam" triggers a dispatcher to assign more work.

"You get so pissed off," Chuck Coles explains. "You're so hungry, and someone calls with the stupidest thing in the world. You have to work really hard to stay in the proper frame of mind. Once in a while, someone is really dying and the switch flips in your mind. You go to work. You go to the hospital. But then you're back to square one again. *Starving.*"

But practiced EMS workers have their tricks. Drivet, for example, has a mental database of every safe, clean place to eat. (He doesn't go by Cisternino's standards, which hold that any place with less than three roaches in five minutes is OK.) One day it seems Drivet will never find food. Abracadabra! His chances of eating magically disappear as he bounces between jobs for hours. Driving to yet another call, he tells his per-diem partner, "If this is a BLS patient"—meaning they can delegate care to the EMT-basics—"there's a chicken place down here, which you can actually eat at and not get sick. They have macaroni. The food is really good, and they turn it over. We all eat there and it's pretty safe. But a Big Mac would taste pretty damn good now."

The patient's problem turns out to be one BLS can handle, and when Drivet gets back in the bus he picks up the conversation precisely where he left off. They decide on McDonald's and Drivet rockets in that direction as his partner's face turns blue-white. "I'm on a suicide mission today," he half jokes. Famished, he needs to eat. "You belted in?"

She smiles weakly and clutches her chest.

Predictably, Dispatch zings them with another assignment: "We have some type of HazMat there. See the Fire Department. We have other units responding."

"Aaaaagh. I hear my Chicken McNuggets calling me!" the per diem cries.

As Drivet gets closer to the designated location, he radios Dispatch for an update.

"We have a seizure there. I don't know if it's related to the HazMat," Dispatch reports. "An officer is experiencing chest pain, and someone else is in seizure."

"Could be the first attack of a neuro agent on U.S. soil. The supervisors will function as our canaries," Drivet says, working hard to keep a straight face. Seeing his partner's quizzical expression, he moves to assure her: "Highly unlikely, though. But, you know, it could mean we're on the lecture circuit."

As the shift stretches on, the balding, bespectacled man's cheery countenance wastes away. His grin flattens. His banter ceases. He looks plain miserable. *I must have raped and pillaged a lot of people in a previous life,* he thinks, *because it sure feels like I'm being punished now.* A coworker offers to give him a hug, to which he replies, "I don't want a hug; I want a cheeseburger."

MR. SANDMAN

Driving home takes additional energy, more than some can muster after the exhausting night tour. Many blue-shirts live outside the city, and a good number live near or beyond the state's borders. One EMS worker saves time by driving a motor home to the hospital, where he lives between shifts.

Fazio starts closing her eyes the minute she gets inside the car. She's tried fighting it but she can't. A physician diagnosed her as having a form of narcolepsy. Fortunately, she carpools. Unfortunately, she's not the only one with a bona fide sleep disorder.

After nineteen years on nights, Drivet just switched to the noon-to-midnight shift, hoping the change might somehow better accommodate his overloaded schedule. So far, it hasn't helped much. "When I worked nights, I used to get five hours of sleep, which was enough," he says. "Now I get three or four hours of sleep, but I toss and turn. I finally get into a restful sleep around six A.M., then I wake up late and rush around. Then I'm so exhausted from rushing around I have to lay down on the bed just to get the energy to drive to work. I know I'm maxed out. My five-year plan is to have one job. I don't care if I have to work a hundred hours a week. I just want one job."

But five hours of sleep was never enough; he's just forgotten how bad it was. He used to set the alarm clock to wake him up after four and a half hours, then sleep through its shrill ring for thirty minutes and wake up thinking, *Dear God, I need more time. I've got to get a different life.* He'd be expected at work and have to race around his condo looking for his pager, his cellular phone, his sunglasses, and the black holster belt that holds his flashlight, scissors, clamps, and other medical tools before dashing out the door and driving his red Saab 75 mph in the express lanes.

One day, when he clocks in for the new shift, he tells Opperman, "Thank God I got that coffee. When I drove through that red light I knew I was tired. I pulled into Wendy's to get a Diet Coke, had thirty-five minutes left, and of course I was late, so I had to drive like crazy."

O'Neill sleeps in parade rest, his body straight—even rigid—and his hands clasped neatly over his stomach. Chronic insomniac that he is, Drivet witnessed this when the two attended a professional conference and shared the cost of a room.

Cisternino is like the silver ball banging its way through a pinball machine. He ricochets between University, college, his other jobs, and teaching in a perpetual cycle with no room for sleep—except for the Zs he can catch between calls, fully dressed, sitting up in the truck. Those few hours a week when Cisternino does get some shut-eye, he says, the innocent faces of HIV victims haunt his dreams.

When Cardona leaves work, at 7:00 A.M., he picks up his sons and drives them to school. He runs home, showers, and changes into civvies. Then he rushes off. Today, for example, he attends a ribbon-cutting ceremony with city officials to celebrate the demolition of the Grafton Street housing projects where he grew up. Then he runs to the credit union, the dry cleaner, the mechanic, and other errands. Not every day is as busy. If he has no other commitment, he tries to make it to bed by 10:30 A.M. He rises three and a half hours later to shower again, iron his uniform, pick his children up from school, grab something to eat, and head back to work.

Some take sleeping pills; others take stimulants. By working overnight, they're fighting an unnatural disruption of the body's biological rhythms, which respond automatically to light and dark. Humans are not naturally nocturnal but are programmed to be alert and lively when the sun shines and to regroup at night, experts say. And researchers have found that night-shift workers have higher rates of cardiovascular disease.[3] The B team's schedule, two nights on, sometimes three, with an additional float day every month, too, alternating with two nights off, keeps everything in flux. Shift work confuses the body, leaving people disoriented and washed out. So do the jam-packed, unhealthful lifestyles many blue-shirts adopt. They push themselves without mercy. They deprive their minds of the chance to relax and cheat their bodies of the rest needed to preserve their health.

Such fatigue, unrelieved by refreshing sleep, can contribute to irritability and impatience, as well as impair motor skills—hazards EMS can ill afford. Emotions are easily triggered. Predictably, relationships suffer. Weariness impairs judgment, too. In the early 1980s, one of their coworkers suffered a fatal car accident on the way home, the blue-shirts recall soberly, even as others brag about driving to and from work in excess of 90 mph.

Several believe they are invincible. Others are convinced they will not live to collect the meager pensions that worry them half to death.

No one ever complains that they feel tired. Their exhaustion is clear, though, in simple exchanges. "It's scary when I fall asleep in the shower," Drivet says with a chuckle. "Your arms are like this," he says, holding them straight out against an imaginary wall.

"It's bad when you fall asleep on the toilet and have that ring around your ass for two days," another volunteers.

"Or when you can't get up from the bowl because your legs are numb," another cracks. Their peers roar at the embarrassing truisms.

The simple act of going to the bathroom becomes hugely complicated when one is always rushed and always on guard. One morning during the witching hour, several B-teamers sit outside writing up paperwork, watching the sunrise, and making plans for the day. "I'm going home to have a BM," one announces. "I'm always constipated at work because I'm afraid I'm going to get called away. I've tried reading. It doesn't work."

"I won't even use the bathroom here," Callahan says. He thinks it's too dirty and prefers to duck into a friend's or relative's apartment.

"Me either!" Cardona agrees. "That one day I got sick, and I just had to, I did a ritual scrub of that toilet seat before I sat down. I hosed it down, and put tissue everywhere."

"You can go in the last stall," Drivet reports, "if you bring your own cleaning products."

"That industrial-size roll of toilet paper, it's like steering a ship," one complains. "And it's abrasive."

"My biggest fear is being shot on the crapper," one confesses. Headquarters is just yards away from street brawls, and drug deals, and the harsh repeat of shots fired. Many worry that the "temporary" building's thin metal walls could not stop a stray bullet. "I won't even be able to wipe myself. '*Don't come in!*' I'll be shouting to the guys as I'm slapping the roll of the toilet paper five degrees port. 'Just give me a five-by-nine [bandage]; it's not for the wound."

One night, nature calls, but it's late and Drivet is nowhere near quarters. His per-diem partner says matter-of-factly, "You could pull over and go to the Amoco station up ahead."

"I could," he agrees. "But I could also have my legs cut off without anesthesia." If he must go, he wants a bathroom in a pre-scouted safe zone. "I have to go, I have to go," he chants, hoping the mantra will get him through the red traffic signal's eternity. Then he gets an idea. He's closer to his other job's station than he is to quarters, so he steers in that direction. When he arrives, he radios Dispatch that he's putting himself out of service "for a personal" and jumps out of the truck. He sprints halfway across the parking lot before he realizes he needs a key.

He jogs back to the truck and tears through his pockets, his canvas portfolio, and other assorted bags. "I hope I have a key," he frets. Desperately he sorts through pens, markers, LifeSavers, medication, house keys, car keys, ambulance keys, and tubes of hand cream (the "manly" kind, for fishermen). A sweat breaks out on his brow. He's laughing, which only makes his task more urgent. "Wouldn't that be awful? This is going to be terrible." He digs through another pile, and tosses his cell phone, gloves, and keys to the ski area aside. Finally, he finds what he's looking for, smiles, and trots off.

"You go, Walter!" his partner cheers.

* * *

"Walter is the kind of guy who does the poopie dance one minute but can don his tactical gear and run two miles with a gas mask on at a minute's notice," O'Neill says admiringly.

LITTLE MARY SUNSHINE

I'm sure if you go out to no-teeth, podunk New Jersey, people root for their patients. But here, you gotta keep something for yourself. You gotta take care of yourself to take care of others. You can't go on to the next patient depressed.

—GEORGE BURR, A RETIRED B-TEAM VETERAN WITH SEVENTEEN YEARS ON THE JOB

Walter Drivet does not feel compelled to indulge in the niceties of patient care, such as ensuring that someone has a blanket, but he is never rude and he is always a gentleman. When he treats children, he speaks to them with respect and tenderness. He does not have to teach one diabetic boy that it hurts less to pierce the side of a finger for blood-sugar testing than the meaty tip, but he does.

If he sees an EMS worker being impolite or judgmental to a patient, he discreetly says, "Thanks for your help. You can go now."

But none of this is about "niceness," Drivet protests. He would sooner stick pins in his eyes than allow anyone to label him "sweet" or "kind." His courteous manners are a strategy to make the job easier, he says. "To do this for nineteen years and not have it destroy my soul, I have to remain objective."

A self-described "caring professional," Drivet says he gives "the best care I can give while I am with them. I don't care about their age, gender, sexual preference, lifestyle, or financial circumstance. When I am with a person, I am very concerned about their well-being, but as soon as they are out of my charge I forget about them. After that, whether they live or die is of no interest."

He sees himself as a "body mechanic," which means he does what is necessary "to be as effective as possible, and then turf them off."

When Drivet was four, his parents divorced. He, his younger brother, and his mother moved in with his maternal grandparents in Bayonne, New Jersey. His granddad was an undertaker, and they all lived in the funeral home. Some of the neighborhood kids used his living arrangements as an excuse for cruelty. But growing up in a funeral home had some advantages, Drivet says. He learned not to fear death. Grandpa Gus assured him that he had nothing to fear from the dead people laid out in different rooms of the house; the living presented much more of a problem.

At six, Drivet got a suit and a job as Grandpa Gus's junior assistant funeral director. He helped carry flowers from the funeral home to the cemetery, cleaned the parlor after services, and did other chores, for which he was paid. (The only thing he couldn't bring himself to do was go into the rooms with corpses at night with the light off.) The experience taught him to be calm and efficient around dying patients, something he usually sees at least once a night in Newark.

"People think that we don't react, that we're unflappable. We have to numb ourselves so we don't become part of that suffering. I don't want to think about my father." When Drivet was a teenager volunteering on his town's emergency squad, he got a call that his dad was ill. Still in his uniform, he drove to the medical center to be at his father's bedside. A doctor, seeing him in medical garb, put him to work. Drivet held his father's head as the doctor inserted a nasogastric tube. Later that night, Drivet's father died of a heart attack.

EMS work can and does change people. Dispatched to a nursing home for a woman having difficulty breathing, Drivet finds a morbidly obese twenty-year-old lying in bed, too weak to sit up. She has a muscle-debilitating disorder that will, in time, kill her. She has a DNR order stapled to her chart. Outsiders might find this sad, even tragic. Drivet does not. "Chronic medical problems are a part of life," says the man who claims to know thirty-five ways to say "I'm sorry for your loss."

"When a person dies, it's a normal part of the life process, and there's a reason why God takes them at that time. Many of the conditions people have are a result of deliberate lifestyle choices," he adds. "For example, the chronic hypertensive who doesn't seek help for ten years and then strokes out." Recalling a sexually active HIV patient he had last night, he explains, "She has HIV; she has drugs"—medicines—"available to treat her, but she won't take them because they have bad side effects and they prevent her from drinking and taking recreational drugs.

"What happened Christmas Eve, now, *that* was a tragedy. It was a holiday, a time of celebration. Two helpless, defenseless people who came out of church, who were not doing anything, were killed by some butthead in a stolen car who ran and fled the scene after, by the way, hitting another car and entrapping people."

The impact threw the victims 150 feet. One woman was dismembered. People on the street became hysterical; some threw themselves to the ground, trying to protect the women.

"The husband comes up to the ambulance and asks, 'Would you like this? Do you need this?' He had his wife's leg in his arms," Drivet adds. "If you take everything to heart, pretty soon your heart breaks."

This summer, Drivet was at work when a friend called in panic. She told him her husband, one of Drivet's best friends, had become deathly ill and was being transported to an area hospital. The circumstances were sudden, suspicious, and grave. (Although neither Drivet nor his friend knew it at the time, the man had suffered respiratory and cardiac arrest only to be revived by a BLS team of firefighters.) Drivet conceived a plan and put it into motion within seconds. Working through Dispatch, he obtained the department director's permission to bring the man to University. He arranged for Dr. Gluckman to assume care. He and Opperman drove to the area hospital. He kept cool even when the doctor, worried that colleagues would think him foolish if the man's problems turned out to be minor, hesitated to release the man. With his persistent diplomacy, Drivet persuaded the doctor to release the man into his care for transport to University.

En route, Drivet attended to his friend's every need, even supplying a joke or two between puking sessions. Although this crisis intermingled his personal life with his work, he managed the situation with self-discipline, emotional disassociation, and skill, a combination that he finds works equally well whether he confronts a one-patient crisis or a whole community in distress. He doesn't want to care. He wants to be high-speed, low-drag. And he is. But it comes at a cost.

Drivet frowns on empathetic EMS workers. "I say no, don't pat patients on the shoulder, because each time you are giving away a little part of yourself and that's a limited resource. And don't hold their hands. It makes it harder on all of us," he explains, "because then everyone will expect it." Being warm toward patients should not be confused with the importance of clinical skills, he says. "It's not hand-holding and clipboard-driving that matter."

His beliefs are popular here, although others, in Newark and throughout the country, believe that making patients, families, and bystanders feel good about their EMS experiences is an important part of the job. The question is, why do so many B-teamers believe that warmth and customer service are separable from and secondary to superior clinical skills?

Paramedic training, which follows the classic physician's model as opposed to nursing's more holistic approach, may be partly to blame. But things are changing in medical schools, where doctors are now taught to treat patients' pain and fear, and to augment the healing process by coaching patients to adopt a positive frame of mind. Youth plays a part in all of this, too. "When I came out of paramedic school, I was a twenty-two-year-old laryngoscope-slinging paramedic," Terry Hoben confesses with an experienced provider's humble maturity. "We take them really young, shove them through the paramedic machine or make them sixty-second EMTs, and spin them out there without any life experience. They come out in their twenties and deal with crisis, pressure, sadness. Making people naked, sticking IVs into them, and pushing drugs is a lot to handle.

"Other professions have some kind of journeyman apprenticeship. Our system immerses them in a double trimester, a few scenarios, and throws them into a clinical experience without the type of preceptors nurses have, or medical-resident mentors. We expect them to be self-motivated, and we set them up for failure. Only the strongest survive. But the strongest are not necessarily the best.

"The hand-patters, the ones who alleviate suffering as well as pain and sickness, those who really care," Hoben says, "we're missing them because we scare them away."

Callousness comes, in part, from the sheer number of jobs. "You go on autopilot. It's second nature. This just happened, now you have to do that," George Burr explains. "The call volume here doesn't give you time to get personal."

Given the number of missions and the intensity with which this team works, it may be too much to ask them to give up their hearts and share their zest for life with patients, too.

CRUSTY SHELL

Armand "What It Means to Be from Maine" Cayer, a twenty-seven-year-old FNG from Auburn, Maine, is still getting used to life in the Renaissance City. He has had to adjust from thirteen calls a month to thirteen calls a night, or more. After a year on the job, the Yankee-pale Cayer now wears a stud in one ear and a thin hoop in the other. He shaves his brown hair short and bleaches its tips. Sometimes he shaves it off altogether. But he's still taken aback by what he calls "the cold, heartless, ruthless way of life" he now witnesses daily. "These people are perfectly willing to kill each other," he says, dismayed. But he also says, "I wouldn't trade this experience at University for the world. I needed to receive that 'welcome-to-the-world' message. I was so naïve."

Recently Cayer watched a volunteer ambulance from someplace outside the city pull up to the ER. "Their truck looked brand-new, like someone washes it every day. It had no dents; the chrome was all shiny. They probably have enough four-by-four bandages, all stacked the same way. There were no rogue spots of blood.

"In walk the volunteers, and the medics refused to speak to anyone on that truck! They came up and said, 'Hi. My name is Fred Smith.' And the medics are like, 'So? You know your name.'

"That just blew me away," he admits. "I was completely shocked. I make it a point to talk to volunteers. There has to be a little bit of common courtesy and decency. It's not like they're taking our jobs. I don't know why we have to be 'We're so great we can't talk to them.' Clearly, some people think their shit don't stink."

Not talking to people is one way the B team says "You don't belong" without actually saying it. Outsiders' opinions do not interest them. War stories do not impress them. They wait for an FNG's moment of crisis and watch. How FNGs fare under fire is what they base their opinions on. Some confess to betting on how long the new guys will last.

It all serves a purpose. It thickens the skin, and makes quick work of those unable to adapt to the streets. Besides, it's not like the old days, when rites of passage included playful stabs or stripping FNGs, wrapping them in a Reeves, and parking them against the fence. One remembers being wrapped in sheets and electrical tape and stuffed into a linen cart that was summarily shoved off the tarmac onto Littleton Avenue. Those who make it through the silence, the hazing, and the streets' surprises learn to trust each other with their lives. Those who survive know their comrades understand how brutal and defeating the job is as well as its power to suck people in. But the team does EMS no favors by blackballing "housewife medics who don't *need* the job," volunteers (which they used to be), and "hand-holders," whose kindness goes farther, apparently, than they can appreciate.

GIVE WHAT'S RIGHT, NOT WHAT'S LEFT[4]

As in all professions, there are rogue members who break their moral contract with society. What is alarming is that they don't seem to know it and they don't seem to police themselves as well as they think they do. Some EMS workers have reported to work drunk, on drugs, or so sleep-deprived that they must ingest stimulants; still, they drive and dispense controlled substances. Some talk of colleagues who unnecessarily stick "asshole" patients with painful needles. Some spray Glade air freshener on stinking homeless patients. Some report coworkers who have been investigated for taking kickbacks from ambulance-chasing attorneys. Some approach patients, who may be upset and unnerved, with the attitude, "You need me. I don't need you."

An elderly woman, depressed by her weakness and constant ailments, cries in the ambulance, "I just want to die." Her blue-shirt replies, "I hope you do," certain that that is a perfectly reasonable response to someone tired of pills, shots, and infirmities. Is this all EMS workers? No. But even the best blue-shirts have their bad days.

EMS workers hate being labeled "lazy." Many feel hurt by public indifference to the amount and caliber of work that they do—labor that few people have the skill or stamina for. But long hours, overwork, and low pay are a poor mix for a society that wants to attract bright, responsible, sociable caregivers to their bedside, or roadside, or cliffside all hours of the day and night. But for a few bozos a noble profession is maligned. Because EMS workers often feel so unrecognized by those they serve, when anyone exposes the profession's ugly underbelly they react defensively and close ranks, which only isolates them further.

But society has moral contracts with other professions that function by virtue of the public's trust, and those who abuse the people they serve are called to account. Cops on the take, for example, or teachers and clergy who molest children—they are more than disreputable; they are criminal. Obviously, not all cops are crooked and not all teachers and clergy are pedophiles. Police community liasons and religious institutions lobby public opinion, reminding people of their contributions and good deeds. And the trust citizens afford them, while not taken for granted, is sustained.

EMS workers have plenty of ways to reach the public, but B-teamers say their triple-header jobs ill afford them the time to speak to church groups and parent-teacher associations or to write editorials. EMS workers from many locales say that they have tipped off journalists numerous times but have seen no effort to penetrate the institutional bureaucracy that hospitals erect to keep the media, and the public interest, at bay. And, people's lack of familiarity with EMS leaves a stunning chasm of ignorance that neither television dramas nor the engulfing blizzards of their own real-life crises can bridge.

HOSANNAS

The Physicians, Nurses and staff at The University Hospital wish all Emergency Service Providers a very happy *EMS Week*.
Thank you for all your hard work and efforts to keep the community healthy and safe.

To show our appreciation, we invite you to see the charge nurse
to receive a coupon for a free donut and coffee at Dunkin'
Donuts on Bergen Street.
Thank you again and keep up the good work.

—ER POSTER TEXT, MAY 23, 2000

EMS Week rolls around every year toward the end of May. Hospitals around the
area host banquets where volunteers, paid providers, and ER staff socialize and
celebrate their lifesaving work. Guest speakers inspire them. They snack on
catered delights or sit down for a formal meal. They imbibe, chow down, and
dance. Exemplary service and outstanding acts are recognized with awards.

The festivities at University Hospital are more subdued. The hospital trots
out its EMS Week poster, a durable, laminated affair replete with ER staff auto-
graphs. This year it also offers a free tour of NorthSTAR and the Trauma Center, and a free lecture on preventing and treating heat emergencies (worth three
continuing-education credits). Management hosts an all-team barbecue in the
quarters parking lot, where guests can take in a pollution-smudged view of the
Manhattan skyline—if they can see past the compound's Dumpsters, chain-link
fence, trash-strewn streets, and tired houses.

The department also gives each guest a fanny pack. But they turn out to be
defective.

There was a time when the department rewarded heroism, dedication, and
innovation with plaques, certificates, medals, and ceremony. The employee-
recognition program commemorated feats such as working thirty-six hours
straight through a 117-degree heat wave.

O'Neill, for example, has earned four Class A awards for actions that the
Policies and Procedures Manual describes as "heroic," reflecting "immeasurable
courage and devotion to duty" and putting a rescuer's "life in jeopardy in order
to preserve another."[5] (Ironically, the manual also states that EMS workers who
take such risks will be considered "private citizens"; they may face discipline,
and jeopardize their insurance, especially if they sustain illness or injuries as a
result.)

The department has also bestowed on O'Neill more than a dozen Class C
awards for "betterment of the Service"; ten Class D awards for exemplary service; three inclement-weather awards, such as one for the time he walked nine
miles through a snowstorm to get to work; one award for helping to orchestrate
a Papal visit; and another for working the Tango and Cash weekend. The
Newark Police Department has also officially commended him for his help ini-
tiating its SWAT emergency response team. The list goes on, literally.

"The fruit salad on my fucking uniform could fill a buffet line," O'Neill admits. Taking a lesson from his mentor Drivet, he prefers to be "a silent professional." Like Drivet, he does not wear his medals except for dress-uniform occasions.

In a public-service job with low pay, meager benefits, and limited opportunities to advance, recognition takes on heightened importance. It's tempting to think that the good feeling that comes from helping people would be sufficient. But it doesn't last long, especially for the veterans who have come to believe that their managers and people in general take them for granted, that the public cares about EMS only when they need it. "If I make a mistake, I'm stink on shit," paramedic Opperman says. "But when I do something great, I'm never gonna hear about it. I need some positive reinforcement."

Several years ago, the department created an annual awards program "to promote espirit de corps" and "improved levels of achievement."[6] But it hasn't been celebrated for years.

Surviving one real-life nightmare to go on to the next is a triumph, but it leaves a mark. And although most would appreciate some recognition from the society that they serve, they have learned to go without it, steeling themselves on admiration from respected peers and loved ones.

One blue-shirt says the ceremonies lost all meaning for him when he discovered that an employee was buying his own medals and decorating himself. Others felt slighted. Because the blue-shirts hold down multiple jobs at various hospitals, they know the effort to which other institutions go to celebrate EMS Week. Punch, cookies, metal folding chairs, and a standard-issue hospital conference room fell short of their expectations, this being the biggest and busiest EMS system in the state.

This past year, some new blood decided to reclaim and resurrect the awards ceremony. They invested several hours planning a ceremony with medals, plaques, certificates, etc. But the festivities did not come off as planned. The supervisor assisting them complained about anglers hoping for a "How Do You Like Me So Far?" award. He never followed through and ordered the actual awards for those who had been selected by their peers. The event was "postponed" again.

For now, the blue-shirts' sense of fraternity remains strong even as morale wavers. Henry Cortacans, Chuck Coles (now a medic), and Rescue responded to a car with three people that flipped on a major city thoroughfare.

"They were trapped. Unconscious," Cortacans recalls breathlessly. "The gas tank ruptured. Everything was soaked, covered, doused with gas. Geno coulda been killed if just one spark—

"Gas was everywhere. One of the patients had a massive hemothorax. They extricated all three of them and deconned the patients right on the scene with the Newark Fire Department. We could never have transported or brought them to the ER like that." Even so, the noxious, throat-choking fumes made Cortacans and Coles tear and cough on the way to the hospital. They managed to intubate their patient anyway. Cortacans was proud of the job and tried to interest an administrator. His boyish face falls flat recounting his boss's response.

"'Oh, yeah? Wow,'" Cortacans deadpans, imitating his boss's apathetic reaction. "He just kept on walking down the hall and out the door.

"*We coulda died! We coulda died! We coulda died!* We coulda been killed in the back of the bus just from the fumes. The ambulance stunk of gasoline for six hours. Anyplace else that would be considered heroic. Here? No one gives a shit."

THE BOTTOM LINE

Put a fork in me . . . I'm done.

—WALTER DRIVET, UNIVERSITY HOSPITAL PARAMEDIC

At forty years of age, Drivet regularly works between 80 and 120 hours a week. He puts in forty hours at his job at University, forty hours directing EMS operations at a popular ski resort, and twenty hours at another busy urban hospital. He also devotes at least ten hours every two weeks to Union County's SWAT team. That means anything from training the crew of tactical medics he commands and giving premission briefings to working with the prosecutors's office and developing projects such as school-violence response.

He also spends time crisscrossing the state from job to job. A sought-after instructor, he teaches, too. The work he loves best is on behalf of a federal entity that fights narcotics trafficking and terrorism. Occasionally he also takes on special details, such as serving as EMS incident commander at special events. He is scheduled to work a fiesta days from now. Although he has no idea where the energy will come from, he's sure he'll rise to the occasion. "If things get out of control this weekend, I'm gonna set my hair on fire and run around like a Roman candle," he says with a mock castanet flourish. "Olé, motherfucker!"

Drivet lives a significant part of his life in his car. He hangs extra uniforms there. And he's been known to shave while he drives. He once messed up his sideburns so badly that O'Neill would not let him out of the EMS compound before evening things out. Years ago, he thought seriously about becoming a doctor or at least a physician's assistant. Having already earned a BS in business administration, Drivet enrolled at Columbia University to bone up on the sciences he would need. While working overlapping jobs, he commuted 130 miles several times per week to complete two semesters of general biology, anatomy and physiology, general physiology, general chemistry, and calculus as well as one semester each of microbiology and organic chemistry. Between his myriad job duties and his family life—he was married at the time—he could not study as intensively as he needed in order to earn competitive grades.

So he put that dream aside, even though he incurred thousands in debt, which he is still paying off. The supplemental education has not been lost on him, though. Drivet loves learning, and part of the reason he excels as a clinician is a profound understanding of pharmacology, biochemistry, and pathophysiology. He adds to his storehouse of knowledge constantly. Between calls he can usually be found poring over texts such as *The Companion Guide to Emergency Medicine* or browsing at an all-night newsstand. He subscribes to thirty magazines, including medical journals, news weeklies, and *Soldier of Fortune*. When he finally sells his condo, a last vestige of married life, he pares down his library and floods quarters with cartons of books on all things medical and military.

Walter Drivet loves life; he loves EMS; he just doesn't want to miss a trick. Being type A is par for the course, he says of himself and his fellow EMS workers. It would have to be.

A CHICKEN IN EVERY POT

> You have an accident scene, and a medic has to stick a needle in someone's chest to relieve a collapsed lung. [They can do that on standing orders, without direct physician oversight.] How do you justify you're paying that guy twelve dollars an hour?
>
> —JERRY JOHNSTON, NAEMT BOARD OF GOVERNORS (IOWA), AND DIRECTOR OF EMS IN HENRY COUNTY, A RURAL SYSTEM IN IOWA

Most of Newark's EMS workers grew up in the U.S., consuming the same media as their fellow citizens and developing the same commercial appetites. They believe in the same American dream as their neighbors from coast to coast. Work hard and you can have it all, or at least a good-sized chunk. They do work hard. But they can't afford a big chunk, much less a healthy slice, on their salaries. EMTs in Newark earn between $14.36 and $19.62 per hour;

paramedics earn between $16.43 and $22.53 per hour. Besides the basic expenses of life, their salaries must also fund job-related parking fees; union dues; pension contributions; health, dental, and life insurance; job-related incidentals; and fitness fees if they use the campus gym.

"How do they live on that?" an EMS supervisor finds himself wondering. "These are people with children."

"No one in EMS is getting rich and living in that big house on the hill," Jerry Johnston says. EMS workers in Tennessee earn between $6 and $8 per hour. Paramedics in Pennsylvania and Texas make $9 an hour. Comparatively, University Hospital's EMS salaries seem generous. University Hospital says it is one of the best EMS payers in New Jersey. But the Garden State is expensive. The National Low Income Housing Coalition says that New Jersey is the least affordable state; $16.88 is the minimum hourly wage one must make to afford a modest two-bedroom apartment. Almost half (forty-four percent) of the state's renters can't afford it, the Coalition says.[7]

Supermarket cashiers and stock clerks here earn more than $16.91 per hour, and their union recently negotiated a 15.5 percent raise on top of that, not to mention a handsome pension supplement, for which there is no mandatory contribution. United Parcel Service package-car drivers earn more than many EMS workers, a fact Cisternino likes to surprise people with.

"UPS will deliver a package under a hundred and fifty pounds from the north end to the south end of Newark overnight, but you have to pack it yourself and take it to them. On the other hand, if you call 911, we come to your home; we'll send at least two people. We package you up. We won't care what you weigh. We'll get you where you are going in less than thirty minutes. We charge more but we earn less.

"What does it take to get a job at UPS?" he asks. "A driver's license and no convictions."

UPS drivers start out earning about $20 per hour to deliver between one hundred and two hundred packages each day. "It's very, very hard work," says Dan McMackin, director of public relations at United Parcel Service. He started on the trucks while working his way through college and says he lost thirty pounds his first two weeks on the job. (He was going to school full time, and also holding down two other jobs, not unlike Cisternino, Drivet, and O'Neill.) "You have to be really sharp. If you're a dunce or you're not committed to serving people, you're not going to make it." Sixty percent of UPS drivers are college-educated.

"We do time-sensitive, extremely important deliveries around the world. It's not just document running. It's everything from medicine to supplies and parts to keep General Motors plants alive," McMackin explains. "Our customers will pay a premium to have their packages delivered the same day."

Cisternino is unimpressed. "Society values its parcels more than its health care," he concludes.

Cisternino's full-time salary at University, where he also serves as a shop steward, is $40,000. "Except for the annual three-percent cost-of-living increase, basically, what I am hired at is my rate of pay for the rest of my career," he explains. The department has no merit increases, and it did away with salary bumps associated with length of stay. "If I left and got rehired, I'd be hired back at a much higher rate, but I'd lose my seniority." (Rank assures his place on the overtime list and allows some influence over his choice of partner and assignment.) He and others who have invested years here were nonplussed to discover that the department bestows signing bonuses on newcomers bereft of similar experience but offers nothing comparable for their troops' loyalty and longevity. This compounds the frustration they feel, because there is no academic or career path; promotions in rank are limited (and generally mean upgrading one's skills from an EMT to a paramedic), and they find it difficult to advance ideas.

For a workforce of approximately 250, "we have three upper-management positions and a few supervisory spots," an administrator states. "Turnover at the upper ranks is slow. While there's not much potential for advancement by promotion, there are ways to enhance and advance one's career . . . but money is an issue."

The ability to increase one's income comes from competing for extra shifts, working special units in addition to one's job, such as Special Operations, and occasional projects that management approves. A self-taught computer whiz who has mastered several programming languages, paramedic Henry Cortacans, for example, designed, built, and maintains the department's Website (*www.uh-ems.org*). Also a lifelong meteorology buff who constructed a substantial weather station on the roof of the urban town house he shares with his parents, Cortacans has worked his forecasting skills into the department's disaster-planning protocols. And he devotes several hours a month to reviewing charts as part of the department's quality assurance. For such tasks, which he performs in addition to working forty hours a week on the streets, the department pays Cortacans at his hourly rate.

In short, pay is commensurate not with increasing experience but with more hours worked. To finance the quality of life they want, almost all the B-teamers have two or more jobs. Cisternino, for instance, works full time at University, holds two part-time medic jobs, teaches, and helps administer the ambulance service at Ramapo College, which he also attends as a full-time student. At the end of the year, he'll clear between $55,000 and $60,000 for his yeoman's effort.

Opperman's base, after nineteen years, is $47,000. He has a pension loan on it and forced savings as well. A husband and a father, Opperman is now down to two jobs, a scant sixty-six hours per week. For years, he worked himself to the max, squirreling away more than $25,000 in overtime to save for a house, which most EMS workers simply cannot afford without multiple jobs. "I just socked it away," he says. "I had no girlfriend, no social life. I just worked and saved."

Cardona almost doubled his salary with overtime last year while still finding time to help build Newark's Hispanic Fire and EMS Association. In the privacy of his bus, he confides in Callahan that his wife, who also has a career, is unhappy that he's working so much. He's torn, because he desperately wants to provide a good life for his sons. Callahan commiserates and urges him to do it now while he's young enough to bear the strain.

Despite their efforts, most earn far below what firefighters and police earn for one job alone. Newark firefighters start out at $28,922; their tuition to the fire academy is paid for, and they earn while they learn. Before ever ascending in rank, they can reach $65,594 per year. Newark police officers collect $31,700 their first year. Their tuition is paid, too, and they also earn while they learn. Patrol officers top out at $61,866 per year. Police and firefighters can retire after twenty-five years, regardless of age, with pensions worth sixty-five percent of their final year's salary and health benefits. Continued service can hike the payout to seventy percent.

EMS workers, on the other hand, have to start the job fully trained and certified. They pay out of their pocket for courses to get and perpetuate their certifications and increase their skills. And they don't just pay once; they shell out every few years throughout their careers. Besides underwriting their professional education, they are expected to pursue it on personal or vacation time. The state's Public Employees Retirement System sets the normal retirement age for EMS workers at sixty. Then it pays vested retirees 45.5 percent of their final average salary.[8] None of the blue-shirts can foresee doing such physical work in middle age. To qualify for early retirement, the blue-shirts must work twenty-five years *and* reach age fifty-five or suffer a quarter of one percent penalty for every month that they are younger than age fifty-five.

State employees, the EMS workers want to participate in the police and firefighters' pension. "We're good enough to provide law-enforcement support and fire standby but not good enough to participate in their pension plan," Heber grumbles. He's happy to help out his fellow emergency-service providers, be it lighting up their crime scenes, repairing their equipment, extricating them, backing up their SWAT missions, or patching up their bullet holes, stab wounds, and burns. He'd just like something that approaches parity when it comes to saving for his old age, especially as opportunities to advance and become supervisors or managers are so limited.

TRAPPED

Seduced by the notion of making a difference, thrilled to develop new skills and exercise autonomy, captivated by the lights-and-sirens urgency of it all, many EMS workers first get involved as teenagers. Some come with the ambition and resources to pursue higher education and thus careers in medicine or other types of emergency management. Others love life on the street and find the work intrinsically rewarding. But their idealism and adrenaline reserves only carry them so far. And time is distorted in the world of EMS. Here, with twelve hours on and twelve hours off, one barely knows whether one is coming or going. Days of the week, weekends, and holidays become meaningless. Adding an extra job, or two, or three, means that months, even years pass by in a blur.

Not infrequently, EMS workers wake up in their thirties, just as their expertise and perspective to do the job well become ripe, to find their youth spent. The psychological and physical toll from a decade or more in the field threatens to force them out of the business. With little opportunity to advance, with families depending on them, their options fade and their beloved careers seem to come to a dead end. It's an intimidating crossroads.

Some EMTs become rescue specialists; some become medics. Some medics become flight medics or deepen their expertise with special emphasis on industrial or wilderness rescue, critical-burn or cardiac patient transport, or weapons of mass destruction response, for example. A few, with natural drive, ability, mentors, and opportunity, are able to build impressively on their early EMS experiences.

Chief Paul Maniscalco exemplifies how blue-shirts can go into the world to make inestimable contributions. The EMS bug bit him when he was a Boy Scout. That's where he first learned CPR, which he later performed on his own father. As a youth, Maniscalco wiled his way to Newark, where he watched University's crews with a buff's enthusiasm. As a teenager, he persuaded Judd Fuller, then course coordinator, to admit him to his first EMS class, although he was slightly underage. He badgered his mom to drive him to campus, where he studied under Fuller and instructors such as Keith Holtermann, then an EMT in the Emergency Department. (Holtermann, who went on to earn master's degrees in public health and business as well as his doctorate, is now the assistant dean of Health Sciences at George Washington University's School of Medicine and Health.) Maniscalco became an EMT while in high school and a New York City paramedic shortly thereafter. As he rose through the Big Apple's EMS ranks to run increasingly challenging operations—for example, the 1993 World Trade Center bombing—Maniscalco chipped away at his studies and sought ways to strengthen the profession and his career.

He presided over the NAEMT and still serves on its executive board. He has published and continues to publish books and articles. He became an expert on how EMS should deal with the consequences of terrorism, i.e., the medical effects, and advises businesses as well as local, federal, and foreign governments. He has always carved out time for pro bono work and to mentor promising EMS workers. A ranking international expert at forty, and poised to complete his Ph.D., Maniscalco credits much of his success to mentors to whom he has continually turned throughout his career.

But the opportunities that have helped make law enforcement, firefighting, nursing, and other helping professions so appealing are underdeveloped in EMS. This troubles Maniscalco and other EMS leaders who believe that America needs a cadre of EMS professionals to work the streets, improve EMS effectiveness through research, and continue shaping the system to meet society's changing needs. With such career-EMS professionals, they argue, one day the industry will be able to reduce and prevent illness and injury, much as firefighters and police have curtailed fires and squelched crime.

Having looked into countless patients' eyes, Maniscalco knows how important it is to have agile, competent, caring people on the front lines. But he also knows that unless something changes, the strains of the job will cause many talented EMS workers to abandon the profession.

"How can you expect these people to go on day in and day out, to expose themselves to unpronounceable disease?" Maniscalco asks. "To get shot at and get shit thrown at them? To get delayed by people who get in the way or jeopardize their safety when they drive? To thrive in bureaucracies that crush them? To work two or three jobs just to put a roof over their family's head, keep food on the table, send their kids to school? And if they get injured . . . you discard them like yesterday's news?"

In communities across the U.S., EMS workers are voting with their feet in favor of careers with avenues for lifelong learning and advancement, such as nursing and law enforcement. Some communities are already struggling to provide residents with an EMS safety net. The problem may seem less dramatic in urban centers like Newark, where droves of ambitious young EMS workers flock in search of the volume and case diversity to jump-start their careers. Ironically, some blue-shirts believe, the more or less steady stream of applicants may encourage management to think of its EMS workers as dispensable, even interchangeable. Management literally shrugs off concerns about the constant churn of street-level medicine: "Sure we need experienced, educated people here to train the younger ones," an administrator says. "But if they leave it's not the end of the world. Others who don't have the experience are willing to go out and get it."

The hospital can put a new crop of blue-shirts on the buses every week, but novices can't offer patients the insights and know-how that truly seasoned EMS workers can. And, to be fair, a blue-shirt's years of service are not sufficient qualification. Some who can't advance in the system or break out of it just hunker down under the strain and mark time until they collect their pensions. Management casually refers to them as "lifers"; they put as much zeal and professional pride into their work as their namesakes.

"We're in crisis! We're in a brain drain!" Maniscalco exclaims. "We lose senior experienced clinicians and rescuers all the time. We have an inability to preserve our history. We don't engender a process to capture the knowledge and pass it down to the youngsters, the rookies. The net result? We're dead-railed. We're a train wreck waiting to happen."

EMS leaders like Maniscalco are working to reframe the profession so those committed to emergent patient care and disaster management can devote their lives to the work. Others, however, continue to view EMS as a way station.

"EMS is a hard job with poor pay. It's gritty. It's dirty. It's all-weather. It offers minimal rewards and no prestige and glamour. It's for young guys," says Dr. Michael Jaker, University Hospital's ER director. "Why should they stay here for twenty years? They shouldn't! It's physically hard. The effort is extreme. You want a sixty-seven-year-old guy carrying you down the stairs? They stay up all night, train rigorously, and work under more and more regulation. They don't have to be up at four A.M., live on 40K a year, and be away from their family. They could use it as a springboard for more education. They can get a master's degree. They can get an M.D., teach, or be an administrator rather than live on a lower-middle-class income for the rest of their life."

But figuring out how to add college or graduate-school courses to the delicate balance of several jobs, recertification classes, and household responsibilities can be overwhelming. Despite the department's affiliation with a large and prominent health-sciences university, there is no clear academic, research, or career path for blue-shirts, and precious little mentoring. One EMT who recently upgraded his skills to become a paramedic slaps the air at the notion of any help or encouragement from management. "You're on your own," he says with a derisive snort.

"Some are frustrated," an administrator acknowledges. "They see others moving ahead, and they don't have any other skills or training. They're stuck in a position of their own creation. If they don't like it, leave. We don't chain them here. We don't force them to work here. A lot of these guys don't live for tomorrow. They don't look at themselves, at where they want to be in five years. They say they want to pay the rent next week." In an industry where people are driven, and many see bootstrapping as a rule, he holds himself up as an example. "I had a full-time job here, a part-time job at another hospital. I went full time to university, plus teaching. And I did all that so I could go someplace in five years. I knew that I didn't just want to be a paramedic for twenty years, not that there's anything bad with that."

Many of the rank and file who can't clear the time or money needed to complete their baccalaureate or advanced degrees are nevertheless eager to innovate, contribute on some level above and beyond the nightly grind and develop opportunities to be useful as age makes fieldwork harder to bear. They volunteer ideas. For example, they have suggested branching into nonemergency medical-transport services for chronic medical procedures such as kidney dialysis. They have volunteered to help management win and carry out EMS contracts in New Jersey's other large municipalities, such as Atlantic City. Sought-after lecturers, they have offered up their countless instructor certifications to staff an EMS training academy. (Less experienced EMS departments and freelancers compete for shares of the training market, education that is state-mandated and often state-funded.) In fact, University once provided the bulk of the state's EMS training, the director says, but that stopped when their grant was exhausted.

Another avenue for EMS workers to improve care, add value to their jobs, build skills, and attract funds to their sponsoring institution is through research. Researchers test protocols and new technologies. They identify problems, such as racial or gender disparities in care. They determine realistic goals for variables, such as response times. They find community weaknesses and propose solutions.

Paramedic Matthew R. Streger, M.P.A., the deputy commissioner of Cleveland EMS and a former University EMT, has had a hand in a retrospective study of charts. For example, Cleveland EMS discovered a significant number of pedestrian-auto accidents at several city intersections. The EMS Department discussed its findings with city administration, which came up with a plan to install speed bumps, signage, and other traffic improvements at three high-risk locations. Cleveland EMS also obtained a grant from the state of Ohio to help raise awareness about pedestrian accidents involving children and how to prevent them. Their campaign to reduce accidents is under way, and they plan to evaluate results.

The need for EMS research is profound, NHTSA says.[9] America continues "to lack adequate information regarding how EMS systems influence patient outcomes for most medical conditions and how they affect the overall health of the communities they serve."[10] Moreover, without research there is no scientific basis for including or excluding new initiatives, from medicines to protocols. Several common EMS practices, originally developed on the battlefield or inside hospitals, remain questionable.

NHTSA urges academic institutions and medical schools to make "long-term commitments to EMS-related research . . . including projects that involve EMS personnel of all levels."[10] But, despite the hospital's affiliation with the prestigious University of Medicine and Dentistry and the large population it serves, which makes for good sample sizes, the department does not drive much prehospital research. A few self-starters, including flight medic O'Brien, have conducted and published research. But they are the exception. "There was an EMS and Pre-Hospital Research Group here, but over time interest waned," says an administrator, who has done research himself. "I think it's important but I don't have the time."

Few EMS workers know how to design, fund, and carry out research. There are programs, such at those taught by the Pre-Hospital Care Research Institute (part of UCLA's medical school), that teach EMS workers how to test ideas, protocols, and technologies inexpensively, but the department rarely sends blue-shirts. Asked why management doesn't back more research or initiatives that percolate up from the blue-shirts, the director says that she has a better grasp of the market than the EMS workforce, which has "very limited employment experience." She explains: "The one thing that makes them effective is their personality; they're type-A, heroic, with egotistic mentalities. They're invincible. They're ballsy. It makes them good at what they do, kind of like trauma surgeons who will cut your heart out, put it in their hands, and squeeze. The downside is, they don't see the big picture. They're very critical. They're shortsighted. They have a very short, narrow scope of education. They get a quick idea and say: 'Let's change the outcome.' It's the lights, the sirens, and the adrenaline pumping. People get their self-esteem from that. You don't see that in the hospital as much, where people are judged by their credentials."

Besides, although she would like to empower the staff to do more, she says, operational costs, an overburdened staff, insufficient space for work and storage, inadequate reimbursement structures, and a seven-figure annual deficit pose too many obstacles. "The hospital is curtailing resources," she explains. "We have to compete for limited space. Space is dedicated to education at the medical school and those bringing in research dollars. I'm losing space to train my own people!" she complains. "Training EMS or paramedics is not the priority."

The busy department operates under real constraints, but the blue-shirts are a can-do group. The initiative-taking and mentoring, which helped to vault University Hospital–trained EMTs like Maniscalco and Holtermann to positions of national and international influence, have flagged and morale has plummeted. Talk in the buses, around the picnic table, and at off-campus get-togethers often addresses plans for the future, plans that do not include University EMS, or EMS at all. Feeling impotent to effect social change or personal growth, the blue-shirts don't encourage each other to stay on the job longer than needed to amass experience, much less the FNGs. Turnover rates are extraordinary.

"We just get shot down, shot down, shot down," Fazio says with disgust. "So now it's like I just do my job and go home. Why should I do anything extra?"

11   *SAY IT AIN'T SO*

It's not a good day at work until you are at
home. And in this current climate of diseases, it
could be fifteen years. I won't know if I'm safe
until I retire.

—KEVEN CLEARY, UNIVERSITY HOSPITAL PARAMEDIC AND
  COMMUNICATIONS CHIEF

HEEBIE JEEBIES

Headed into the West Ward to treat a "woman, sick," Callahan and Cardona
park and collect their gear. The two climb the stoop and squeeze through a
doorway to enter a first-floor apartment. Inside, a mocha-colored woman
slouches in a big, cushy chair. Her hair is damp; her eyes are closed; her mouth
is open. Her arms dangle. One hand hangs near a plastic jug of water. The
other rests on a pack of cigarettes. Her legs, limp as noodles, flop open at the
crotch.

"Inhale, outhale," a skinny black man in a dirty white T-shirt chants.
"Inhale, outhale."

"This vomit came from her mouth!" an elderly woman yells, pointing
down a dark hall. Callahan and Cardona keep their eyes trained on their
patient. She does not look good.

Cockroaches walk unabashedly along a dingy orange carpet. One stumbles
into a toddler seated on the floor. Unmolested, it simply adjusts its route.
Another crawls up a speaker tower.

"She been having nosebleeds all day long," the elderly woman reports.

"All *week* long," the gaunt man corrects her. "Her temperature keeps risin' even though we got a fan on her at night."

Quietly, family members enter the room and take discrete positions against paneled walls decorated with honor-roll certificates, public-school diplomas, a crucifix, a horseshoe hung with its ends pointed down, and portraits of Malcom X and Nelson Mandela.

"I can't breathe," the patient sighs, and her eyelids flutter.

Callahan looks to see if she is straining and using her diaphragm muscles to breathe. She's not. *But something's not right*, his radar warns.

Bending on one knee, he wraps his fingers around her wrist and measures her pulse.

"She got meningitis, tuberculosis, and liver cirrhosis," the elderly woman reports.

"Did the doctor tell you that, ma'am?" Cardona asks the patient.

She doesn't respond. But the elderly lady says, "Yes, he did. Doctor told her that two months ago." To make *sure* the partners listen, she adds, "I'm her mother. I know."

Hearing the multiple diagnoses, Callahan wastes no time setting up his portable oxygen tank and strapping a mask on the woman's face. She needs the supplemental oxygen, and he and Cardona need protection from her. Meningitis and TB, potentially fatal maladies, spread through the air if conditions are right. The apartment is dark, humid, crowded, and dirty, ideal breeding conditions for infectious disease. Newark is among the top twenty-five cities with active cases of TB.[1] Both EMTs should be wearing their particulate filter masks, but they don't want to make the patient feel ashamed. Both have the right to be treated prophylactically for meningitis and TB exposure, but they won't seek it. The department tests them for TB every six months anyway, they figure.

By now, both partners are itching to get out of the close, dank apartment. Cardona can practically feel the lethal organisms multiplying around him. But he also sees a half-dozen children in the room. "Did anybody tell you how contagious meningitis and tuberculosis are?" he asks incredulously. "You guys got kids in the house!"

"These are my grandchildren and great-grandchildren. This is my house," the elderly woman explains as she waves her arm behind of her. Ashtrays overflow. Clothes are stacked in piles. "My daughter's got six kids of her own—little babies. She's only visiting."

"Is she HIV-positive?"

"No!"

Callahan gives Cardona a look that says, *This girl is really, really sick*. The woman reminds him of another patient. *One just like her, one who died. She was pregnant with twins. They tried to take the twins at the hospital, but they weren't old enough.* Callahan has a bad feeling.

"You got ALS coming for me?" Cardona radios Dispatch.

"Yeah, MIC 1 is coming out of East Orange."

While Callahan sets up the stair-chair, Cardona continues his interview. The patient is thirty-eight years old. She is not likely to be pregnant. She has no phone. Although she takes medication for hypertension, her blood pressure is 92/38. Her heart is pumping overly fast at 116 beats per minute. The nose-bleeds, her companion now says, have actually gone on for one or two months.

Before they leave, Cardona ventures down the hall to inspect the vomit that the patient's mother keeps talking about. He passes a kitchen ripe with garbage.

Puddles of crimson blood have splattered across the bathroom's black-and-white tile floor. Meatball-sized clots congeal in the shimmering mess.

"She drinks a lot?" Cardona asks. It's not uncommon for cirrhosis patients to vomit clots.

"Yes, she's a heavy drinker," the mother nods. Having just had a hip replacement, she stays behind with her brood but limps to the door with the EMTs as they carry her daughter to the ambulance. "I'm the closest thing to her. I want to know what's going on." Wagging her finger at adults on her stoop, she warns them, "Don't let any kids in the house."

The skinny man comes along for the ride. He brings a sandwich wrapped in paper.

"How many times you vomited blood today?" Cardona asks the woman as they loaded her into the bus.

"Three times," she says, opening her eyes for a moment. They are large, moist, and brown.

"Was the last amount of blood the most?"

"Yes," she answers lethargically.

"Do you have blood in your stool?"

"Yessss," she replies, and drifts into a feverish sleep.

Callahan makes good time and arrives at the hospital before the medics ever catch up. He got the heebie-jeebies during this job. When Cardona peels off his gloves, he shudders and hopes he got nothing else.

SKEL JUICE

Cardona and Callahan hike through several hallways and courtyard apartments before finding their next patient doubled over in a stairwell. The bushy-haired, saffron-tinted, forty-three-year-old woman can't spell her own name. She reeks of alcohol and complains of daylong stomach pains. A bystander suggests that the woman might be pregnant. But when Cardona asks her, she screws up her face with the effort of thinking, and her lip trembles when she admits she does not know. She does not resist when the partners lift her to her feet and guide her through the maze of apartment buildings, hallways, and courtyards where she makes her home. As they wind their way through Escherlike staircases, a team of resident security guards flies through the halls. By the time the EMTs make it to the street, they hear the sharp staccato of gunfire. Pow! Pow! Pow! *It could be a quick dash to the bus,* they think, *but this woman weighs at least three hundred pounds, is unsteady on her feet and increasingly agitated.*

"Don't let them tie me down when we get there," she begs.

"Why would they do that?" Cardona asks, as Callahan looks up and down the block for signs of danger.

"The people at the hospital think I'm craaaaaazy," she whines. Tears spill from her eyes.

"Why would they think that?"

"Because I used my knife to try and stab myself in my heart."

Moments pass with no firefight, so the partners stride to the bus; each has one arm around the woman. As they enter the bus, Cardona offers her a seat on the bench and leans over to buckle her seatbelt. She gives him a menacing wild-eyed stare. *Better keep my distance from this one,* he thinks. Besides, the potent stench of aged urine makes his eyes smart.

The sounds of street battle erupt again. Police cars come screeching from all directions. Dispatch blasts a warning, albeit belated. In the past, Callahan has had to huddle with patients behind cars for protection. He prefers not to tempt fate again and drives off without waiting for Cardona to complete his paperwork in the compulsively neat style that has become his trademark.

The woman denies having any medical problems. She does take "little yellow pills," but she doesn't know what they are for; she can't find them, and she can't remember when she last had them. She doesn't know her Social Security number. Her stomach hurts. She closes her gray, watery eyes, jiggles her knees, bends her head into her lap, and grips her badly scarred shins.

"Honey, you're not bleeding vaginally, are you?" Cardona asks.

"Something's coming out of me. I don't know what it is," the woman cries. Realizing that some peculiar process is under way, she lifts her large hands with their raggedy cuticles to her face and moans, "Oh God, *something's coming out of me!*"

Cardona takes one look at her huge pendulous belly and braces himself for the inevitable exam. Having delivered dozens of babies, he doesn't fear labor and delivery. But he knows how much more complicated the process can be when a woman takes poor care of herself. He breathes an audible sigh of relief when Callahan turns into University's driveway, one second later. By the time he has unbuckled the woman's seat belt and raised her to her unsteady feet, Callahan appears with a wheelchair.

"I got a chair for you and everything," Callahan coaches. When she stands, the odor around her is so pungent that the time-tested EMT almost faints. But he doesn't. "Everything's going to be all right," he coaxes her chivalrously. "Let's go, sweetie."

They're almost home free, but as they pass through the ER corridor the woman's distress is renewed. Several uniformed Newark police officers and undercover cops hang out in the hallway, waiting to speak with crime victims, or for their prisoners to undergo treatment. They lean against the corridor walls, swap jokes, and kill time. But the woman imagines they're laughing at her. She begins to quake and cry. By the time Cardona and Callahan comfort her, transfer her to a nurse, and depart for their next call, they've forgotten to disinfect the bench where the woman sat in urine-and-who-knows-what-else-soaked panties. Later that night, they'll both sit in that seat. So will several patients. And tomorrow day workers will use the same bus. Hopefully, she had no hepatitis, some strains of which can survive in dried blood, urine, and other bodily fluids for days.

Until recently, no self-respecting B-teamer would sit for more than a moment on a patient-care bench without first covering it with a sheet. The vinyl bench is damp and sticky in the summer and as cold and clammy as snakeskin in the winter. The linen is a psychological buffer between their patients' misery and sticky remnants, even though they know it can't shield them from pathogens. It's a comforting touch to those stuck hours on end in the box's cramped quarters. This spring, however, the department forbade workers from using the linens themselves. They have no need for it, an administrator says. There is no sleeping on the job. Their uniforms are sufficient to keep them warm. Without linen, their favorite asset, all illusions evaporate. Cooties are loathsome. Skel juice is worse.

GOLDEN AGE

Cardona zooms across town, sans safety belt, to help care for a man who was robbed, then shot, while visiting friends in a neighborhood senior citizens' club. The bullet entered the man's back and exited under his left armpit. A recent widower, the man weeps, "Please let me die."

"That's up to the doctor," the medic, a per diem, says. "Nobody dies in my bus." The man does not die, but he sure does bleed. Everywhere. Despite the towel-thick pressure bandages, his blood seeps through and drips onto the stretcher, onto the floor. Calmly, the medic asks for a sheet, drapes it over his lap protectively, and searches for a vein to draw blood and start fluids. When they arrive at the ER, Callahan and Cardona pull the patient out of the bus. The medic grabs the clipboard and paperwork with his bloodied gloves and briefs the ER staff, "One shot, close range, upper thoracic. Blood pressure 150 palp, rate 100, strong radial pulses."

The ER has a small, tile-floored room complete with showerheads, hoses, and bottles of powerful disinfectant. Most items contaminated by body fluids land here, where the EMS workers scrub them briskly. They scour stretchers and truck interiors outside. Cardona lends the medics a hand cleaning their truck. But no one catches the blood on the clipboard. Callahan cleans the stretcher. He's pretty thorough, finding a half-dozen bloody streaks concealed on an obscure inner rail. But spots of the viscous fluid do squeak by unnoticed. With any luck, this patient's blood is free of HIV and hepatitis.

Years ago, when infectious-disease transmission was less understood, EMS workers did not wear gloves. In fact, coming back from a job up to one's elbows in blood was a badge of honor. More than one EMS worker at University has hepatitis as a souvenir of the days, including EMD Lorraine Murray, one of the first female blue-shirts on staff. "My hands were *always* cut and nicked from carrying patients," she recalls. "And nine times out of ten, my ass was in the back of the box with the patients."

After Murray was diagnosed, she says she was asked to prove she contracted the disease on the job. A five-foot-three-inch, 127-pound spitfire with hazel eyes, a second-degree black belt in Isshinryu Karate, and a monogamous marriage, Murray replied, "You have to be kidding! How else would I get it?"

"Back then," she says, "nobody thought of suing the hospital. If you contracted something it was just part of the job. All I wanted to do was recover, and I did. I went back on the street, but when I got sick again, a doctor told me I could die. I had small children and a husband. I didn't want to die of hepatitis. I spoke to Judd Fuller; he had just started REMCS, so I went to work for him."

Although she became ill, Murray counts herself fortunate. Emergency workers have sued municipalities for keeping from them evidence that suggests they might have "hepatitis, cardiac arrhythmias, pulmonary abnormalities, hypertension and other conditions."[2]

Today EMS workers are trained, and retrained annually, to reduce the chance of becoming infected. But some patients are walking, talking biohazards. The emotional strain and rapid pace of the job increases human error. And cost-saving measures may be shortsighted. One glove manufacturer at a major EMS trade show claimed she would be thrilled if all of her customers were EMS workers hired by fire departments. "They don't skimp on quality to save money," she says. For exactly that reason, Drivet buys his own gloves. Heber does, too, and he wears two pairs at once. "I'll be damned if I'm going to get some damn disease because of these chintzy pieces of garbage," he vows.

Maniscalco and others believe that the financial pressures on EMS as an extension of the medical system are as inappropriate as having police charge by the bullet and firefighters charge by the bucket.

ODDS ARE . . .

When B-team paramedic Daniel R. Gerard, Sr., became chairman of the NAEMT paramedic division, colleagues flooded him with stories about EMS workers who became sick, injured, or killed in the line of duty. Gerard wondered how his coworkers fared compared with their emergency-response colleagues in law enforcement and firefighting. He was dismayed to learn that national data on EMS workers do not exist. Between one and two million people work and volunteer as EMS workers in the U.S., a NHTSA specialist estimates.

Although the NAEMT worked with Congress to have EMS workers included in the public-safety officer's death benefit, no government agency or professional association tracks EMS worker illness and injuries, much less compares data with their emergency response colleagues.

"The National Fire Academy can tell me, down to a firefighter, how many get killed or injured on the job. The National Institute of Justice can tell me, down to a police officer, how many police get killed or injured in a year. The Federal Bureau of Investigation can even tell me how many police dogs were killed in the line of duty," he says. "But even the National EMS Memorial can only venture rough numbers about EMS workers. They are still getting reports of people to add to the list—people who died in the line of duty two, five, even ten years ago. Why can't anyone tell me what our cost is? We're going into the same situations that police and firefighters are, and some others as well."

Gerard hypothesizes that EMS workers have nearly the same rate of injury as their public-safety colleagues. EMS workers were among those emergency responders who lost their lives during World Trade Center rescue missions in 2001, for example. Not infrequently, they arrive at dangerous scenes and treat and transport patients without police or fire-department assistance. And patients do not always advise EMS workers when they carry infectious disease; some do not even know how sick they are.

At a recent national EMS conference, Ann B. McGowan, an instructor at Texas A&M, rattled off more than twenty distressing diseases EMS workers risk exposure to, from encephalitis and bubonic plague to scarlet fever and rheumatic fever. Blue-shirts do not have the option of refraining from treating contagious patients.[3] To withhold care is to risk being sued for abandonment. The best they can do to guard against contamination is to follow industry guidelines, treat all patients as potentially infectious, and wear gloves, face shields, particulate masks, and occasionally gowns, too. But even those precautions are no guarantee.

NHTSA cites studies that show contaminated-needle sticks occur between six and nineteen times for every thousand ALS responses,[4] which raises the specter of occupational hazards such as HIV and hepatitis. According to another study, fourteen percent of EMS workers have been exposed to hepatitis B— three to five times more than the general population.[5]

The dangers can also be insidious. More than one-third of health-care-worker exposures come from personal belongings most likely tainted on the job, McGowan says. EMS workers, for example, routinely step in blood, spit, phlegm, vomit, urine, feces, mucus, rodent waste, etc., only to later yank their boots off with their hands.

Cautious EMS workers remove their boots and uniforms before entering their own cars. Some bear the expense and inconvenience of having everything laundered outside their homes. Others devise personal protection strategies. For instance, Drivet declines to lend his stethoscope. He purposely buys himself a fancy pen, which discourages him from lending it or chewing on it and unthinkingly ingesting whatever germs it picked up during his EMS travels. He never eats, drinks, or lies down in the back of the box. And he keeps the skin on his hands supple, with a "manly" moisturizing cream, so it won't crack and compromise its function as a natural pathogen barrier.

Still, EMS workers get sick. University's blue-shirts have been treated with courses of noxious medications for job-related TB and HIV exposure. A few have contracted hepatitis. They have broken bones; torn tendons, ligaments, and cartilage; ruptured discs in their back; and suffered surgery. Get them talking about their infirmities and they can wax on for hours; it's amazing they're not all using walkers.[6] In 1999, University EMS workers filed 209 claims, ranging from encounters with acid and broken glass to carpal tunnel syndrome and electric shock.

The department awards blue-shirts between 96 and 112 hours of sick time per year but ties the benefit to its Attendance Abuse Control program. It expects EMS workers to report for duty unless they are seriously ill or injured. If a blue-shirt takes roughly half of the allocated time, he or she can expect "formal counseling," a prelude to discipline. For absences of more than two days, management requires proof of illness from the EMS worker's personal physician. (It also reserves the right to reject any such verification.) Newark police and firefighters, on the other hand, have unlimited sick leave.

* * *

For years, the Department of Labor has surveyed job-related illnesses, injuries, and fatalities using a Bureau of Census Occupational Coding Manual. Among other professions, the manual codes police and firefighters' incidents, so that the consequences of their work can be distilled and examined. It lumps EMS workers, however, with a motley assortment of jobs from artificial-limb fitters and animal technicians to water-pollution specialists and food-service technicians. But surveys beginning in 2003 will use the Office of Management and Budget's Standard Occupational Code Manual, which assigns EMTs and paramedics their own code.[7]

The new government statistics should provide insights, which Gerard hopes the industry will use to improve job safety, worker longevity, and benefits as well as to reduce injuries, sick-time usage, and other costs. For example, EMS workers suffer a preponderance of lifting, moving, and vehicle-collision injuries. It seems that extra training to better help EMS workers protect themselves is in order. "We do preventive maintenance for ambulances," Gerard reasons. "Human resources are even more valuable." But training is costly, so he and his coworkers need facts to help make the case.

But many states do not report incidents involving their public employees to the federal government, so Gerard and his fellow EMS advocates still have much work ahead. He has already begun his research by surveying each state to find out whether and how they collect injury data, if they collate and publish it, and what they do with the information. So far he is unimpressed. New Jersey's Department of Health and Senior Services, for example, tracks only a portion of ambulance crashes—those that occur while EMS workers are transporting patients in vehicles that it specially licenses, a fraction of those operating in New Jersey. All other injuries EMS providers suffer go unaccounted. And if volunteer EMS workers trip and drop a patient down a flight of stairs, the state has no sure way of knowing that the patient was hurt, much less the EMTs, Gerard says.

Gerard hopes to raise awareness of the dangers EMS workers face and help them achieve parity in terms of protective equipment, training, pay, disability provisions, and pensions. That's the only way, he fears, people will feel safe enough to stay on the job and make careers of EMS.

BATTLE SCARS

From rubberneckers and onlookers to idle gossips, people are curious about the EMS workers' worst experiences. They think nothing of prying. Usually they get nothing in return. Blue-shirts have no interest in feeding the outsider's hunger for vicarious gruesome experiences. Most will decline the offer to chat casually about events so scarring as to interfere with their sleep; cause them to self-medicate with drink, drugs, sex, or comfort food; and turn away from family and friends.

Given time, wherever they serve, EMS workers encounter events that forever rock their world. The lives they see cut violently short are too dreadful for polite society's consumption. If they talk at all, it is to each other, and occasionally to their spouses.

One August morning, Cisternino spots a fire about 0400 hours and radios it in. When he gets back to quarters, Piumelli asks him about it. Their brief conversation sparks a ghoulish walk down memory lane. "Remember the Carlton Hotel fire?" Piumelli asks Heber, who instantly nods. "All it was was this fucking garbage fire, but people panicked. This guy leaps off the Carlton, hits me on the helmet, drops at my feet, and breaks every bone in his body. Another one hit the air-conditioner and split right in half. Remember those people hanging from sheets?"

Piumelli is on a roll now, thinking back to other sickening sights. "The worst had to be that guy who offed his wife in bed. He found out she was cheating, stuck a shotgun under her chin, and took her whole head off. Then he blew himself apart. I remember getting there and seeing the cops running out vomiting—there's nothing like seeing a job when a cop pukes his brains out. Her scalp was stuck to the wall. I can still see her hair rollers in it."

"What do you think the last thing to go through her mind was?" Cisternino asks with a small smirk and a big twinkle in his eye. Piumelli just waits patiently for him to spill. "Her nose." Cisternino earns some chuckles as well as a groan or two. Piumelli and Heber have their arms folded behind their heads and their feet up on chairs. They lean back against headquarters' leprous blue walls, which peel with paint.

"Remember that guy they threw out of a car? They stabbed him, they shot him, and then they lit him on fire?" Heber asks. "I doused him with an extinguisher but he reignited. His body rekindled." B-teamers between calls drift in and out of their nostalgic exchange, lazing around an old conference table; it replaced the picnic table, which took too much abuse and finally crapped out. The thick cigarette smoke does not deter Newark's ambitious mosquitoes, which find plenty of meat.

"There are some people it's best not to fuck with," Heber says somberly. "They like to de-head you and put your body in one place and your head in another."

"Oh, yeah," Piumelli responds. "Remember those people hacked up with machetes, their blood on the ceiling?"

By this point they're both laughing.

"Remember the Night of the Living Dead?" Heber asks. "Back in the late 1980s, this man got electrocuted at like five A.M. up in the north. We had BLS, ALS, Rescue, and a supervisor go, but we couldn't find any body.

"Some citizen told us, 'He's on the railroad tracks.' So we looked. He had jumped over the fence and it was like a forty- to fifty-foot drop. But as he fell, he hit the catenary lines. The wires broke the fall and electrocuted him, but he was not dead.

"He starts walking up this abandoned staircase, eighty percent covered with third-degree burns. Opperman jumps over the fence to help the guy. We're using our hydraulics to cut the gate's steel-plated hinges off so we can get in. Opperman tries to get the guy to lie down, but he just continued walking up toward us like Frankenstein.

"We're trying to cut through the fence when we see this smoke coming out of his mouth. His skin is peeling; he has red bleeding wounds under charred tissue. He's a black man but his skin is burned white. He tries talking, but only moans come out, and smoke.

"And when you get burned like that, you do nerve damage and skin damage so your body swells. His arms were up like a robot, like the living dead." Heber pauses a minute, reflecting. He shakes his head as if *he* doesn't believe his own stories.

Opperman recalls that event, too—every detail, from the man's smoking dreadlocks to his plaintive cries for help. Thieves often sneaked into the area, trying to steal copper to resell at recycling plants for quick cash, he explains. He imagines the man took a tumble during just such a caper. "Instead he got fried really good," Opperman says. "I swear to Christ, it scared the shit out of me. I wanted to run back over the fence." But he didn't. He did his job. He treated his patient, and now he bears the scar.

"Remember that guy stabbed twenty-four times?" Heber asks, dredging up another memory. "Musta been a mob hit."

"Yeah, I remember," Piumelli says. "They took a razor and sliced him every two inches—just superficial slices so he'd die in pain. They poured salt in the cuts."

All this and Heber swears the only thing getting to him after nineteen years on the job is the night shifts. He realized it was time to get off the BLS truck when he saw a rat nibbling from a pan full of grease on a patient's stove. Disgust must have showed on his wholesome, freckled face, because he remembers that one of the family members said, "He's got to eat, too." EMD Lorraine Murray had a similar experience. Her patient told her it was better to feed the rats than risk getting bit.

Another apartment Heber visited was full of naked females; it wasn't a brothel, it was just how the mother and her daughters lived—watching television, cooking, and wandering about. The very last straw for him was watching a twelve-year-old girl give birth. "You are trying to tell me that you did not know she was pregnant?" he remembers asking the child's family. "All the people in the apartment were like, 'This is great!'" Heber has three children at home, two of them daughters. After a while, he just couldn't fathom or tolerate some of the lifestyles he encountered. *You fucking people need to jump out the window, all of you.*

"That's why I don't miss BLS," Heber says. "I've seen it. I've heard it." Although Rescue may be more gruesome, to him it's less insane. Sometimes floating between such calls can leave EMS workers feeling that they are driving through one enormous, open-air asylum.

SAY "CHEESE!"

Some EMS workers keep photos of odd and incredible scenes. They are religious about protecting the images and do exploit the celluloid horrors for gain. Used primarily for teaching purposes, the photos bear witness to the carnage that is their daily bread. One underground scrapbook has a snapshot of a human head so twisted and crushed that it seems more like a meatball with hair, teeth, and eyes. In the shot, the head sits on some train tracks, severed from a torso equally warped and distorted by the unstoppable mass and velocity of the train that destroyed it.

Field supervisor Victor Mendez carries a photo in his briefcase, whipping it out at the end of a story as proof of his experience. Supervisors at University retain their EMS certifications. When the field is hopping they pitch in, too. Dispatch needed someone to go to "a possible miscarriage" one afternoon, but there were no blue-shirts to send. Mendez, a much admired and decorated veteran, volunteered. When he arrived at the patient's apartment, her mate answered the door and pointed to the bathroom. There he found a woman squatting over the toilet. She was weak, sweating, and exhausted.

Mendez helped stand her up so he could walk her to the bedroom, where she could rest until an ambulance arrived. When she got on her feet, he looked in the toilet. A bowl of blood and fecal matter stared back. As he led her down the hall, a wail came from the bathroom, which instantly froze him. Mendez handed the woman off to her mate and sprinted back to the bathroom. He rolled up his sleeves, tugged on some gloves, and dug into the mess. He didn't have time to feel sickened. Deep in the foul soup, he felt a baby and lifted it out.

As soon as he saw the child's face, however, something yanked it from his hands back into the toilet bowl.

Mendez tried again, and the same thing happened. He couldn't call for help on his radio, though, because both hands were now polluted. He tried a third time, carefully running his hands through the opaque, bloody broth and along the bottom of the bowl. His breath caught when each hand felt a head. *They must be twins*, he thought.

Holding both heads in his hands, Mendez brought them up though the filthy stew to see a baby's face and a blank sphere of flesh the size and shape of another head attached to it. Stunned, he didn't know what to make of it. When the head with the face announced it was here to stay with a high-pitched scream, it reminded him to pull and twist until he had the whole infant out, and its blank, bulbous sphere, too.

When an ambulance finally arrived, the crew whisked the odd newborn and mother to the hospital. There, pediatricians explained the faceless head as a growth, which they punctured, drained, and surgically removed. The baby lived. Mendez keeps the photo as a memento.

CROSSING OVER

Cortacans has had the spirit-crushing experience of finding a palm-sized baby wrapped in a towel inside a patient's apartment. "The mother was doing hard drugs every day," he says of the crack-cocaine addict who delivered at twenty-one weeks. (It usually takes forty weeks for a fetus to reach full term.) "Its eyes weren't even fully developed," he recalls incredulously, "just mucous membranes."

The baby's heart rate was fifty, compared with an average newborn's heart rate of about 160. So Cortacans began CPR and called for paramedics. Vincent Cisternino and Danny Gerard responded. Using their smallest laryngoscope blade and shaving the endotracheal tube even thinner, they managed to intubate the infant and get it to the hospital alive. It takes the best that medical science has to give a one-pound infant a chance at survival. This baby weighed less than one pound. Doctors pronounced it dead while its heart was still beating.

Their nights are filled with the grisly, the weird, and the unbearably sad.

Deaths from drugs and gangs and other illicit activities do not bother the team much. As Cardona says, "They're in the game."

One incident that haunts Fazio was the time she was called to an elderly couple's home to find them sprawled face-to-face on the living-room floor, bleeding out. "The man had ten stabs, four in his abdomen, two in his chest," Fazio recalls. "Their arms were sliced with defensive wounds." The man's wife had also been cut to shreds. "The wife wouldn't let us touch her until she told the cops who did it," Fazio recalls. "She said her niece and the niece's boyfriend attacked them for twenty-three dollars and car keys."

Fazio also pronounced a woman she found disemboweled. It wasn't the blood all over the floor or the entrails that struck her as much as the face of the dead woman's seven-year-old daughter. The little girl's blank and lifeless eyes had the same thousand-yard stare of battle-hardened combat veterans. "I can still see the cop trying to carry the daughter out of the room without slipping in all the blood."

EMS workers do not see death as a gentle good night. Drivet says, "The death process can actually be very painful. It's not just like the movies. They seize. They get expressions of panic." About ten years ago, Drivet treated a railway worker who got caught between two train cars as they coupled. Although the man suffered a mortal injury, his death was not instantaneous. "Don't let me die," he begged Drivet. "Don't let me die." The man's coworkers were trying to reach his wife, but the man had minutes before his organs began failing from the crush injuries. Officials decided to pull the trains apart. The man "was conscious one minute, dead the next," Drivet recalls. "All his blood just literally poured out of his body. We just laid his body on the backboard . . . all of his intestinal tract and abdominal organs fell out.

"That was one of the few times they brought the Critical Incident Stress Debriefing people in. When we told them the story, they cried and said, 'Oh my God, that's terrible!'

" 'Why are these people here?' I asked my partner."

THIN SKIN

It's not always untimely or violent death that can make the work so disturbing; it's knowing what patients endure. One night Fazio tries treating a man with diffuse scleroderma, an autoimmune illness that mummifies people while they are alive. The man's skin is so stiff that she can't get a pulse. She can't give him an IV, either, because his veins are too tough. *He's going to drown*, she thinks. *His epiglottis will harden and he won't be able to swallow and he'll drown on his own secretions.*

Cardona still hears the screams of violent mental patients he transported to a hospital for the criminally insane at a previous EMS job. The building was stashed deep inside a heavily landscaped, bucolic campus. All pretenses stopped at the front door. "As you go up in the elevator the screams are so terrible, they are unreal. They stay in your head forever," he says with a shudder and a vacant look in his eye. "You can't go in there with a stethoscope around your neck; you can't have a pen in your pocket. They make four or six police officers go with you.

"Those patients are permanently committed. They're not going anywhere ever again. They live out their lives in four-point restraints; twenty-four hours a day they're fastened on beds, mattresses really, that are almost flush with the floor," Cardona explains. "They live in cells that look like cages in a zoo. The windows are just one little slit. It's the same on the doors.

"I used to read the commitment papers on the way out there. They sedated the patients to the point of unconsciousness. Half the meds in that place aren't even in the book," he says ominously. "I've tried looking it up."

Child victims, all agree, are the most distressing. EMT Joe Grassi found a dead newborn, still attached to its umbilical cord, inside its mother's pajama bottoms. She lay in bed watching TV throughout her labor and estimated the time of birth for him as "somewhere between *The Honeymooners* and *Seinfeld*."

Something is really wrong here, too, he remembers thinking as a shiver rippled across his body. He sensed an oddity but couldn't pinpoint it. Police, Division of Youth and Family Services, and other authorities were called in on that job. He later learned that the patient and everyone in the household, from youngsters to young adults, were all born of incest.

Vince Callahan still gets chilled when he thinks of the two boys whose unsupervised play ended with them mangled and twisted inseparably inside elevator-shaft machinery.

Normally mild-mannered, even Callahan loses it occasionally. "*Get the baby, you idiot!*" he screamed one evening from inside his bus as he spotted a toddler stumble into the traffic a block away. The idiot, a woman, couldn't hear him because his windows were up. Fortunately, she turned around and casually scooped up the youngster. Callahan wiped sweat from his brow, pent up from wondering what to do next—honk, jump out of the bus, or what.

Just the other night, Callahan and Cardona responded to a "sleep in the street" to find an exhausted thirteen-year-old boy who had run away from home and been selling himself as a prostitute.

The other night Callahan brought a three-month-old girl to the hospital. She was so badly burned that the skin from her belly to her toes was falling off. "She was in agony; she was in so much pain," he recalls. "We put some nice, sterile, dry dressings on her and gave her some blow-by oxygen"—EMS workers don't always put masks on struggling infants' faces. "That baby grabbed my hand and went right to sleep."

The father blamed his seven-year-old son, but the story didn't ring true with Callahan. The baby's suffering and the father's behavior depressed him to the point that momentarily he questioned life itself. He questioned the job, too. When he returned to quarters he found an empty bathroom stall and cried. "I know we come out tough and bold like it does not bother us, but I'm not too proud to say I break down like a kid."

"Seeing these kids makes you live your life fuller," Callahan says soberly. He tries never to leave his home angry. Cardona says he kisses and hugs his children even when they are asleep. Piumelli tells his wife and young sons to be careful every time they walk out the door. Everyone who stays on the job finds ways to cope: some are healthful; some are not. Those who can't, quit. Several on the team have seen new people walk off the job the same day that they start. One had his car stolen. One was mugged. One witnessed the carnage of a high-speed multi-car collision.

Brutal jobs live crouched in the back of the blue-shirts' minds, sometimes stoking post-traumatic stress disorder (PTSD), which NHTSA says affects emergency workers at least twice as much as the general population.[8] When Piumelli began working in Newark, twenty years ago, PTSD did exist, but mental-health professionals attributed the condition primarily to war-zone vets. Now the department attempts to fashion a constructive relief valve by importing EMS workers trained in psychological debriefing. Research is inconclusive, however, as to whether it works.

For years, EMS workers were left to fend for themselves. "Have a drink and get the fuck back to work," Piumelli laughs at the tactic old-timers used before there was a recognized need for debriefing. Back then, hard drinking helped hard living, even if that meant coming to work blind drunk. (Among themselves, some who outgrew the practice still look back on it as a hoot instead of a gross dereliction.)

A few EMS workers with great longevity remember gambling away their paychecks playing cards or sending someone to place bets at the track. Sometimes, they say, EMS workers were tempted to use drugs, which they "found" on patients. At least one used drugs secreted from the narcotics kits. And, some admit, there was a time when snorting cocaine in the bathroom was de rigueur.

The American Psychiatric Association now defines PTSD as a debilitating state that can affect "people who have survived earthquakes, airplane crashes, terrorist bombings, inner-city violence, domestic abuse, rape, war, genocide and other disasters both natural and man-made." The nature of the job injects EMS workers into all of these scenes regularly. And in dense population centers they parachute into such crises all the time. Naturally, it can get to be too much. Even the most powerful mind-body connection can't repress all the symptoms and co-morbid problems: Depression. Substance abuse. Nightmares. Insomnia. Dizziness. Headaches. Stomach aches. Chest pain. Emotional numbness. Irritability.

For years, O'Neill thought he could handle the job's pressures because he grew up as a tough Jersey City kid and survived a severe Catholic school. However hardboiled, O'Neill could not assimilate the sights, the sounds, and the inevitable losses without getting a bad case of PTSD, which he neither advertises nor hides. "The winter of 1989 was bad. It seemed like every time we came on duty, three or four kids would die in a fire," he remembers. "Eventually, I fucking snapped."

At the time he was in paramedic school, completing a clinical rotation in the hospital's neurological intensive-care unit, a place others call "Heads in Beds" and he calls "the Cabbage Patch" or "the Ventilator Farm."

"I was just coming off a stretch. I wasn't sleeping. I wasn't eating. I had 'an event.' Something short-circuited. I just froze in place. I couldn't tell you where I was, or how the fuck I got there or why I was wearing a scowl. I stared at the wall for hours. Someone found me and said, 'You look like you're in rough shape.' Next thing I knew I was in the Employee Assistance Program, whose advice for a long happy life was intense therapy.

"After only three visits, EAP referred me to some 'practitioner' who worked out of the basement in his house. I didn't take time off work. I didn't want the 'psycho' stamp. Then I hurt my back on the job and found some relief by washing my Flexaril [a muscle relaxant] down with Coors Light."

O'Neill had seen at least one colleague claim PTSD and manipulate management into doling out some cushy perks. Presuming they could not afford to treat everyone this way, and worried they would use a similar time-off request as an excuse to get rid of him, O'Neill found another way to cope. "I figured I had to pull myself up by my bootstraps or get myself a new line of work. To prevent nightmares, I would self-medicate because the anesthetized brain doesn't dream. That worked for about five years." He had plenty of company. The team often went drinking after work. The high-spirited group also took trips to amusement parks, helped organize educational symposiums, and participated in ambulance rodeos.

O'Neill met his wife, a former EMT, at a backyard barbecue. She and Drivet saved his life, he says. Quietly, consistently, and discreetly they coached him to get help. Drivet helped O'Neill check himself into a rehabilitation center, where he spent twenty-one days in recovery. He has now been sober for more than seven years. He knows the day and hour of his last drink. He sincerely regrets the pain he caused others, the years that he wasted, and the debt he accumulated. But O'Neill has moved on, corralled his demons, and found more constructive ways to channel on-the-job stress. And he keeps an eye out for hard drinkers who might be getting themselves into trouble, unwittingly.

Several others have been detoxed and dried out, too. Some never went the way of drugs and alcohol but fell headlong into agonizing depressions. "I never picked up the drinking, nicotine, or caffeine habit," one confesses, "but every time I'd go to sleep, I'd have weird dreams—nightmares. I'd wake up screaming."

He'd see himself caring for one patient and finding another bleeding out near the hospital. While struggling to treat both of them, he'd see a cop get shot. He'd race into the ER yelling "Gotta Go! Gotta Go!," rushing to transfer his patients so he could return for the officer. But no matter how hard he tried, he couldn't rescue them all.

"Somewhere in my head a voice kept telling me to calm down, but it was no use." Overwhelmed, he'd wake up half-frozen, soaked in his own sweat. "Oh man, I'll *never* forget that dream," he says morosely.

The depression also caused a type of paralysis. He says he had to drag himself to work on many occasions, fighting the fear of having to do CPR on a child, the disgust of getting drenched in the spittle of drunks, and the revulsion of getting soaked with someone's "piss."

He visited with a psychiatrist but says, "I pretty much had to work it out myself." That is common among the troops. Many feel alone or that no one understands. A good number are convinced that no one would believe their stories if they ever decided to spill.

As time passed, so did this EMS worker's despair. But some have not been able to cope. Some held on longer than they should have, only to take their own lives. At least one committed suicide.

"We're so emotionally damaged from the shit that we see all day, we're a psychiatrist's wet dream," one surmises.

There is always an exception to the rule and Billy "the Squirrel" Heber is it. At forty-four, Billy Heber is the team grown-up; not the team father, not the team boss—just an elder who has learned how to work EMS in Newark and live a good life. Married to his high-school sweetheart, Heber makes his family his priority. He and his wife, an ER nurse who works part time, have a comfortable house two counties away with an emerald tree canopy bedecked with bird feeders and terraced gardens they built themselves. A hand-hewn staircase leads down to a shimmering, bass-filled lake and small private beach (he hauled the sand himself). "When I go home I open the garage, walk right out onto the deck, and overlook the lake. Sometimes, I'll even go fish for a little while still in uniform. It's so quiet up there. All I have to deal with is the bears and the snakes.

"I have great stress relievers," he adds. Besides his passion for fishing, he belongs to a model railroad club and enjoys "playing on the computer," and when spring first thaws the lake, he is outside working on his vegetable garden. A proud father of three, Heber cheers his kids at their athletic events and marching-band practices, too.

Bill Heber is an exception. "I haven't gotten hurt on the job. I haven't called out sick in over a year," he says. "I have over fifteen hundred hour's sick time banked." Although some of his robust health may come from good genes, it must also be due to his principles and philosophy. "The job is a commitment and you should keep it," he says. "My concern is for me to survive here and go home and relax." He works one job, carefully budgets his earnings, and sleeps well.

DARK HUMOR

A man falls sixteen floors onto concrete. The medic relays the information by radio. The ER doc asks, "What is your ETA?"

"My ETA to what, lunch?"

"You're not bringing him to the trauma center?"

"With what, a shovel?"

—A CONVERSATION TWO B-TEAMERS SAY THEY HAD AT WORK

On Christmas, BLS trucks worked more than twenty jobs a shift. One job involved a man who hanged himself outside in brittle cold. During one rare moment of downtime, someone brought up the half-frozen suicide victim, asking, "If ya had beat him with a stick, do ya think maybe candy would have fallen out?"

Like their hospital-based colleagues, B-teamers can tell sick jokes and laugh at them. In the confines of their work, they don't have to explain that their humor is not meant to be mean-spirited or disrespectful. It's just a device to trigger emotion. When they laugh, they breathe. And tears roll down their faces. And for a moment everything is all right with the world.

A man is shot in the thigh one summer morning around 0500 hours in a neighborhood known for drug trafficking. BLS is on scene shortly; it takes Cisternino and Fazio a few minutes longer. Cardona packages the patient. When the ALS truck arrives, they pop him inside and try resuscitation. Cardona cuts off the man's pant leg in search of wounds to patch; liters of blood splash onto the floor. Gunshots clipped the patient's femoral artery, and he has bled out entirely. There is no blood left in his veins, and therefore no way to start an IV. Fazio checks the skin inside the pouches under his eyes and his nail beds, too.

They are both ghostly pale, a sign that even his capillaries have drained. Cisternino does his best to start an IV in the man's jugular, but it's no use. "Attention Kmart shoppers, we're out of blood in Aisle Three."

Occasionally, circumstances, though tragic, throw the human condition into such stark relief, humor is an automatic relief valve. What are EMS workers to think when they find someone dead on the toilet from having strained too hard?

Sometimes, humor and creativity join by way of song. To the tune of "Kumbaya," a few blue-shirts crafted their own verses: "Someone's seizing, Lord, send MIC 3. Someone's dying, Lord, send MIC 3." They have rewritten "The Twelve Days of Christmas," too. The chorus merrily repeats the city's twelve most diseased and dangerous addresses, places the B-team won't otherwise even whisper lest the capricious Gods of EMS get angry and send them there.

"Anyone tells you they're not superstitious?" Fazio says skeptically. "They haven't been doing this long enough." Some of her iron-clad rules include: never compliment a medic on his or her IV skills; never get out of the bus between jobs; never open the pediatric kit or make a dead baby joke. "If you do, you are knocking on the web of fate. 'Hello? We haven't seen a dead baby in a while.'

"Never say, 'Wouldn't it be funny if this was a fill-in-the-blank?' Because it *will* happen and it *won't* be funny. And never, ever say the 'q' word [quiet], because mayhem and bedlam will ensue."

Black humor is also a talisman. "You look for excuses to explain why the patient died or got sick so you can say, 'Yeah, they deserved it,' because it distances you," says George Daniels, the B team's longest-serving member. "We saw one guy get creamed on a highway, and then we saw he was dressed in black.

"See?" Daniels asks. "He deserved it!

"It's hard to deal with someone's death," he explains more soberly. "We don't want to feel that grief. We don't want to believe that what happened to them could happen to us. We don't want to get sucked into that misery. It's not very pleasant. If you don't get it out of your system, you eat, drink, and take drugs."

Commedienne Joan Rivers brings a broader social perspective: "Better to let people who work in these dark professions blow their off-color steam occasionally, than to force them to suppress it, and exacerbate the crippling post-traumatic stress syndrome that so many already battle as a result of the work they do.

"The most awful jokes cracked about the most sacred things give people a chance to laugh riotously, and the line between laughter and tears is blurred. It may sound scandalous, but it's a valid excuse to roar. Dark humor is a powerful, immediate, and essentially harmless tool that knocks the stuffing out of the world's absurd cruelties, if only for a few seconds—time enough to pull oneself together and head out to the next crisis."

Only by witnessing the breakneck pace and torrent of tragedies can outsiders begin to appreciate the experienced EMS workers' sometimes cynical perspective. "Something happens and I say 'it's very bad,'" Drivet explains. "Everyone else says, 'No, it's a catastrophe.' I say '*No*, it's bad on a sliding scale,' because we have seen so much terror, panic, and pain."

12   DAWN

*W*hen spring rolls around the following year, at shift's end one morning, what's left of the B team wrings chart-writers' cramps from their hands and adds pale blue clouds from their cigarettes to a glorious sunrise nestled inside a chiffon confection of pink and peach haze.

The picnic table has long since splintered and been carted away. Members sit on office furniture rejects or on bus bumpers, or lean against the building. There has been talk of creating "a smoking area," but that has yet to come to fruition.

Billy "the Squirrel" Heber has done more than seed his country garden with vegetables; he has abandoned the B team in favor of a day shift. It has taken two months for the man who worked the graveyard shift twenty years to reset his internal clock. He loves it, but says, "I miss Geno."

Five more years and Heber will have the twenty-five years' service required for early retirement—but he'll have to work ten to win his full pension. He is putting his credentials in order and planning for a second career in state or county emergency management.

Eugene "Geno" O'Neill is busy breaking in his new partner, rescue specialist Joe "Lee Harvey" Grassi. (His nickname is an irreverent homage to his ability to get the job done despite having often been paired with do-nothing, undirected partners.) O'Neill is unhappy about the nine pounds he's gained, although he still cuts a dashing and muscular figure. "All the kid wants to do is eat," O'Neill grumbles about Grassi. "It's either that or I'm eating out of depression. I miss Billy." That's something he never thought he would say.

"Emotionally, I am actually reaching the terminus of my life in the field," O'Neill admits. "I can do more for EMS as an educator, or maybe even as a psychologist, than I can as a provider." To that end, O'Neill has created a niche for himself as lead instructor for domestic preparedness and hazardous-materials mitigation. He has raised awareness of on-the-job-dangers to the point that all staff get some training in dealing with dangerous substances, including weapons of mass destruction. And, on behalf of an administrator he meets with the state police for all matters regarding terrorism.

If the department does not promote him, sooner or later he will move on. He wants to finish his degree, earn more, and deepen his expertise. He may pursue emergency management, take a position preparing the country to deal with terrorism and its medical consequences, or explore psychology and help other EMS workers adjust to the profession's great strains.

Vincent Callahan and Benny Cardona are still riding BLS. Benny Cardona wants to stay in Newark and have a career where he feels useful, challenged, and able to earn enough to indulge his young sons. With his criminal-justice education and his security background, he believes that becoming a Newark police officer would be a dream come true. It might, but Cardona has a real talent for treating patients on the town's tough streets. Fazio and Cisternino have been rooting for him to become a paramedic. Either way, his commitment to the people of Newark shows. He takes a leadership role in the Hispanic Fire and EMS Association and organizes a candlelight vigil for Newark police officers, firefighters, and EMS workers who have lost their lives in the line of duty.

Callahan wants to stay in EMS but worries that that may be too selfish. He feels pressure to earn more for his family. He can't switch over to EMS in Maryland, where he lives, without losing seniority. But he's dog-tired of traveling several states every week. When separated from the son it took fifteen years to have, he misses the little boy badly. He doesn't want to call the child on the phone ten times a day. He wants to be there for school plays and basketball practice. Although Callahan leans toward the Muslim faith, his wife and son are still practicing Baptists. Either way, the family is God-fearing and observant. "It kills me," he says, "the church deacons think he has no father."

A relative has been tempting him with talk about careers in network administration. If he leaves EMS, it will be a great loss to the people of Newark. But he wants his son to have all the advantages, including a college education, which is hard to save for on take-home pay of $370 per week.

Callahan's sincere commitment to community and his passion for helping young people distinguish him. He would make an exemplary teacher or principal, which might allow him the home life he dreams of as well as the chance to do meaningful work without aggravating his asthma or his many knee and back injuries.

Vincent Francis "Fester" Cisternino works with the B team only occasionally. He graduates from college with a hard-earned B.A. in Psychology and East Asian studies but finds himself busier at the end of his final undergraduate semester than perhaps ever before. He has won one of the coveted spots on NorthSTAR and has taken on its challenging curriculum, too. "It never was the speed, lights, or sirens that attracted me to EMS; it's the challenge," Cisternino explains. "Give me the patient with little or no chance of survival, their illnesses or injuries are so catastrophic, they're not expected to survive. Give me that patient. That's what really pumps my adrenaline. It's dealing with the worst of the worst."

NorthSTAR's patients are more taxing, but the perpetual student is already studying so he can challenge the nursing boards. He had added a strand of nursing-related courses during his studies, and although it afforded him knowledge, he got a disturbing glimpse into the profession. "You know what they call a cut? A cut is not a laceration anymore. It's a 'temporary interruption in skin integrity,' " he told Drivet one night when they were working together.

"Get out of here!" Drivet said, staring at him suspiciously from the corner of his eye.

"And when someone is choking, they call it 'ineffective airway clearance secondary to increased mucus product.' "

"That is so unsat!"

It is unsat, but it pays more. And Cisternino has plans for graduate school. He's already completing applications. He hopes to become a physician's assistant, a forensic psychologist, or perhaps even a health-care attorney.

Tracey "Ma Barker" Fazio is missing, as well. She married a fellow paramedic; bought a home with two wooded acres in the gentle hills of Pennsylvania; adopted a wildly affectionate mutt with Rottweiler, pit bull, and Australian cattle dog in his blood; and bore her first child, a son. Having worked her way up from an online fantasy game player to senior game master, her native creativity is beginning to pay off, literally. But it does not promise financial salvation. Fazio will return to University when her maternity leave expires, but she also plans to challenge the nursing exam, become an R.N., and work in a Pennsylvania hospital. "If I'm gonna be abused, I might as well do it for two times the pay." Her days as a paramedic are numbered.

Walter "the Commander" Drivet makes it to the very final stage of the NorthSTAR competition but does not get one of the slots. His many admirers are devastated; they grumble and mumble about departmental politics, although

Drivet keeps dignity and his head high. He harnesses the deep disappointment and uses it as motivation to get on with his life. He accepts a full-time offer from another busy urban hospital and shifts to part-time at University. Within months he resigns altogether. His new employer awards him a significant pay increase and ample, paid time off to serve his county and country.

He continues as Union County Commander of Tactical EMS Support for Emergency Response/SWAT. He oversees much of the ski resort's rescue operations. And, increasingly, he teaches for the Casualty Care Research Center, a division of the Department of Defense's Uniformed University of the Health Sciences. Given his choice, Drivet would be "fast-roping out of helicopters and killing terrorists," but he'd gladly settle for full-time work supporting federal law-enforcement agencies on their various missions, a long-sought goal he may well yet achieve.

Tommy Opperman takes a few months off so he and his wife can welcome their second daughter into the world. He spends the summer playing with his children, building a deck off the back of his hilltop home, and romping with Seamus, his dog. The fresh air and simple life do him good. "This is the first summer in memory," he says, that he's not been shot at or "had some asshole beat the crap out of me."

After a nineteen-year track record working BLS, Rescue, and ALS, the thirty-eight-year-old has experience, knowledge, and an exceptional ability to explain complex physiology and pharmacology. But management has blocked his ambition to mentor new medics even though his University coworkers elected him Paramedic of the Year in 2000, and his colleagues at the rural medical center where he holds his second job voted him Paramedic of the Year in 2001. Not easily intimidated, Opperman feels comfortable speaking his mind. Some coworkers have nicknamed him "the conscience of the place" because he stands up to management when he feels it is necessary. Others call him "Captain Misery."

A future in EMS is important to the decorated veteran, who worries that when he returns to work management will weigh his characteristic forthrightness more heavily than his many contributions and deny him the opportunity to become a supervisor. "I love being a paramedic, and it kills me that I can't finish out my career," Opperman worries. "I've got a heart condition, hepatitis, a bad back, shitty wrists, and a fucking attitude." He also has at least seventeen more years on the job before he can collect his pension.

Henry "Scrappy" Cortacans gets engaged. With a wedding to pay for and a new home to buy, Cortacans cannot resist another employer's offer to double his salary. He resigns from his full-time job at University to become aquatics director for a growing concern. But he continues to work at University as a per-diem medic and Webmaster.

Cortacans didn't make the move to the private sector purely for money. He endured skepticism, criticism, and insufficient resources while crafting a place for the department on the Web. He hoped next to develop some Web-based training, making it easier and less costly for blue-shirts to obtain the continual education they need to maintain their certifications. But, he reports, management said it could not afford to pay him for his effort, nor would it sanction any efforts on his part to obtain grant moneys.

EMT Che-heibe Scott resigns, too. He finds better hours, a larger salary, and a career track working with The Sharing Network, a company whose business is organ donation.

EMT Juan Ortiz leaves the Dispatch Center to return to the streets. This time, he practices EMS in University's Camden division. A bilingual EMS veteran with seventeen years' experience on the ground and on the mike, he also angles for a supervisor's position.

William "Buzz" Busby still calms distraught callers and overtaxed caregivers with his compassion-rich caramel tones.

"It's light outside," one B-teamer notes. "We can now go into our coffins." Two, who have been staging a sword fight with a garbage picker and a broom handle, put down their makeshift sabers and prepare to swipe out. Day-team blue-shirts trudge in, rubbing sleep from their eyes and slurping coffee from portable mugs. Barbed wire and broken glass reflect the morning light.

"Hello, day-pukes," a B-teamer shouts, and raises his hands in greeting. The day-pukes wave back wordlessly. One smirks and flips them the bird.

13   *SEE YA AT THE BIG ONE*

RISE AND SHINE

At 0700 hours on September 11, 2001, former partners Gene O'Neill and Billy Heber spend a few minutes catching up with each other inside the Rescue office. Then, with sun glare in his eyes and a cigarette in his mouth, O'Neill heads home to take care of his children so that his wife, a state police dispatcher and former EMT, can get to work. Heber and his new partner drive the Rescue truck to a garage about twenty miles away for repairs.

At home, O'Neill showers, prepares breakfast, and sees his daughter off to school before dressing his three-year-old son and driving him to day care. Having had only had four hours' sleep over the past forty-eight hours, he can hear the bedsheets calling.

About 0850 hours, Heber and his partner sit outside the garage while a mechanic works on their truck. Heber, an outdoorsman, and his new partner, an artist who loves to hike, admire the cloudless sky, which is almost painfully blue. They are inhaling the first crisp scents of fall when another mechanic approaches and asks if they heard about the plane crashing into the World Trade Center's North Tower.

A practiced skeptic, Heber's first reaction is: *Bullshit*. But the thought passes when he reads the mechanic's strained face. He asks for details, but the mechanic doesn't have much more to tell him other than that one of the towers is aflame. Shocked, Heber does not immediately hark back to the 1993 terrorist attack, when management summoned him from his day off and arranged for him to hitch a ride to Manhattan with an ambulance and take over operations based from the mass-casualty response unit (MCRU). He and his coworkers spent fifteen hours supporting WTC rescue operations there.

A history buff, he first thinks of the summer day in 1945 when a B-25 bomber crashed into the Empire State Building. *But that can't be*, he reasons. *It sits in one of the most restricted airspaces in the country*. And he is certain the landmark is covered by radar. Heber and his partner search out a TV in the waiting room, where a crowd is already gathering.

This can't be a mistake, he ponders. Then he sees the footage of the first crash and watches, dumbfounded, as a jet crashes through the South Tower, too. *It has to be a terrorist act*. Memories of 1993 kick in. Momentarily, all he can think of is "the hole," an image so raw and powerful in his mind that he still likens it to a volcanic crater. Since then, cadres of University's EMS workers have taken Department of Defense courses and other specialized training to help address terrorist attacks. Heber phones headquarters and asks whether the EMS Department is mobilized to respond.

A manager tells Heber that New York City officials have not yet asked for help, but University anticipates the request and preparations are under way. After working the 1993 WTC rescue operations together, Drivet and Maniscalco agreed that New York and New Jersey would benefit from a predetermined agreement that assured each state's commitment to rapidly deploy assets should the other experience an overwhelming event. Working with state police and other emergency-management officials, they roughed out procedures, which later became a formal memorandum of understanding. University EMS was designated the frontline contact for New Jersey's EMS assets.

Heber predicts that the MCRU will be indispensable. He and another EMT designed the one-of-a-kind vehicle in the mid-eighties after researching what other large cities had available or wished they did. The white MCRU, shaped like an old bread-delivery truck, is twenty feet long and eight feet wide. Albeit unglamorous, it is as potent a tool as a dusty bottle that washes ashore replete with a genie. It brims with almost anything an EMS worker could want. Besides having deployed it at the 1993 WTC attacks, blue-shirts have used it to treat patients at such calamities as a chemical dump fire, a chemical-factory fire, and plane crashes. During one storm, which killed a nursing home's power supply, blue-shirts used the MCRU to supply oxygen to respirator-dependent patients. One of the truck's most ingenious features is an oxygen manifold that

Heber developed, which enables the truck to oxygenate fifty-six patients simultaneously. (Many ERs can't match that.)

The manager makes arrangements to retrieve the MCRU, which is at another off-campus garage being serviced. Heber and his partner jump in the Rescue truck and race the eighteen miles back to quarters. As they get closer to the complex, through their windshield they watch the Twin Towers burn. They and other blue-shirts en route to Newark notice that hundreds of drivers throughout the area are pulling off the roads to stare at the view.

Meanwhile, O'Neill has just reached his son's day-care center when an administrator calls on the cell phone, briefs him, and recalls him to duty. Despite having had a hand in the 1993 WTC relief effort, O'Neill, too, is fleetingly incredulous. He flips on the car radio and hears a major broadcast station confirm the news. Instead of crawling into bed where he belongs, O'Neill kisses his towheaded son good-bye and points his truck toward Newark. He knows he may never see his boy again but calls on SWAT-team training to detach from his emotions and focus on what must be done. En route, he phones his wife, immensely relieved that she no longer works as a field EMT. He also calls his parents in Delaware.

Firefighters and hazardous-materials experts from several New Jersey counties hear the reports, too, and feel fortunate that federal experts have visited to begin training them how to deal with weapons-of-mass-destruction attacks. They start calling in specially trained crews and organizing their equipment. Leaders will take teams to a staging area the state has designated near the Holland Tunnel. From there, it's a short hop to lower Manhattan.

A recently appointed emergency-management coordinator from Hoboken, New Jersey—a transportation hub where trains, buses, and ferries bring tens of thousands of commuters to and from lower Manhattan every day—anticipates that some victims may appear in town. Hoboken's proximity to Manhattan and commuters' familiarity with it make his concerns a real likelihood. Phone lines are available only intermittently. He reaches out to a county HazMat team; he phones various emergency agencies. The neighboring town of Weehawken has its own ferry slip and its own concerns. People from nearby towns, such as Bayonne and Kearney—in fact, everyone from the surrounding area, it seems—are headed to Jersey City and Liberty State Park, which officials have designated as casualty collection points.

He calls the captain of the local ambulance corps, also his OEM deputy, and asks, "What can we do to get additional support in case thousands show up here?" It isn't an unrealistic scenario. Hoboken routinely has thousands of commuters during rush hour, and it received patients from the 1993 attacks. The captain reaches out to the local hospital and to the New Jersey First Aid Council, both of whom agree to marshal resources and assist Hoboken.

GET READY, GET SET

O'Neill and Heber arrive at quarters. Management has activated the Special Operations Group and sent EMS workers on the Urban Search and Rescue Team to join their colleagues at Lakehurst Naval Air Station. It put more dispatchers on duty to handle the deluge of calls and help coordinate response efforts from around the state, which means hundreds of buses. It calls blueshirts in from home in order to have enough staff to mount a response and still meet Newark's routine demands.

EMS workers can see the WTC smoke plumes from quarters. They have flashbacks to 1993 and remember that their MCRU, a seemingly bottomless treasure chest, did exhaust some supplies and equipment, which they could not replenish. This morning, they stockpile the MCRU, their ambulances, and a support vehicle with supplies. Heber trebles the MCRU's normal inventory, including twelve extra H-tanks of oxygen, dozens more triage tags, Tyvek protective suits, particulate masks, gloves, and other supplies and equipment to help keep rescuers safe.

Theoretically, hazardous-materials experts will decontaminate patients before EMS workers ever touch them, but there are no guarantees. Heber would feel safer if he had the same protective equipment that the HazMat technicians do. He works quickly and confidently but not without frustration. *Government-issued equipment intended for all emergency responders is stashed in the fire department,* he thinks, *inaccessible thanks to interagency politics.*

At about 0945 hours, EMS workers assemble in the conference room to await orders. An administrator enters the room with nerve-agent antidote kits, describes the signs and symptoms of chemical weapons effects they might encounter, lectures on antidote usage, and gives everybody two kits. One blueshirt who has never seen the materials listens incredulously as he is directed to self-medicate with injections of atropine and sodium chloride in the thigh. He is grateful to be prepared but can't help asking himself, *OK, am I a soldier now, going to war?*

A TV in the background shows the South Tower collapsing just after 1000 hours. *How many rescuers are in that?* one blue-shirt wonders. *Oh my God, this is our worst nightmare!* The briefing is mercifully short. The bottom line, one surmises, is "Watch yourself."

Heber will work as logistics leader. O'Neill will serve as decontamination officer. The blue-shirts hustle about the tarmac, trying to shake off disbelief and adjusting to the sudden sensation that they are now a platoon.

INTO THE BREACH

The department readies its task force: a command car, two ALS ambulances, four BLS trucks, the MCRU, and a support vehicle. Solemnly, O'Neill walks from bus to bus, emphasizing to the blue-shirts that they will be driving *toward* terrorism, an unknown quantity of victims, and as yet unidentified threats. They might not all come back. If anyone chooses not to go, no one will think the worse of them, he says. Everyone understands they have families to protect. He wishes them well. He thinks of his children.

Shortly after 1020 hours, University's task force departs for the Holland Tunnel staging area. A command car leads the lights-and-sirens convoy. Via radio, the blue-shirts learn that the Pentagon is aflame; a plane has crashed in Pennsylvania; and possibly other planes have been hijacked. A few rescuers hear one of their colleagues already at Ground Zero shriek over the radio "Oh my God, I'm going to die!" as the North Tower, shrouded in menacing, black smoke, implodes, crushes his vehicle, and cloaks him in powder. Tense moments pass before they confirm he survived.

With little traffic and lots of speed, what is normally a thirty-five-minute trip takes half the time. Just before reaching the staging area, however, authorities reassign them to Hoboken.

WTC victims and others are scrambling out of New York City. Some of the first casualties to flee are rescuers who escaped the crushing collapse by ducking into an underwater transit station and piling on one of the last trains to leave the WTC for Hoboken. Based on experience from 1993, officials estimate that between two hundred and a thousand people will self-evacuate and try to arrange transport connections home from Hoboken. The station will soon be inundated. Emergency responders and staff from a local hospital have begun to organize, but they will need help. Besides, the disaster managers know that terrorists laced explosives with cyanide in 1993—intending to wipe out the first wave of rescuers and incite even more terror. They want to ensure that anyone contaminated with chemical, biological, or other dangerous substances is cleansed before going further in state and possibly endangering others. A bulletin comes in over the radio: victims leaving Manhattan by ferry and headed for Hoboken are covered with an unknown powder.

CONVERTING CHAOS

The University team arrives at Hoboken terminus at about 1040 hours. Ambulances are scattered about. Dozens of ghostly pale, ash-covered people swarm without an obvious direction. *Near-riot conditions,* one blue-shirt thinks. *People are upset they're not being treated on a timely basis.* Boats that ferry commuters between New Jersey and New York are massing just off the piers with victims. Eye-blinkingly bright emergency-vehicle lights flash incessantly across the river. Volunteers and self-proclaimed experts from around the area have begun to descend. The air tastes of chalk. A group of firefighters is hosing down victims; their command officers have set up a post in a nearby tavern. Municipal police are stationed close by, too, but there is no discernible incident-command post where police, fire, and EMS can strategize together. "Incident command" is a predetermined organizational strategy and hierarchical template that the emergency services use to "control, direct, and coordinate responders and resources." It allows law enforcement, firefighters, EMS, and other disaster-management professionals to converge upon a scene and clarify who is in charge of what, who reports to whom, and how responsibility is divided and delegated, so no one person is overwhelmed—at least theoretically.

The local ambulance squad and hospital have already set up a treatment area under a couple of blue-and-white tents in an intersection near the terminal. *We'll have to move that,* one blue-shirt notes right away. *It inhibits emergency traffic.*

A contingent of medical staff from the local hospital has come to the scene. *They're not used to the masses coming at them,* one thinks when he sees ten or more hospital staff clustered around one patient while dozens are waiting. The hospital workers seemingly lack an understanding of field triage, too. For example, one classifies a particular patient "green," which means "walking wounded" or not seriously sick or injured. The hospital worker explains that the patient is walking and talking. An EMS worker clarifies that although this is true, the patient is also short of breath, which their ABCs[2] have taught them is a significant compromise.

Why don't they stay at the hospital, where they're needed? some blue-shirts wonder, anxious about turf wars and how hard they might have to work to persuade those on hand to let them lead. *Why has the town has leapfrogged over the prehospital, disaster-management system, which has worked so hard to adapt the military model for civilian application?* Although the local emergency squad had set up a field triage unit, when the local hospital sent its physicians, nurses, and supplies, everyone's efforts merged. It strikes the blue-shirts that they are looking at a MASH unit operating inside a small American city. They don't know that one of the on-scene physicians, a surgeon, is a reservist with the Third Battalion of the Fourteenth Marines—a Desert Storm vet who has brought his battlefield experience to the incident.

The infamous notion of "home rule" is already influencing decisions about just who is in command of what. Police, fire, and medical workers, officials from New Jersey Transit, which runs the terminus, and University EMS engage in a brief but tense power struggle. Everyone claims jurisdiction. Everyone clamors to be heard. Some voices are low; others are urgent; and still others are shrill. There are questions about letting victims into Hoboken, because the contaminants are still unknown. People are afraid of making mistakes and losing their jobs. It won't be the first time today that the reservist-surgeon uses his experience to bridge the prehospital pros with their hospital counterparts; he translates values, quells disputes, and redirects emphasis on the victims.

When he discovers the MCRU, he considers it "a beautiful thing." Impressed that it can treat a hundred patients at once, he tells colleagues, "It's well stocked. It's well equipped. It has all these great O_2 lines, all these toys and things we can use to protect ourselves. And it has the best technicians one can imagine. I can't say I've see anything like it outside the military." Authorities have told him to anticipate up to thousands of patients. When he shares this with the University blue-shirts, he sees that they don't panic but consider how to adapt. He finds that comforting, and he lobbies to integrate them into the chain of command. Within a few minutes, but not without some displays of temper, ego, and anxiety, all the rescuers agree to a plan and a workable system soon emerges.

New Jersey Transit will close the terminal to further commuter and pedestrian traffic. Police will coordinate getting victims off of the boats and keep the crowds orderly. Cortacans and several others will work a forward triage area, routing victims in need of decon and treatment one way and everyone else out of the area. The firefighters will continue their gross decon until HazMat experts arrive. And since the MCRU has proven itself hundreds of times, the hospital staff and emergency squad will shift their treatment area over to University's triage, treatment, and transport system, and, in so doing, clear a path for emergency vehicles. Rescue specialist Joe Grassi will set up a staging area for emergency vehicles.

One of the first tasks is to segregate victims from the regular mass of commuters. Those who fled from lower Manhattan have inhaled smoke and been showered with residue and debris from the towers. The rescuers have some indication that asbestos is present but are not sure whether chemical and biological weapons are at work as well. For the victims' health, to ensure the safety of hospitals where some will be transported, and for families to whom the victims will soon return, the rescuers decide to decontaminate all the casualties.

Afterward, people who decline treatment can go home. Others who need medical care will get it.

GETTING ORGANIZED

O'Neill takes charge of the medical aspects of decon. Soon, Essex County's eight-member hazardous-materials team arrives from nearby Nutley, New Jersey. Their convoy includes a decontamination trailer and built-in shower, a HazMat response truck, a pumper with 200 gallons of water and more than a mile of hose, and emergency vehicles piled with other equipment. Tom Nicolette, their team leader, spots O'Neill and thinks, *This is a take-charge guy. He's the boss.* O'Neill is calm, and it's clear that this helps keep everyone around them composed. *Thank heaven.* Nicolette has known at least one administrator "who tends to scream over the radio, bark out a lot of nonsense, and generally make people want to tear their hair out."

O'Neill and Nicolette are talking through how to set up the decon system each feels is necessary when Rich Kozub, the HazMat team leader from Middlesex, arrives. Like their medical colleagues from University, both Nicolette and Kozub's teams have been training to handle such events for several years thanks to government grants. The three men are seasoned and their paths have crossed before. They talk easily with one another.

Kozub rattles off his equipment list, which leaves O'Neill and Nicolette temporarily speechless. Kozub has encapsulated suits with their own air supplies. Kozub has devices to sniff out chemical weapons from mustard to sarin gas.

God, am I glad to see these guys, O'Neill thinks. *They lead two of the most capable HazMat teams in the state.* He was prepared to oversee the decon operation, but he recognizes the two groups' expertise and welcomes the notion of a coalition. *With these guys on our side, we can get just about anything done.*

In the same measured tones of voice they might use to coordinate a multi-car collision, they discuss what needs to be done, examine the layout, and within two to three minutes rough out a strategy. They will stick with the gross decon firefighters are conducting temporarily until Kozub's team can set up their equipment, which is bigger, faster, and more sophisticated.

Victims have little choice about whether to wait like cattle or get soaked to the skin. As they approach, firefighters instruct them to knock the dust off of themselves. Then a half-dozen firefighters, using hand lines, hoses, and nozzles, rinse people two at a time. Some waiting and watching on line ask if the water is cold. It is. Stoically, no one complains. Fortunately, Kozub has brought portable water heaters, which will soon be online with the rest of his equipment. There is no drain, but a private company sucks pools of contaminated water up into its trucks. A few people ask why decontamination is necessary. Neither the HazMat technicians nor the EMS workers have substantive answers. The rescuers worry that asbestos, concrete dust, pulverized glass, and other irritants will complicate some people's breathing. Biological or chemical contaminants are concerns, too, although some argue that any such threats would have vaporized in the heat of the impact.

"We're not a hundred percent sure what's involved," Kozub explains. "The information from New York suggests possible asbestos. We want to wash off as much as possible. If it's wet, it won't aerosolize. You don't want to be breathing this stuff in.

"When you get home, launder your clothing and shower some more so you can get it all out of your hair and off your face and skin."

Discreetly, Kozub's trained techs have begun walking through the crowds with chemical and biological weapons detectors. Thankfully, results come back negative and continue to do so.

Within minutes, Kozub's three navy blue decontamination tents, about twenty by twenty feet each, rise, inflated by a special pump. It's just after 1115 hours when they switch over to his system. Throughout the rest of the day, Kozub, O'Neill, and Nicolette regroup in brief stand-up meetings.

In the interim, Heber and a few other EMS workers have been constructing the MCRU's hourglass-shaped triage, treatment, and transport area near the station's bus terminal. Heber has already sent over a stack of backboards (the MCRU carries fifty) and stair-chairs (the MCRU carries ten) to the forward triage area others are setting up by the piers. He has extracted an incident-command bag, which contains colored and labeled vests to show which EMS worker is in charge of what; customized incident command forms; two cell phones; six portable radios; a mobile base station, which he can set up in two minutes; and an electrical adapter. By plugging the base station into one of the onboard generators or even a nearby building, EMS workers can stay in contact with headquarters without being battery-dependent.

At the tip of the triage area he has organized six stretchers, which he connects to decon via crime-scene tape. That's where paramedics, assisted by the local emergency squad, will quickly examine patients fresh from decon. The medics will classify those who need treatment by color-coded triage tags—green tags for the walking wounded (those not seriously hurt), yellow for patients who are moderately ill or injured, and red for those with serious or critical problems. (Black tags are also on hand—for the dead, the mortally wounded, or those so badly off that to care for them when others have a better chance at surviving would breach triage protocol and medical ethics. Heber's crew has set up a morgue area to address that potentiality.)

Triage teams are trained *not* to treat patients, just to classify them for the most efficient use of resources. Still, Heber designed each of the MCRU's four triage bags to carry one hundred sets of gloves, oral airways, bandages, and packs of roll gauze. That way, EMS workers can at least position a patient's head for optimal breathing, insert a simple airway, and control bleeding until others move them to the treatment zone, into which triage funnels.

Any patients who need to go to the hospital can be rolled directly from Treatment to Transport, the next linear section and one nearest the ambulance staging area.

Nicolette watches briefly as Heber and the EMS workers on his team unload the MCRU. It's like watching a magician pull scarf after scarf after scarf from his sleeve. Each of two ALS medical footlockers has enough supplies to treat fifty patients, including epinephrine and albuterol vials to ease breathing for people in respiratory distress; two airway kits with enough equipment to intubate twenty-five patients; eight multilator bags, *each* of which contains twenty-five adult oxygen masks, ten adult nasal cannulas, ten pediatric masks, and ten nebulizers to aerosolize breathing medications; four portable suction units; one hundred bags of intravenous saline; one hundred bags of Ringer's lactate; a case of sterile water; mini-drips; and four biohazard containers for used needles.

Each of two ALS trauma footlockers can treat up to one hundred trauma patients.

Each of the eight BLS footlockers has hundreds of bandages and dressings as well as cravats, bundles of rolled gauze, tape, and burn sheets.

The MCRU also carries six H-tanks of oxygen, each of which has 6,900 liters, and two M-tanks with 3,000 liters apiece. The M-tanks sport quick-connect valves for portability in the event Heber wants to set up treatment areas away from the truck. The block manifold he designed can draw from all six H-tanks simultaneously and distribute high-flow oxygen to both sides of the vehicle. (And then there are the extra tanks Heber loaded on board.)

They stuff two pounds of shit into a one-pound bag, Nicolette marvels. *I don't know how they do it.* Everything that has earned a place on the carefully designed, space-conscious truck is the product of research, testing, and trial and error.

The first patients trickle through the system, but Heber knows there are more to come. He doesn't know that means thousands more.

Updates from New York stream in; the news is not good. O'Neill speaks with his colleagues on the other side of the river. Kozub has contacts with the Army

Corps of Engineers. They learn that officials have abandoned New York City's Emergency Command Center on the twenty-third floor of Seven World Trade Center. There are five inches of ash on the ground. Ambulances staged near the complex have been crushed by debris. The rescuers presume they have friends and coworkers in New York's emergency services who are already dead. They labor to suppress the foreboding sense of personal tragedy and loss, determined to carry on and deal with the immediate challenges.

O'Neill spots a free fighter group of F-15s circling overhead and thinks, *We're in the shit!* Then, he sees an A-10 Warthog (Thunderbolt) blow by at some sixty meters' altitude. *That's a ground-to-air tactical aircraft! It's a low-flying tank killer. It's a titanium bathtub. If they have deployed that kind of airframe, we're in a goddamn ground war.* He watches it cruise over the Hudson River and imagines it searching for a target, waiting for an assignment. *What is he looking for? Are we in danger of being overrun?* For the first time, O'Neill begins to estimate the threat level on a personal basis and urges everyone to keep their eyes open.

Blackhawk helicopters buzz overhead.

WELCOME TO NEW JERSEY

Authorities designate two piers to receive boats—one for small craft and the other for large. *It's quite an assortment,* Kozub marvels. Like Heber, he conjures up a historical reference. The scene reminds him of everything he has ever learned about Dunkirk. *People used anything that floated to get soldiers across the channel,* Kozub remembers. Now he sees a small armada of yachts, rowboats, power boats, patrol boats, ferries, and tugs charge across the glittering river. Wide-eyed passengers eager to get home stare at the terminus as they approach. Just hours before, it bustled with commuters rushing between newsstands, snack shops, and various routes to New York. Now emergency workers in white Tyvek coveralls await them with wondering eyes. The boats teem with victims and others desperate to escape Manhattan.

O'Neill, Nicolette, and Kozup also stage a forward triage center here to screen passengers and get a quick assessment of what's to come. Using crime-scene tape, rope, and wooden horses, they erect a makeshift holding pen and a decontamination corridor to corral disembarking passengers. Paramedic Henry Cortacans, his colleagues, some HazMat technicians, and several nurses from the local hospital wait with stretchers and long boards from the MCRU.

Cortacans prays his sister will appear on one of the boats; she works for a hotel based in the WTC and hasn't been heard from. Every time he uses his cell phone to dial her, he hears, "All circuits are busy." Rumors add to his anxiety. People are saying that Washington, D.C., is on fire; that the Sears Tower in Chicago in down; that Los Angeles just blew up. *This is insane*, he thinks. He can't stop thinking of a fellow paramedic who just joined the Port Authority police last year.

Police allow only one boat to disembark at a time. "Welcome to New Jersey!" an officer's voice booms through a megaphone to the approaching passengers. "When you get off the boat, go down the corridor. You'll go to Decontamination. Then you can leave or get medical assistance. Anyone with obvious injuries, you get off first."

Between 300 and 350 people struggle down the gangplank. Among them, a pregnant woman with a broken leg has her arms wrapped around the necks of two men in suits. People with burns and ugly lacerations are escorted off. Cortacans encounters elderly people and victims with terminal illnesses who tell him they can't afford to get wet and catch pneumonia. Frustrated that he doesn't have time to talk to each patient, he tells the fragile ones that it's in their best interest to get on a stretcher and "let these fine gentlemen take care of you."

Police ask passengers who were anywhere near the WTC to follow the corridor that runs across the broad, sheltered plaza that the train station and ferries share. They permit others to filter into the station and try to arrange transportation to their various destinations. Some, overwhelmed by the crowd and convinced that no local transportation will be available, just take to the streets.

For every two boats in the slips, six more wait to unload. Suddenly, the decon line has a thousand victims waiting. *This is nuts*, Cortacans tells himself. *This is nuts!*

At this pace, O'Neill and his colleagues imagine they will have to process five hundred to a thousand patients an hour for who knows how long. It's a staggering number. Except for the first WTC bombing, the department has planned its mass-casualty-response efforts to suit factory and large transportation accidents. If the pace holds up, they'll rip through the fourteen hundred triage tags they brought almost immediately. Fortunately, some thirty ambulances are queued up in the staging area; each should have tags that the rescuers can poach.

Ash-covered victims whisper to one another. Some cry. Some shake. Nicolette overhears some talking; they waited hours to escape Manhattan by boat. Heber, waiting in the treatment area, spies the first group of patients come off the ferry. Everything is powdered—hair, clothing, purses, computers. Largely silent, their faces etched with dismay, victims file slowly down the corridor, beneath a small tunnel, and into the decon area. *This is the weirdest thing. Everything is moving along as planned but it all feels surreal,* he thinks. *The patients have to be terrified. Crisis teams in hospitals are going to be overwhelmed with civilians and volunteers. It's going to be amazing.*

ALL WET

Having anticipated a weapons-of-mass-destruction event, Middlesex County HazMat used federal grant monies to purchase its inflatable decontamination tents two years ago. Each tent divides inside into three aisles separated by floor-to-ceiling curtains. Males go on one side, females on another, and HazMat techs escort those who can't walk down the center. With all three tents in operation, the rescuers can wash about eighteen patients simultaneously.

Most patients go through decon fully dressed. Because some will surely go to hospitals, HazMat techs strip them down to their bare flesh and cleanse them. (Hospitals cannot afford to take potentially contaminated victims, lest they risk affecting other patients and their medical staff as well.) The tents have a roller assembly in the middle aisle so techs can slide through patients in wheelchairs, stair-chairs, stretchers, and backboards. Economy of movement becomes very important in a long operation.

About noon, O'Neill sneaks a peek at lower Manhattan. *It's still a goddamn smoke column,* he marvels. *It looks like a goddamn tombstone.* Then the entire system blinks when someone finds a suspicious package and authorities began yelling, "Get the fuck out of here! Everybody run!"

Nicolette climbs up on his pumper and shouts for his crew to stay close. He spies O'Neill and Kozub, who have suspended operations while everyone takes a minute to figure out it's a terrible hoax.

Rescuers estimate that at least five hundred people bolt. One woman is trampled. Hundreds avoid decon, triage, and treatment altogether before dozens of EMS workers, firefighters, and police join hands, literally, and form a human chain to corral and calm the victims and reset the system.

Drivet and O'Neill talk by cell phone. O'Neill wishes his friend and mentor were by his side, which he expresses with typical terseness: "We're deconning thousands. Get your ass over here!" Although Drivet is now a per-diem employee, because he has worked many drills and real mass casualties, and started the Special Operations Group, the rescuers know he can make a valuable contribution and they welcome his participation. *This is a hugely tremendous task,*

Drivet considers as he drives toward quarters to check in and then on to Hoboken. *It may be the biggest job of my career. We'll just have to take a bite out of each corner until we eat the whole thing.*

An emergency radio chronicles a state police chase; officers are pursuing a van that may contain chemical weapons. They stop it not far from the day-care center where O'Neill's son is playing. O'Neill looks into the terrified eyes of mothers clutching their babies. Their uncertainty is palpable. *No one is safe,* O'Neill realizes. *In all my seventeen years on the job, the highs, the lows, all the education, all the life experience, I've never cried on the job.* Nevertheless, his eyes water. Even though he and his colleagues have an effective system in motion, the scene sometimes becomes overpowering. Cortacans spots a side of O'Neill he has never seen, much less imagined. It awes him to see a battle-scarred veteran shed a tear. Cortacans loses a tear or two, too. Throughout the day, almost everyone feels overcome, at least for a minute.

Throughout the long day, which stretches until 0100 the next morning, few victims complain. One doesn't want to ruin his eight-hundred-dollar Italian suit. Another, who claims to work for a senator, threatens to call his powerful boss. A woman frets over an expensive pair of shoes. Tired of waiting and eager to get home, victims surround the agitators in their midst and move them through decon before police get involved. (Because the area is under a state of emergency, the HazMat officials can order people to comply and even have police handcuff them if necessary. And police can force those they take into custody to be decontaminated lest they pollute the jail.) For the most part, the crowd is compliant and cooperative, almost too good. *People are not looking anywhere in particular,* Kozub notices. *It's like they're not really here with it; they look like zombies; they've all got the thousand-yard stare.* Disturbed, he tries to keep an eye on the small groups of glassy-eyed victims as they move through the tent showers.

As patients enter, they give their computers, cameras, and other valuables to technicians, who store the possessions in what Kozub calls "huge Ziploc bags." One woman hands over a purse into which chunks of concrete have fallen. The techs give each patient a triage tag that approximates their treatment priority. (Medically trained triage pros will examine each patient again after the HazMat teams decontaminate them.)

Patients walk deeper into the tents, which are well lit thanks to another generator. Shower booms run overhead. Warm water deluges between three and six people per tent. Neither soap nor other cleansers seem necessary, because the pollutants appear to be nonreactive powder. Pipes inside the tent stretch all the way to the river, where they dump the spillage. "There's no other means to contain it," Nicolette explains.

The one-minute showers allow crews to clean approximately three hundred patients per hour. Hot-air generators help dry the victims, although technicians wheel in linen carts filled with towels, sheets, blankets, and surgical scrubs, from infant size to six extra-large, for those who want a change of clothes.

By design, it's an assembly line. Mechanization helps make the process efficient. But the plight of the people before them is not lost on the rescuers. The scene before them reminds some of refugee camps. O'Neill sees too many people with unanswered questions clouding sorrowful eyes. He spies a boy, bald from chemotherapy, crying on his way through the showers, and trying to shield his small head from view. The scarf the child wears to conceal his naked scalp, his Jesse "the Body" Ventura bandanna, has gone astray in the commotion. O'Neill, the medal winner, tough, gruff, and infinitely cynical, kneels and offers the boy his University Hospital baseball cap.

Wet, well-dressed businessmen ask how they can help instead of how to get home. "I can do this for you," one says, grabbing an armful of garbage bags from one of the techs who patrols the tents picking up refuse. "You go do something more important." The man, who looks like a Wall Street titan to Kozub, spends hours stooping and collecting garbage so his guys can catch a break.

Some victims help carry patients and equipment. Others distribute towels. When some of the women emerge from the showers, their clothes, now sodden, cling. Some outfits are even transparent. It astonishes Kozub how everyone instinctively protects others' dignity. Men avert their eyes while handing the women towels, or drape them over the women's shoulders. Kozub doesn't hear one off-color remark.

Every half-hour, it seems to Kozub, some now-decontaminated patient asks, "What do you need?" And as the day runs on and on, he tells them: towels, garbage bags, garbage cans, etc. Miraculously, a huge truck with supplies arrives from Home Depot. Later, he needs propane to keep the shower water warm. Someone shows up with thirty propane canisters. A security officer from nearby Stevens Institute of Technology practically begs to assist. Kozub asks for paper towels and is rewarded with case upon case, bundle upon bundle.

Kozub brought five 10-gallon water coolers. But the warm September day and the rescuers' exertion has depleted reserves.

New Jersey Transit makes its staffs available. Electricians stay on hand to help whenever the slightest glitch occurs. "We get it, find it, build it," Kozub marvels. "Everyone is helping everyone."

HEY, LOOK ME OVER

As patients emerge from the decontamination tents, a crime-scene tape and rope corridor leads them to the triage area Heber set up near the tip of the MCRU. Most people refuse medical aid. But there are people with shortness of breath, cuts, abrasions, inhalation injuries, burns, and fractures. One woman learns that her husband has most likely died and succumbs to heart-wrenching grief and distress.

EMS workers take red-tagged patients, those with burns or cardiac and respiratory distress, to a fifty-by-twenty-foot area adjacent to the MCRU and demarcated by red cones. Here, the MCRU has resources to care for up to twenty critical patients in four rows of five. One paramedic can attend to two patients if necessary. But local physicians are on hand, as well. The yellow treatment area, set apart by yellow cones, flanks the red and can also accommodate twenty moderately injured patients. One University EMT can handle two patients. But local nurses are working here, too. For the most part, yellow coded patients get breathing treatments and splints.

The green area, bordered by green cones, is adjacent to the yellow zone. It holds even larger numbers of patients because they don't need oxygen. Here, EMS workers and their hospital-based colleagues use cases of saline to flush soot and debris from patients' eyes. They cleanse and bandage minor lacerations.

Heber has everything running smoothly, but his job does not stop here. He watches patients progress through the line. If need be, Heber can open up the other side of the truck and care for twice as many; like the Rescue truck, the MCRU can work from either side or both. He keeps an eye on supplies. He uses his mechanical skills, because one small or annoying thing keeps breaking or falling apart. He's constantly on the move, looking 360 degrees all the time. It seems like there are never enough lizard luggers (people who lift and carry).

The blue-shirts in the treatment area are experienced in working under trying circumstances. They know that their hospital-based colleagues are skilled, too, but those who perform wonders inside an ER seem to them less adept in the field. Under the strain, the traditional rivalries they've worked hard to suppress begin to emerge. "Nurses can't start IVs in the field to save their life," one medic grumbles. Surely some can, but it's not as easy as doing it in familiar, controlled clinical settings. So some patients get pierced again and again.

The blue-shirts' goal is to stabilize and transport—rapidly. With some three hundred patients an hour and a line stretching as far as the eye can see, pressure mounts. They become increasingly frustrated with bottlenecks they attribute to the hospital staff. Some feel pushed to the side by doctors and nurses who seem to look upon the situation as if they had brought the hospital to the transportation hub so they can function as they normally do. The MCRU's natural effi-ciency begins bogging down. "This isn't where we should be hooking them up to heart monitors and giving them nitro!" a blue-shirt protests. "We ought to just get them into the buses where they can get going." There are plenty of ambulances ready to transport patients to area hospitals and treat them en route, but the EMS workers can't very well tear patients away from their hospital-based colleagues.

One self-important volunteer swaggers into the Treatment Area boasting what strikes the paid EMS workers as empty credentials, questioning the system, and generally stirring things up. A blue-shirt speaks to him bluntly: "You need to stop what you are doing and get out of this area, because you are causing the entire treatment area to get out of control."

"Well, I *am* an EMT instructor," the man rebutts. Unfamiliar with the MCRU system, perhaps he does not realize a proven system is in place and working, albeit top-heavy with helpers. The man has his own views of disaster management and says so. "I *teach* Mass Casualty Incident Management."

"That's nice," the EMS worker retorts. "How many MCIs have you been on?"

"I've been to five," the man brags.

"OK, well, I've been to more than a hundred, so I guess that makes me in charge."

Freelancers! he fumes. That's his term for people who converge on a scene, disregarding or ignorant of the incident-command system, a hierarchical tem-plate that trained emergency workers in police, fire, and EMS apply (at least the-oretically) to establish order over chaos. The University EMS workers know that most freelancers' hearts are in the right place, but this is neither the time nor the place for handholding, social work, résumé-building, or ego-stroking. Freelancers add confusion to already hectic scenes. Out of step with everyone else, they risk getting hurt and adding to the patient load.

At about 1400 hours, Drivet arrives and joins the EMS branch staff. The whole scene is S-shaped—it's impossible to take everything in at once. Drivet paces the area to make connections and get a sense of operations. Amongst the rescuers he notes frayed tempers, and he sees that stress and exhaustion have worn the edge off of everyone. And they're still spooling up to handle more victims. Putting his diplomatic skills and life experience to work, he starts to deflate tensions and assuage feelings so operations can run without disruption. He listens to disparate parties who have been seething and competing to be heard, to exercise their ideas of what is best. And then he directs them in ways they feel good about.

Drivet deputizes a volunteer who is pursing her graduate degree in emergency management. She admires his "low-key, steady-as-she-goes" manner. He gives her a handful of markers so she can have rescuers write "doctor," "nurse," "medic," "EMT," "volunteer," and other such titles on their white-suits, making the caregivers easy to recognize, organize, and delegate to. He has her establish an incident-command organization just for the volunteers. By coordinating them and assigning them specific chores, she harnesses dozens of people who might otherwise be in the way and has them distribute towels, help victims dress, give directions, offer food and drinks, and carry out other supporting activities.

One fatigued blue-shirt thinks, *Drivet is fresh and full vigor. Look how he's able to regroup the troops!* Comparing himself with Drivet, the EMS worker realizes that he is tense from stress, which may be affecting his decisions. But there is precious little time for introspection; the site is still inundated.

With all the patients to care for, no one has yet organized a rest and rehabilitation spot for the emergency workers to grab a few minutes' peace and reset themselves. Although few feel comfortable taking a break, adrenaline reserves can be exhausted. Those in chain of command try to keep an eye on the workers and rotate them out for short intermissions. A few restaurants have opened their doors so that workers can eat, use the bathroom, or just grab some quite time. Not many leave the scene, though. Some are too tense to eat. Still, others guzzle bottled water and devour the pizza slices, sandwiches, and slices of watermelon that area restaurants, delis, and stores have been delivering with steady generosity. But relief is sporadic. When O'Neill finally takes a short break late in the day, he prefers to climb into an empty ambulance, lock the door, and cry. *There's a point where you either have this cathartic episode or you have a psychotic break,* he knows. Then he wipes his face and gets back to work. Deliberately, he seals off thoughts of friends in New York who may be dead. *When there's enough downtime, I'll deal with it,* he thinks.

O'Neill checks in with his wife. She can't get away from her job either but arranges for her parents to retrieve their children so she and her husband can continue to work.

Officials reroute some of the incoming vessels to Liberty State Park, on Ellis Island, where other EMS workers have set up another casualty collection point. That will give the Hoboken crews a bit of respite. As evening approaches, Heber and company shift the treatment area closer to the terminus to take advantage of its lighting. The line of victims still snakes back to the piers.

*   *   *

Cortacans's fiancée reaches him by cell phone and reports that his sister is safe in a Brooklyn hospital, albeit with a broken arm. Cortacans feels an immense rush of relief. He also feels ill as well as immeasurably angry at what has happened; he needs an outlet. During a short break, he hunts down an American flag. He strikes gold on a neglected shelf in the train station and carries his treasure back to the MCRU with pride. The blue-shirts hang the enormous old flag over the truck. "That's right," some people roar from the crowd. "*Represent!*"

"*Fuck, yeah!*" the exceptionally polite Cortacans tells himself.

Ironically, low tide makes it impossible for the boats near Ellis Island to dock. They all turn around and head back to Hoboken.

Twilight arrives and Cortacans watches somberly as the Manhattan skyline gradually lights up—except for lower Manhattan.

Eventually the victims stop coming. Sometime between 2000 and 2100 hours, the rescuers begin to shut down the system and clean up. University EMS brought enough supplies to decontaminate ten thousand patients. Thirteen hours later, there is nothing left. Rescuers figured they used extra supplies on some patients and not enough on others. When they write up their reports, most feel confident that eight thousand patients is a conservative estimate.

Before September 11, most domestic preparedness programs theorized that mass-decontamination programs were not possible, O'Neill thinks. He stares at the exhausted blue-shirts, firefighters, and HazMat technicians, awed that they have just conducted perhaps the largest mass decontamination in history.

Weariness now has new meaning, but there is still sufficient energy to laugh when Drivet distills the day's events to a simple "My feet hurt so much!" At midnight, he heads over to the Port Authority's makeshift emergency operations center to relieve an administrator who has been there all day. He works until 0930 hours, drives home for four hours' sleep, and returns to the EOC.

By 0100 hours, Heber has returned the MCRU to HQ and is restocking it. *The best part was that everyone in EMS came out of this unhurt,* he reflects. He takes a lot of pride in running a safe operation. *I never thought I'd see two thousand patients in a single day. Being accustomed to working in chaos has its benefits.* Only a fraction of those treated went on to area hospitals: three red patients, twenty-two yellow patients, and eighteen green. He doesn't yet realize that two EMS workers he and the blue-shirts have worked with, two who became Port Authority police officers, went down with the towers and died.

Four agencies that never worked together pulled this off, Nicolette marvels on his drive home. *You would think we did this three hundred times before!* By 0130 hours, he steps over his threshold, takes a shower, talks with his pregnant wife, drinks a glass of chocolate milk, and falls dead asleep.

O'Neill gets home about 0145 hours on Wednesday. (Hoboken's emergency-management coordinator is still on the job, having city services cleanse the terminus, decide what to do with massive amounts of contaminated towels, deal with the Porta-Johns they imported, and handle other tasks as well as taking stock of resources that might be needed the following day.)

It's 0200 hours before Heber phones his wife. He hasn't spoken with her since he left home for work twenty hours ago. He didn't call for days after the first WTC bombing. His wife and children spent the day sticking as close to their normal routine as possible. They ate dinner and did homework. Then they went to church. After twenty years in the business, Heber and his wife have learned to trust one another. She trusts him to take care of himself. He trusts her to look after the family.

On Wednesday morning O'Neill meets with a colleague to update a presentation, naps briefly, and reports for duty at 1500 hours, where he joins others in a task force headed into Manhattan. There, they take over for colleagues who have staged the resources New Jersey has been sending its neighboring state—a situation the department has long been prepared for. "We've discussed it," a blue-shirt explains. "If and when their [New York's] resources are wiped out, we're going to be there to help them pick up the pieces."

O'Neill works until 1200 hours on Thursday, drives home, kisses his family, showers, and conks out for four hours. When he awakens late that afternoon, he regroups with his family for a few slices of pizza and a piece of birthday cake. Today is O'Neill's thirty-fifth birthday.

This evening he makes his way far into upstate New York. Tomorrow morning he will speak about domestic preparedness to rescuers attending an annual conference, and then he will haul himself back to the job.

GLOSSARY

AIDS	Acquired Immuno Deficiency Virus
ALS	Advanced Life Support
AVL	Automatic Vehicle Locator
BLS	Basic Life Support
Blue-shirt	An ALS or BLS EMS worker who wears a blue-collar shirt and works the streets
Catheter	A device that provides access to veins
CISD	Critical Incident Stress Debriefing, a process to vent stress, raise and answer questions, and obtain support associated with traumatic incidents
CPR	Cardiac Pulmonary Resuscitation
CVA	Cerebral Vascular Accident, also known as a stroke or brain attack
DOA	Dead on Arrival
DNR	Do Not Resuscitate, a doctor-prescribed order instructing rescuers not to attempt to reverse death with drugs, CPR, defibrillation, etc.

DYFS	The Division of Youth and Family Services
EAP	Employee Assistance Program
ECG (EKG)	Electrocardiogram
EDP	Emotionally Disturbed Person
EMD	Emergency Medical Dispatcher
EMT	Emergency Medical Technician
EMS	Emergency Medical Service
EOC	Emergency Operations Center
ER	Emergency Room
ETA	Estimated Time of Arrival
FNG	Fucking New Guy
GPS	Global Positioning Satellite
HIV	Human immunodefficiency virus
IV	Intravenous, a delivery system that allows EMS workers to infuse fluids and medications directly into a patient's veins
KED	Kendrick Extrication Device, a splinting tool used to protect the spine and internal organs of trauma patients who are injured but do not show signs or symptoms of life threat
MCRU	Mass Casualty Response Unit
MIC or MICU	Mobile Intensive Care Unit, an Advanced Life Support or paramedic truck
MICP	Mobile Intensive Care Paramedic
NAEMT	National Association of Emergency Medical Technicians
NHTSA	National Highway Traffic and Safety Administration
PTSD	Post-Traumatic Stress Disorder, a combination of mental, emotional and physical symptoms suffered by people who experience severe trauma and extraordinary stress
QA	Quality Assurance
Reeves	A brand-name carrying device, a large plastic sheet reinforced with wooden slats
REMCS	Regional Emergency Medical Communication System, the official name for the E-911 Dispatch Center at University Hospital
Ringer's Lactate	An electrolyte-rich fluid paramedics sometimes infuse patients with
SOG	Special Operations Group
SWAT	Special Weapons and Tactics
TB	Tuberculosis
Vollies	Slang for "volunteers"
White-shirt	A supervisor or manager
World Trade Center	WTC

NOTES

INTRODUCTION

1. *Emergency Medical Services Agenda for the Future*, DOT HS 808 441, NTS-42, National Highway Traffic Safety Administration, U.S. Department of Transportation, 1996, 61.
2. Katherine Traver Barkley, *The Ambulance* (Kiamesha, NY: Load N Go Press, 1990), 153.
3. "Twenty-five Years on the Front Line," edited by John A. Rupke, M.D. (Dallas, Texas: American College of Emergency Physicians, 1993), 8.
4. Except for first responders, all certified prehospital caregivers are emergency medical technicians (EMTs). Their levels of training and titles vary from state to state, however. In fact, NHTSA says there are forty different variations. In New Jersey, EMT-Basics provide basic life support (BLS)—that is, what they have learned in their 120-hour class, ER internship, and continuing-education courses. New Jersey has no EMT-Intermediates. In other states, however, EMT-Is have additional training and might insert airways or start intravenous lines. The EMT-Advanced, also known as "paramedic," is trained to the highest level of prehospital care. They can administer dozens of drugs

and execute several invasive procedures. All EMS workers operate under a physician's medical direction.

5. The hospital and the EMS workers dispute the number of missions. EMS workers count every assignment that causes them to turn the wheel and rush to a job, regardless of whether they eventually assume care of a patient or get canceled. They literally take their lives in their hands each time they venture out of headquarters onto the congested city streets, which are plagued by stolen cars and drunk or otherwise reckless drivers. And, not infrequently, two-person crews transport more than one patient for the sake of expedient care. The hospital claims that the actual number of patients treated and transported is closer to thirteen to fifteen patients per shift, which by most standards is still a considerable load.

CHAPTER 1

1. New Jersey paramedics can dispense forty drugs and perform several invasive procedures.
2. Because they work in proximity to live weapons, tactical medics must know how to handle weapons and make them safe.
3. Facts that illustrate Newark history from the 1930s through 1966 here were gleaned from *Newark*, a book that chronicles the city's development over its first three hundred years. John T. Cunningham, *Newark* (Newark, New Jersey: The New Jersey Historical Society, 1966), 299–315.
4. Cunningham, 299.
5. Debra Lynn Vial, "When Newark Tore Itself Apart," *Bergen Record*, July 6, 1997. Obtained online at www.bergen.com.
6. Laurie Goodstein, "Rebirth Is Slow at Ground Zero of Newark Riots," *Washington Post*, May 7, 1992, A27.
7. Goodstein, A27.

CHAPTER 2

1. Some states, however, do enhance EMT training, permitting them to start intravenous lines, etc.
2. Neither doctors nor nurses are required to spend time on an ambulance as part of their education and preparation to work in an ER.

CHAPTER 3

1. EMS telemetry is based on technology NASA created to monitor astronaut health from Earth. In some EMS systems, *telemetry* means the transmission of a patient's physiological data—for example, an individual's cardiac rhythm as read by a cardiac monitor. In Newark, *telemetry* means everything involved in keeping paramedics in voice contact with supervising physicians. University Hospital's Newark paramedics are so experienced at electrocardiogram (ECG) readings that physicians here rarely require transmission. Paramedics do attach each patient's ECG strip to his or her chart.

2. John Erich, "Wheels of Fortune," *EMS Magazine*, Volume 29, No. 11 (November 2000), 43–66.

3. Members of the National Emergency Numbers Association listserv discussed the matter of 911 calls coming from patients inside hospitals and other health-care facilities in February 2002 after one member shared a Chicago-area article reporting one such incident [Jon Davis, "Call placed from hospital emergency room," *Daily Herald* (January 30, 2002)]. Other emergency medical dispatchers from elsewhere in the country shared similar experiences, which some believe reflect endemic ER overcrowding. One reported calls from an inpatient who could not get her hospital staff's attention to discharge her. Several mentioned calls from distressed, sometimes disoriented patients in nursing homes and mental institutions. Some patients had actual, real-time emergencies; others were reliving past traumas through active hallucination. The emergency medical dispatchers discussed strategies for managing such dilemmas.

4. Emergency medical dispatchers discussed such a caller and the dilemma posed for busy call centers in the National Emergency Numbers Association listserv on January 3, 2002.

CHAPTER 4

1. The National EMS Memorial continues to compile a registry of the profession's line-of-duty deaths (*www.nems.org*).

2. New Jersey State Police, *1999 Uniform Crime Report: Section VI: Crime in the Cities*, obtained online at www.state.nj.us.

3. This figure reflects Callahan's take-home salary, which after eighteen years on the job, he says, is approximately $39,000. It does not include uniform allocations, a taxable sum that the department gives EMS workers to help subsidize the cost of required gear; nor does it reflect one-time salary adjustments, which the union can sometimes eke out during contract negotiations.

Several years have passed since the department did away with longevity or merit increases. Salaries now increase only by cost-of-living adjustments.

4. The Association for Children of New Jersey, *Newark Kids Count 2001: A Profile of Child Well-Being* (Newark, New Jersey, 2001), 48.

5. www.guide2newark.com/factsandfigures.htm.

6. *Webster's Encyclopedic Unabridged Dictionary of the English Language,* (New York, NY: Portland House, a division of Random House Value Publishing, © 1996), 1334.

7. Samuel Shem, *House of God: A Novel* (New York: R. Marek Publishers, 1978), x.

8. The department forbids such visceral exhibitions of camaraderie, instructing endangered employees to alert Dispatch, which will, in turn, notify superiors and police. But the EMS workers whose lives are at risk in such dynamic circumstances feel safer knowing the team's self-reliance is paramount.

9. Theoretically, once these patients enter the health-care system someone in the emergency department endeavors to teach them how to take advantage of the diverse health and social services that the city offers. Ideally, such mechanisms will prevent them from relapsing into successive crises and flooding EMS and the ER with wave after wave of urgent care requests. Something is broken, however. The knowledge doesn't sink in, and the vicious cycle continues.

CHAPTER 5

1. Final Report: Mobile Intensive Care Unit Pilot Program, "The Effects of MICU Paramedic Service in New Jersey:" New Jersey State Department of Health, Emergency Medical Services Program, May 1979, 10.

2. Code is slang for "clinical death," i.e., when the heart stops beating and the lungs stop breathing. EMS workers also refer to "biological death," which occurs four to six minutes after clinical death—when cells begin to die irreparably from lack of oxygen and fuel. "Legal death" occurs when a paramedic, physician, medical examiner, or other authorized person makes an official pronouncement.

3. *Emergency Medical Services Agenda for the Future*, p. 22.

4. One supervisor compares the job divisions of EMS to "the social classes of the 1890s. BLS is at the bottom, the backbone of the system, followed by the Rescue guys, ALS, and then the supervisors. Everyone always wants to aim higher. For example, female ALS won't date male BLS." He points out that such separations between ranks, genders, teams, races, etc., "are probably the reason that everyone [in EMS] thinks they're alone."

5. Richard Beebe, MEd. R.N., NREMT-P, "Size Matters," *JEMS*, Vol. 27, No. 1 (January 2002), 22–33.
6. *Size Matters*, p. 26.

CHAPTER 6

1. State of New Jersey Department of Health and Senior Services, Division of Alcoholism, Drug Abuse, and Addiction Services, *New Jersey Alcohol and Drug Abuse Data System*, January 1, 2000, to December 31, 2000, County of Essex, which breaks out admissions to treatment programs by municipality and primary drug.
2. Centers for Disease Control and Prevention, *HIV/AIDS Surveillance Report*, "Table 4: AIDS Cases and annual rates per 100,000 population, by metropolitan area and age group reported through June 2001, United States," Vol. 13. No. 1 (Atlanta, Georgia) 8–9. Also available at cdc.gov/hiv.

CHAPTER 7

1. Shem, pp. 43, 382.
2. *Newark Kids Count 2001*, p. 7.
3. *Newark Kids Count 2001*, p. 28.
4. *Newark Kids Count 2001*, pp. 22–24.
5. *Newark Kids Count 2001*, p. 7.

CHAPTER 8

1. *Newark Kids Count 2001,* p. 21.
2. Ehrich, pp. 43–66.

CHAPTER 9

1. BLS workers also have their charts audited, but the requirements are somewhat less rigorous, in keeping with the lower level of training and responsibility. The review process, however, is similar to that of ALS.

CHAPTER 10

1. B. Karlsson, et. al., "Is there an association between shift work and having a metabolic syndrome? Results from a population-based study of 27,485 people," *Occupational & Environmental Medicine*, Vol. 58, No. 11 (November 2001): 747–52. Obtained through the good offices of Terri Brownlee, M.P.H., R.D., L.D.N., a content contributor to Nutrio.com and director of the Duke University Diet & Fitness Center.

2. Rosmond, R., et. al. "The influence of occupational and social factors on obesity and body fat distribution in middle-aged men" *International Journal of Obesity* 20 (July 1996): 599–607. Obtained initially through the good offices of Terri Brownlee, M.P.H., R.D., L.D.N., a content contributor to Nutrio.com and director of the Duke University Diet & Fitness Center and from the Nature Publishing Group, Specialist Journals, UK.

3. Raffaello Furlan, Franca Barbic, Simona Piazza, Mauro Tinelli, Paolo Seghizzi, and Alberto Malliani, "Modifications of Cardiac Autonomic Profile Associated With a Shift Schedule of Work," *Circulation* (Journal of the American Heart Association), 102 (October 2000): 1912–16.

4. The expression "Give what's right, not what's left" came from a billboard outside the Parsippany Baptist Church in Parsippany, New Jersey. The pastor's wife thought she borrowed it from one of her many quote books. All my efforts to identify the author have been unsuccessful.

5. "EMS Employee Recognition Program," #42062-3300-102, *University Hospital–Emergency Medical Services EMS Policy and Procedures Manual*.

6. This information was obtained from the Department of Treasury, Office of Pension and Benefits, State of New Jersey.

7. Ellen Simon, "Union Reaches Deal with Supermarkets," *The Star-Ledger*, April 14, 2001, 19.

8. *Emergency Medical Services Agenda for the Future*, p. 13.

9. *Emergency Medical Services Agenda for the Future*, p. 4.

10. *Emergency Medical Services Agenda for the Future*, p. 26.

CHAPTER 11

1. Centers for Disease Control and Prevention, *TB Surveillance Report*: Table 36: Tuberculosis Cases in Select Cities: 2000 and 1999.

2. "City Accused of Concealing Responders' Health Problems," *Journal of Emergency Medical Services* (October 2001): 14.

3. EMS workers are obligated to care for their patients, as opposed to police and firefighters, whose primary focus is on law enforcement and firefighting.

For example, in Chapter 4 firefighters were first on-scene after a vehicle struck the Good Samaritan on Routes 1 and 9, but they did nothing for him. EMS workers found the man lying unattended in the road. Newark police officers ticketed a young man for speeding, although they knew he was transporting his ill and elderly mother to the hospital. One issued a summons and the other sat in the radio car while a two-person team of EMS workers struggled mightily to get the large and clearly distressed woman from the car to their bus. New York City police officers crossed their arms in front of their chests and did nothing to help the bicyclist whom I mentioned in this book's Introduction. In each of these situations there was the risk of infectious-disease transmission, but only the EMS workers incurred real exposure.

4. *Emergency Medical Services Agenda for the Future*, p. 26.
5. *Emergency Medical Services Agenda for the Future*, p. 26.
6. None of the EMS workers I spoke with envisioned living long enough to really enjoy retirement; they shared the belief that some job-related illness or injury would catch up with them eventually and contribute to early death.
7. The government will begin publishing results from the new occupational code in the latter half of 2004.
8. *Emergency Medical Services Agenda for the Future*, p. 26.

CHAPTER 13

1. Edited by Bruce D. Brown, M.D., FAAOS, et al., *AAOS Emergency Care and Transportation of the Sick and Injured* (Sudbury, MA: Jones and Bartlett Publishers, 1998), 824.
2. ABC stands for Airway, Breathing, and Circulation, universal EMS treatment priorities.

ACKNOWLEDGMENTS

I have many people to thank for the privilege of recounting what happens in the back of an ambulance and where EMS workers tread. Throughout my reporting, I was fortunate to make many learned friends who patiently educated me—more than I could hope to name here.

Watching the B team in action was more eye-opening and inspiring than I had imagined. The crews I rode with and everyone I talked with were stupendously generous. Even for a group of savvy, battle-hardened veterans, having a critical journalist look over their shoulders was not easy. They answered infinite questions; they subjected themselves to constant scrutiny. They allowed me to chronicle the times when they felt drained, hungry, cranky, and woefully unappreciated in addition to some of their many heroic acts. Some are intensely private people, but they made themselves accessible to help cast a light on EMS, a profession they love unabashedly and invest in although society consistently underestimates its value.

My thanks are insufficient, but nevertheless, I begin by expressing my gratitude to them. Walter Joseph "The Commander" Drivet is an unsurpassed paramedic, leader, colleague, and friend. He inspires excellence, loyalty, and humility; the funniest man I know. Eugene J. O'Neill brings smarts and wit to the team, and through him, I also learned and laughed. Vincent Callahan's miraculous ability to constantly tap into his heart makes the EMS experience humane. Benjamin Cardona, who commits his considerable talent and energy to make Newark a better place for his family, patients, and his colleagues in the emergency services, is nothing short of inspiring. William Heber is a brutally honest, inventive, and extraordinarily buoyant man with many unsung talents. Vincent Francis Cisternino is a profoundly intellectual and spirited paramedic. Tracey Ann Fazio's clever pluck, compassion, and good nature clearly mean a great deal to her patients and coworkers. Tom Opperman's resolute effort, proficiency, and courageous candor distinguish him. I am grateful to Che-heibe Scott and Ennis Terrell, as well.

I am indebted to Daniel R. Gerard, Sr., M.S., M.I.C.P., R.N., an EMS visionary. One of my first EMS instructors, a recent chair of the NAEMT paramedic division, one of the most passionate EMS devotees I have ever met, and a loyal friend, he graciously answered questions day and night, steered me around pitfalls and potholes, and provided me with access to many EMS leaders.

I appreciate the many contributions of other University Hospital EMS pros who generously shared their experiences, particularly: Supervisors Mario Piumelli, Victor Mendez, Tom Tryon, and Terry Hoben, Air Medical Coordinator, everyone at REMCS, and the men and women of the A, B, C, and D teams (blue-shirts *and* white-shirts).

I am especially grateful to the people of University Hospital for their fortitude. Allowing me to observe and report on real EMS has, at times, made managers there uneasy. As a friend of EMS and an admirer of University, I believed from the start that the profession and the department were strong enough to withstand scrutiny. If the EMS profession's or characters' imperfections seem magnified on these pages, and therefore embarrassing to the institution, I wish to reassure readers everywhere that, after a year watching University EMS professionals, I am confident that the people who live in and visit Newark, New Jersey, are in superior hands. I hope that this up-close look will result in greater public awareness and support of EMS and only enhance the performance of their capable specialists.

I would never have started down the EMS road at all if not for Dick Richards and the many wonderful people at the Chatham Emergency Squad. I thank my instructors at Saint Barnabas Medical Center, where I learned how to become an EMT. Despite his international standing and ferociously busy schedule, Chief Paul M. Maniscalco, a tireless, articulate, and effective EMS advocate, made room for frequent and frank consultation.

* * *

I made inroads into the complex profession with the assistance and insight of several EMS experts, including Carol Bacon, NorthSTAR flight nurse; Joel Bunis, M.I.C.P.; Tom Chetney, M.I.C.P. and supervisor; Joe Dyl, M.I.C.P.; MaryAnn Ferrara, president of the New Jersey First Aid Council; James Fitzsimmons, police lieutenant and OEM coordinator, Hoboken, New Jersey; John S. Fitzsimmons, director of EMS at Lincoln Regional Hospital in Fayetteville, Tennessee; David Garmon, M.Ed., NREMT-P, CCEMT-P; Frank Goodstein, mobilization coordinator for the New Jersey First Aid Council; Mike Helbock, president of EMT-C; Jerry Johnston, director of EMS, Henry County, Iowa; Jeanne Kerwin, director of EMS for Atlantic Health Care and its dispatch center; CENCOM Central Communications director Gareth Williams and supervisors Lisa Marie Gerard and Jim Grissom; Meredith Moss, EMT and emergency-management graduate student; Gerard C. Muench, Jr., M.P.A., M.I.C.P.; Billy O'Brien, NorthSTAR flight medic; Mike Sturgill; James Troisi, EMT instructor; Bill White, president of the National Native American Emergency Medical Services Association, Inc.; Robert K. Waddell II, director, EMS Systems with EMS for Children.

A. J. Heightman, M.I.C.P., edits *The Journal of Emergency Medical Services* and helps direct EMS Today. He made it possible for me to attend the conference and benefit from countless, informative interviews with EMS experts from around the world who actively shape the profession.

I thank the National Association of Emergency Medical Technicians for welcoming me to their conference and introducing me to ardent EMS workers across the nation.

I deeply appreciate Police Officer Debbie Conte and the Al-Atiyat family for sharing their stirring experiences and poignantly illustrating the value that EMS brings.

I am grateful to comedienne Joan Rivers, whom I heard expressing support for police and emergency workers on her radio program. She graciously helped me explain the dark humor that EMS workers invoke to cope with the nightmares that are their job.

Prior to publication, I shared drafts of the manuscript with civilian and EMS readers I deeply respect: Fern Abrams; Diana Buffum; Andrew Forrest; Yolanda Fundora; Dr. Patti Murphy; Marg Smith, Esq.; Matthew R. Streger, M.I.C.P., M.P.H.; Dr. Richard Wein; and Pam Winnick, Esq. Each of them as well as the EMS workers portrayed took considerable time to help me clarify this complex field and decide how to present it.

Professor Sam Freedman, of Columbia University's Graduate School of Journalism, encouraged and helped me develop one passionately sincere paragraph into this tale of modern EMS. I hope always to write books that do him proud. I thank my agent, Jane Dystel; Joe McNeely, an associate publisher who originally championed this book; and Patrick Jamison, whose advice on discipline carried me page after page and who coined the subtitle. Marc Resnick, my editor at St. Martin's Press, expertly shaped this book into a streamlined, power-packed read representative of EMS itself.

Professor Freedman once compared the ups and downs associated with writing a book to riding a powerful roller coaster. As usual, I found him to be dead-on. Thankfully, I had an intrepid, loyal, insightful, and infinitely patient partner, my husband, Gerald M. Karam, friends who supported me in the most imaginative and generous ways: the Behrles, the Gerards, the Chases, Terry Edwards, the Halfins, my sister, Alison Abrams, and my constant companion and clown Maybel.

With great respect, I thank each and every University Hospital blue-shirt and white-shirt for taking the time to share his or her views on EMS.

INDEX